Comparative Pharmacokinetics

Principles, Techniques, and Applications

Comparative Pharmacokinetics

Principles, Techniques, and Applications

JIM E. RIVIERE
North Carolina State University
Raleigh, North Carolina

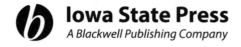 **Iowa State Press**
A Blackwell Publishing Company

Jim E. Riviere received his DVM and his PhD from Purdue University. He is presently Burroughs Wellcome Distinguished Professor of Veterinary Pharmacology and Director of the Center for Chemical Toxicology Research and Pharmacokinetics, College of Veterinary Medicine, North Carolina State University, Raleigh.

© 1999 Iowa State Press
A Blackwell Publishing Company
All rights reserved

Iowa State Press
2121 State Avenue, Ames, Iowa 50014

Orders: 1-800-862-6657
Office: 1-515-292-0140
Fax: 1-515-292-3348
Web site: www.iowastatepress.com

∞ Printed on acid-free paper in the United States of America

First edition, 1999

Library of Congress Cataloging-in-Publication Data

Riviere, Jim E. (Jim Edmond)
    Comparative pharmacokinetics : principles, techniques, and applications / by Jim E. Riviere. — 1st ed.
        p.   cm.
    Includes index.
    ISBN 0-8138-2931-3 (hardcover); 08138-2138-X (paperback)
        1. Pharmacokinetics.   2. Veterinary pharmacology.   I. Title.
    RM301.5.R58   1999
    636.089′57—dc21   98-31926

The last digit is the print number: 9 8 7 6 5 4 3 2 1

Contents

Coauthors, **vi**
Preface, **vii**

1. Introduction, **3**
2. Principles of Drug Movement in the Body, **11**
3. Absorption, **21**
4. Distribution, **47**
5. Renal Elimination, **62**
6. Hepatic Biotransformation and Biliary Excretion, **81**
7. Compartmental Models, **107**
8. Noncompartmental Models, **148**
9. Nonlinear Models, **168**
10. Physiological Models, **189**
11. Dosage Regimens, **202**
12. Simultaneous Pharmacokinetic–Pharmacodynamic Modeling, **215**
13. Study Design and Data Analysis, **239**
14. Population Pharmacokinetic Models and Bayesian Forecasting Applied to Clinical Pharmacokinetics, **259**
15. Dosage Adjustments in Renal Disease, **283**
16. Interspecies Extrapolations, **296**
17. Tissue Residues and Withdrawal Times, **308**

Index, **319**

Coauthors

The numbers in parentheses indicate chapters

Gui Lin Qiao, *DVM, PhD* (6, 12)
Research Scientist
Center for Veterinary Medicine
Food and Drug Administration
Rockville, Maryland

Patrick L. Williams, *PhD* (8, 9)
Polytheoretics, Inc.
Wake Forest, North Carolina

Adjunct Associate Professor of Pharmacokinetics
Center for Chemical Toxicology Research and Pharmacokinetics
College of Veterinary Medicine
North Carolina State University
Raleigh, North Carolina

Tomás Martín-Jiménez, *DVM, Diplomate ACVCP* (14)
Assistant Professor
Department of Veterinary Biosciences
College of Veterinary Medicine
University of Illinois
Urbana, Illinois

James D. Brooks, *MS* (Illustrator)
Research Associate
Center for Chemical Toxicology Research and Pharmacokinetics
College of Veterinary Medicine
North Carolina State University
Raleigh, North Carolina

Preface

This book is written for both the generator and the user of pharmacokinetic data. However, it also is written to present the author's perspective of how pharmacokinetic concepts may unify many topics in comparative medicine. The book is essentially a single-author text, with five of the chapters coauthored by close colleagues. This approach has some immediate strengths and weaknesses. Of necessity, the book will be biased by the author's perception of the discipline that was developed from experience applying these principles to problems encountered in the laboratory. The approach is also influenced by efforts spent in attempting to teach these concepts to the uninitiated, in both a university and a professional setting.

The writing of this text has been greatly facilitated by the author's participation in the Food Animal Residue Avoidance Databank (FARAD), a comparative pharmacokinetic database originally codeveloped with Drs. Art Craigmill and Steve Sundlof. The compilation, maintenance, and access to this databank has provided many applications for the techniques presented in this text. It must be stressed that this book is intended to illustrate concepts and is not an exhaustive review and presentation of the comparative pharmacokinetic literature. The FARAD *Comparative Pharmacokinetic Handbook* series could be consulted for this purpose. Rather, experimental and field data are quoted to illustrate pharmacokinetic concepts or to demonstrate how pharmacokinetic parameters can be used to quantitate clinical events. Wherever possible, examples from the author's laboratory using therapeutic drugs, pesticides, and toxicants will be used throughout the text to illustrate concepts and provide threads of homogeneity to the presentations. I am indebted to my former and current graduate students (Drs. Ronald Baynes, Michael Carver, Shao Chang, Robert DeWosken, Donita Frazier, Mark Heit, Tomás Martín-Jiménez, Jean Luc Riond, and Shelly Vaden) and my postdoctoral fellows (Drs. Lynn Dix, Patrick Williams, and Gui Lin Qiao) for their constant stimulation and for generating the experimental data used to present these ideas.

There is no optimal organization for a text such as this. The major difficulty in structuring this book was to select the optimal sequence of topics since many have origins in both biology and pharmacokinetics. Basic principles and background physiology are presented so that the latter chapters on modeling have a basis in reality. Many concepts are only introduced in these initial physiology-based chapters on disposition since their fuller development requires modeling concepts. Every effort has been made to cross-reference these ideas. This is made evident with the concept of clearance—a parameter required to understand both renal and hepatic elimination. This parameter is independently developed in multiple chapters using the context of that discipline. Although repetitious to some readers, the intent is to develop an understanding from multiple perspectives, which ultimately should aid in the proper use and interpretation of this parameter. A similar situation exists with the volume of distribution. The book ends with a discussion of the application of these techniques to selected common problems in an attempt to reinforce the basic concepts covered earlier in the text and reaffirm linkages between modeling concepts and the underlying biology. My goal in adopting this approach is to provide the reader with a sense of the practicality of this discipline since it is often presented in a manner devoid of biological context. In this light, mathematics is kept to a minimum whenever possible. With today's extensive use of computers and user-friendly software, model derivation and data analyses that once required an extensive background in calculus are no longer needed. However, because the language of pharmacokinetics is the rate of movement of compounds in the body, its grammar is that of differential calculus. The presentation will be held to concepts as much as possible so that the reader has a basis when selecting models to use in available software packages. Derivations of equations are kept to a minimum. More extensive mathematical background is required only for a few advanced sections in some of the chapters, which could be bypassed without negative effect if these processes are not being directly studied. In general, knowledge of high school algebra should be sufficient to understand the concepts presented. The reader is directed to more advanced or comprehensive texts when complex models are required to analyze specific experimental scenarios. In many instances, such models are in the "libraries" of many modern software packages. This book will serve as a bridge to these texts and software packages as well as to the open pharmacokinetic literature.

The present text was inspired by Professor Desmond Baggot's beautiful 1977 book, *Principles of Drug Disposition in Domestic Animals*. I encountered this text in the formative stages of my career and was greatly influenced by its seamless blending of comparative physiology and pharmacokinetics. The present book builds on this approach and updates it to modern methods of pharmacokinetic analysis, while hopefully still maintaining its roots in the underlying physiology that defines the processes of drug disposition. I also thank my mentor, Dr. Gordon L. Coppoc, for originally encouraging and supporting me to become involved in pharmacokinetics during graduate school, and for providing the intellectual climate that shaped my career.

I would like to personally acknowledge a number of individuals who made this book possible. My strongest thanks goes to my close friends and colleagues Drs. Gary Koritz and Arthur Craigmill, who graciously "volunteered" to review draft copies of this book. Their comments were an education in themselves, and hopefully their efforts made this text more readable and accurate. I also thank these two individuals for their continuous encouragement throughout the writing of the text, and for their analysis of the sample data set in Chapter 13.

Similarly, thanks go to Drs. Jim Caputo, Mark Papich, and Gui Lin Qiao for contributing their analysis of this data set to Chapter 13. I thank Drs. Steve Sundlof and Scott Brown for their friendship and unique professional relationship. Finally, I thank the staff of the North Carolina State University Center for Cutaneous Toxicology and Residue Pharmacology for making the research presented here possible. In a similar vein, I acknowledge the financial assistance of the U.S. Department of Agriculture, National Institutes of Health, Food and Drug Administration, Department of Defense, Environmental Protection Agency, Becton Dickinson, and Cellegy Pharmaceuticals for supporting my pharmacokinetic research over the years. Appreciation goes out to Gretchen Van Houten and Judi Brown of Iowa State University Press for agreeing to publish this book and providing support throughout the project, and to my editors Lynne Bishop and Jane Dugan for their expert assistance in polishing this text.

This book would not be possible were it not for the sacrifices made by my children, Brian, Christopher, and Jessica, throughout and especially during the completion of this text. Similarly, I owe a unique debt to my spouse, soul mate, and colleague, Dr. Nancy Monteiro-Riviere, both for professionally offering advice and for providing research problems to apply pharmacokinetic techniques and, more importantly, for providing endless love to support me in this endeavor.

Comparative Pharmacokinetics

Principles, Techniques, and Applications

1

Introduction

Pharmacokinetics is best defined as *the use of mathematical models to quantitate the time course of drug absorption and disposition in man and animals.* With the tremendous advances in medicine and analytical chemistry, coupled with the almost universal availability of computers, what was once an arcane science has now entered the mainstream of most fields of human and veterinary medicine. This discipline has allowed dosages of drugs to be tailored to individuals or groups to optimize therapeutic effectiveness, minimize toxicity, and avoid violative tissue residues in the case of food-producing animals.

What differentiates this discipline from other fields of pharmacology and medicine is its focus on quantitating biological phenomena using various mathematical models and restricting its purview to the movement of drugs and chemicals into, through, and out of the body. The subsequent effects of these drugs on biological processes fall in the realm of pharmacodynamics, which generally is not included in most basic pharmacokinetic experiments. There are numerous applications of pharmacokinetics in clinical practice, some of them unknown to the practitioner because the terminology has been incorporated into the lexicon of general medicine.

Since the publication of the last comparative pharmacokinetics text by Baggot in 1977, there has been explosive growth in all aspects of this discipline. The primary pharmacokinetic models utilized by comparative and veterinary pharmacokineticists are the so-called classic open compartmental models presented in Chapter 7 of the present text. These models, first clearly elucidated by Teorell in 1937, have been the mainstay of pharmacokinetics for much of this decade. However, the use of noncompartmental models, especially those based on statistical moment analyses, has recently taken hold. This popularity can be linked in part to a superb suitability for analysis by digital computers. Paradoxically, many of the properties that make the analysis of serum pharmacokinetic data amenable to exponential equations result from a few mathematical peculiarities in the solution of these compartmental models. Newer noncompartmental approaches to data analysis share many of these attributes and thus also share the same limitations of the classic modeling approaches. These intricacies will be completely explored in this text.

Pharmacokinetic principles have become widespread in the discipline of toxicology, an application termed toxicokinetics. There are no fundamental differences between pharmacokinetic and toxicokinetic principles except that the latter often deal with higher doses of chemical, which may saturate metabolizing enzymes and in some cases may damage eliminating organs, thereby altering the disposition of the toxin. However, the principles involved are identical, and the concepts presented in this text are applicable to both fields.

Physiologically-based pharmacokinetic models have become routine in many fields of pharmacology and toxicology. These models, unlike the others mentioned, build on the basis of sound anatomical and physiological principles and, although data-intensive, may allow the best opportunity for true mechanism-based interspecies pharmacokinetic extrapolations. Individual organ function is easily scaled across species and *in vitro* data may be extrapolated to the whole animal.

In fact, much work has focused on quantifying *in vitro* to *in vivo* correlations. *In vitro* studies may be conducted with very simple subcellular, single cell, or tissue culture systems or more complex perfused organ preparations (also referred to as *ex vivo* models). The goal is always to extrapolate the drug concentration profile in the more simple *in vitro* experimental environment to that which actually exists in the cells or tissues of whole animals. Such an extrapolation (albeit very crude) is made daily with the use of minimum inhibitory concentrations (MICs) to estimate the efficacy of an antimicrobial drug against a specific bacteria in a human or animal patient.

In drug development and biochemical toxicology laboratories, extrapolation is often from a simple receptor or subcellular fraction assay, which detects drug or toxin binding, to the dose of drug that would be required to achieve this effective concentration *in vivo*. Alternatively, DNA binding or cytotoxicity screens may detect potential adverse events associated with a specific chemical. This defines a hazard in the risk assessment process. However, sufficient exposure in the intact organism is still required for this hazard to be realized as a risk. Pharmacokinetics is often the bridge in this extrapolation. In fact, sophisticated concentration-response relationships, obtained from *in vitro* bioassay systems, may be defined and then linked to the *in vivo* dose-response profile using integrated pharmacokinetic-pharmacodynamic modeling techniques.

The extrapolation of pharmacokinetic parameters across species is a major focus of research. This is true in laboratory animal medicine and especially so in exotic animal and zoo animal medicine. Many "classic" compartmental pharmacokinetic studies conducted in multiple animal species have been extrapolated using the techniques of allometry. This is often employed when laboratory animal toxicology data must be extended to humans to put into perspective the relationship between the expected toxic dose and therapeutically useful doses. This concept of a "therapeutic window" framed by a minimal effective therapeutic dose or resultant concentration and maximally safe toxic threshold is found in many areas of medicine and is implicitly based in pharmacokinetic methodology.

The fields of clinical pharmacology have grown in both human and veterinary medicine. Subpopulations of patients based on age or disease processes are routinely defined and dosages of drug appropriately altered. Part of the growth of this discipline was facilitated by the routine application of pharmacokinetics in clinical patients. This led to the development in the early 1980s of so-called population-based pharmacokinetics, which merges the estimation of pharmacokinetic parameters with simultaneous clinical estimates of physiological parameters and population variability. Its application to defining disease-induced changes in drug disposition and probing the nature of pharmacokinetic variance are widespread. In veterinary medicine, these same principles are needed to extrapolate dosage regimens for extralabel drug use.

This proliferation of pharmacokinetics throughout these diverse fields has been fueled by the explosive growth in analytical methodologies using principles of both chromatography (high-performance liquid and gas chromatography) and immunology (radioimmunoassay, ELISA). Not only has the cost per sample of these procedures plummeted, but their availability and sensitivity have increased tremendously. For many drugs, simple disposable card-type assays are being developed that will provide the clinician instantly with estimates of drug concentrations. In veterinary medicine, such assays are available to monitor milk and urine for the presence of violative drug residues.

With the drug concentration data now readily available, complex mathematical modeling that was once restricted to the esoteric and truly "user- *un*friendly" and even "user-adverse" mainframe computers can now be routinely done on nearly any available personal computer using one of a myriad of simple-to-use pharmacokinetic software packages (e.g., CONSAAM and SAAM, PK-Analyst, P-Pharm, Win-Nonlin). In fact, this is one of the developments that highlighted the need for this text because, parallel to this proliferation of tools to conduct pharmacokinetic analyses, many workers have failed to study its basic principles and often inappropriately apply models to experimental and clinical situations.

OBJECTIVES AND PHILOSOPHY

The purpose of this book is to provide an overview of the discipline of pharmacokinetics for the student, researcher, and comparative medicine clinician. The text presents an overview of the basic processes of drug absorption and disposition and then details how these processes can be quantitated using different pharmacokinetic approaches. The book is directed toward both the individual responsible for doing the analysis and the user of the pharmacokinetic information generated. To properly employ pharmacokinetic information, the limitations of the specific model that generated the pharmacokinetic parameter estimates must be appreciated. Are the parameters compatible with the model in which it will be used to make predictions? Many pharmacokinetic parameters are model-dependent, and serious errors may occur if the inappropriate parameters are used. *A pharmacokinetic model is simply an artificial mathematical link to the underlying interaction of a drug's pharmacology with an animal's physiology* (Figure 1.1). The nature of the link will determine the types of parameters calculated.

A common misconception is that if one specific model fails to adequately predict the data or experimental scenario, then the process being studied is assumed to not be

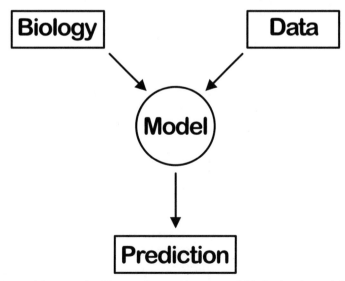

FIGURE 1.1. Conceptual framework of how a pharmacokinetic model links the observed data to the underlying biology controlling drug disposition.

amenable to pharmacokinetic analysis. Often, the fault is that insufficient data have been collected to properly define the model and its so-called inference space. The "links" were not properly constructed. In other cases, incomplete understanding of the disposition processes involved resulted in construction of a woefully inadequate model in the first place. The limitations of specific models and techniques must be appreciated before extrapolations can be made.

This book is also written for the individual who never plans on actually doing a pharmacokinetic study but wants to understand more about the time course of drug movement throughout the body. The primary goal of pharmacokinetics is to generate parameters that are mathematical abstractions that quantitate physiological processes as an aid to better understanding drug disposition. Mathematical modeling generates parameters that may vary as the physiology varies as a result of disease, age, sex, or drug-induced toxicity. The parameters are mathematical constructs that reflect changes in underlying physiology. There is no absolute value of any parameter that exists independent of the model; parameters are defined by the model and reflect the nature of the mathematical links to the physiology. Models may be classified as mechanistic (e.g., compartmental and physiological), which represent some abstraction of the underlying physiologic reality, or as empirical (e.g., noncompartmental, neural-net analysis), which are restricted to predicting observed data. Alternatively, models may be classified as deterministic and thus purport to have exact predictability; or stochastic, which incorporate a level of statistical uncertainty in the predictions. An understanding of how models and links are derived is necessary for a thorough understanding of drug disposition and ultimately drug efficacy or toxicity.

There are many misconceptions as to what a pharmacokinetic study actually entails. Many workers in veterinary medicine believe that measuring drug concentrations in plasma or blood and plotting the resulting concentration-time profile comprises such a study. Similarly, some feel that if parameters such as peak concentration, time to peak concentration, and the area under the concentration-time curve are recorded, a pharmacokinetic analysis has been performed. As will be stressed throughout this book, the problem with such studies is that they are descriptive only for the experiment performed and are difficult to use for extrapolation to another animal or clinical conditions. Although such types of studies are useful, they must be categorized as descriptive and do not constitute a pharmacokinetic analysis.

A pharmacokinetic study in the context of this book is defined as an experiment in which some type of mathematical model is fitted to the drug concentration-time profile in blood, tissue, and/or excreta. This opens the possibility of correlating model parameters to physiological processes or using them for interspecies extrapolation. In these types of analyses, parameters such as half-life, volume of distribution, and clearance are calculated in addition to the descriptive parameters mentioned above. A separate chapter will be devoted to the physiology underlying each type of parameter. Similarly, the major types of modeling paradigms adopted will be developed and compared. The "core" of the book is Chapter 7, which develops the basis for most of the subsequent chapters. Whatever type of model is employed (linear versus nonlinear, compartmental versus noncompartmental), *a model is only a tool to estimate drug concentrations and generate parameters that are useful for further analyses and quantitating the biological process under investigation.* Models are neither correct nor incorrect, but should be judged only as to how accurately drug concentrations are predicted under new exposure conditions.

The selection of a model relative to its use for prediction of future events is an important decision. Figure 1.2 depicts how three radically different mathematical models may fit the same limited data set. The three models are statistically equivalent in ability to describe the observed data, and thus all are mathematically appropriate. However, only the

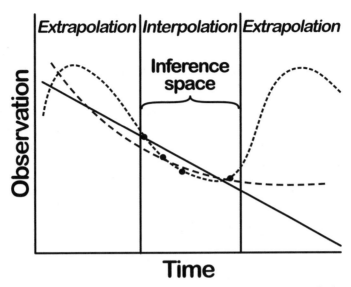

FIGURE 1.2. Illustration of how three very diverse mathematical models may adequately describe the same limited set of data yet result in very different values when predictions are extrapolated beyond the models' inference space. Linear (—); sinusoidal (– –); exponential (- - -).

exponential model has a relatively direct link to biological reality. All three predict very different drug concentrations for times beyond the actual data collected. Within the observed time interval, all models accurately interpolate drug concentrations at times between collections. This is defined as the inference space of the model. However, extrapolation outside of the observed time window requires knowledge that the model has biological reality at these time points. Collection of as few as two additional data points would expand the model's inference space and help select the more predictive model. It is surprising how often this simple limitation of fitting equations to data is overlooked.

Completely independent of the model selected, it is the fitting of the model to the data, for the purposes of the investigator, that must be optimized. This is where statistics interfaces with pharmacokinetics. For example, three different approaches and sets of sampling intervals are used in studies to estimate a peak drug plasma concentration, to determine a dosing interval for chronic treatment, or to estimate the tissue residue withdrawal time in a food-producing animal. Although the underlying models may be very similar, or even identical, these three cases require optimizing estimates of different components of the model, and thus the experimental time frame may be very different, ranging from minutes to hours to days. The drug concentration ranges for these three applications are also likely to differ by three to four orders of magnitude. Failure to select a specific model appropriate to the proper experimental frame of reference may lead to serious errors in extrapolation. These aspects of experimental design and data analysis will be extensively reviewed at the end of the text.

Semantics plays a very important role in this interface between statistics and pharmacokinetics. Serious errors have occurred when the same term in both disciplines refers to two different items. Examples include the use of the Greek letter ß which in statistics may refer to the probability of a type II statistical error or the slope of a regression line, while in pharmacokinetics it specifically refers to the terminal exponential slope of the plasma drug concentration versus time data from a two-compartment model following intravenous drug administration. Standard practices for fitting mathematical models to the same data set in both disciplines may be very different. For example, the modeling approaches used in pharmacokinetics often are based on additive exponential functions simply because the resulting parameters then have physiological meaning; that is, they can be linked back to the animal. Such exponential functions are but a subset of those available to the statistician and may not even be the best for fitting to a specific curve. Nevertheless, they are used because they can be incorporated into models that physiologically and pharmacologically make sense. Even if exponential equations are used by both disciplines, pharmacokinetic analysis often employs the principle of superposition and thus curve "stripping" to analyze the data, a restriction not present in a pure statistical model. Neither approach is right or wrong as each has its merits. Problems arise only when parameters from one model are mistakenly used as input into another.

Recent advances in *in vitro* technology and the ease of conducting large-scaled pharmacokinetic trials have resulted in a plethora of readily available data that would appear to span all levels of biological organization. This is especially true in comparative pharmacology and risk assessment. The combination of such diverse data requires that certain assumptions be fulfilled and the limits of the mathematical bridges employed to link the data sets be strictly defined. Even when done properly, some combinations of diverse *in vitro* and *in vivo* model systems result in the generation of so-called emergent properties, the hallmark of complex system behavior. In other cases, nonlinear systems dynamics or "chaotic behavior" may take hold, making extrapolations possible but difficult unless the behavior is clearly understood. Thus, as will become evident throughout this text, pharmacokinetics and other forms of mathematical extrapolations may be used in many scenarios, but they must be applied in the proper context and the assumptions and defining rules inherent to each system closely tested and followed.

TARGET AUDIENCE AND APPLICATIONS

The focus of this book is to present the basic concepts of pharmacokinetic principles to the scientist or practitioner with a strong biological background. The mathematics should be tolerable to such an individual as it will not go much beyond what he or she has already encountered in related disciplines. The most obvious user of pharmacokinetic principles is the basic scientist studying drug or chemical disposition in animals. Simple pharmacokinetic studies are often used to describe the blood or tissue concentrations seen after drug administration. These parameters provide the basis for determining differences in the rate and extent of drug absorption, distribution, or elimination. They allow for the development of simple mathematical models to interpret the time-dependent nature of numerous biological phenomena. These strategies will be completely developed.

Pharmaceutical scientists use pharmacokinetics in many industrial and regulatory settings. Parameters are derived to define the shape of an efficacious drug's blood concentration versus time profile (area under the curve, peak blood concentration) so that other products may be formulated to "copy" this profile, in pharmacokinetic jargon, to be "bioequivalent." Similarly, drug absorption is assessed in simple model systems to select candidate drugs for development and determine the purity of a drug formulation. Pharmacokinetic parameters are calculated to extrapolate from preclinical and clinical trial results. Similarly, toxicologists in these environments must use pharmacokinetic principles to interpret the dose that produces a toxicological "event" in an animal study relative to its potential to do the same in a clinical setting at therapeutic doses. Many practices of risk assessment use similar extrapolations.

The field of pharmacokinetics and its concepts have become especially important as a consequence of the dramatic and almost radical changes that occurred at the end of this decade relative to the regulations surrounding drug use in veterinary medicine. For most of the recent past, the operative concept was that a single dose of drug listed on a product label was optimal for all therapeutic uses. Very recently, however, the legal concept of

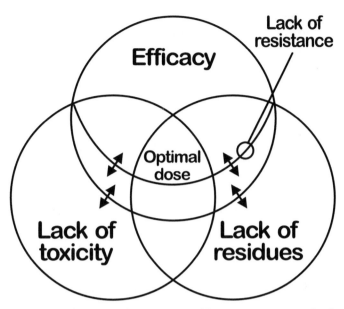

FIGURE 1.3. Illustration of the food animal veterinarian's dilemma in optimizing the dose of a therapeutic drug.

"flexible or professional labeling" and the passage by the U.S. Congress in 1994 of the Animal Medicinal Drug Use Clarification Act (AMDUCA) legalizing extralabel drug use forever eradicated this fallacious ideal of a single optimal dose. The veterinarian must now select a drug dose based on numerous factors inherent to the therapeutic scenario at hand to maximize therapeutic efficacy and minimize the likelihood of drug-induced toxicity or induction of microbial resistance. Unlike human medicine and companion animal practices, food animal veterinarians face the further restriction that proper withdrawal times must be determined to ensure that drug residues do not persist in the edible tissues or by-products (milk, eggs) of treated animals long after they have left the care of the veterinarian (Figure 1.3). As will be demonstrated, the withdrawal time is in reality a pure pharmacokinetic parameter since it can be calculated solely from knowledge of the legal tissue tolerance and the drug's half-life or rate of decay in that tissue.

Yet it is not only the food animal veterinarian who faces these challenges. The laboratory animal and exotic/zoo animal worker must often extrapolate drug dosages across species with widely differing body sizes and physiology since there are very few approved drugs for the treatment of such animals. Pharmacokinetic principles and techniques are ideally suited for this application. Practitioners are often faced with disease processes (e.g., renal failure) that are known to affect the disposition of a drug. Knowledge of how such a pathological process affects a drug's clearance or volume of distribution is sufficient to adapt a dosage regimen appropriate for this condition.

Other scientists who deal with drugs in both *in vitro* and *in vivo* systems may not be interested in constructing complex pharmacokinetic models but rather in the relationship between the administered dose and the effect. The link between dose and effect, however, is the drug concentration at the site of action (the so-called biophase), which is the essence of a pharmacokinetic study. These data are necessary to link these different systems in order to determine whether a drug concentration threshold exists for drug action or toxicity, or to study the time course of drug effect. Pharmacokinetics provides the parameters to serve as experimental endpoints and to extrapolate beyond the individual experiment to the target population.

To pursue these varied goals, this book starts with the biology and progresses to the presentation of the different modeling approaches used in pharmacokinetics. The book concludes with elements of experimental design and data analysis followed by some specific applications to select fields.

SELECTED READINGS

Baggot, J. D. 1977. *Principles of Drug Disposition in Domestic Animals: The Basis of Veterinary Clinical Pharmacology.* Philadelphia: W.B. Saunders Co.

Bourne, D.W.A. 1995. *Mathematical Modeling of Pharmacokinetic Data.* Lancaster, PA: Technomic Publishing Co.

Boxenbaum, H. 1992. Pharmacokinetics: Philosophy of modeling. *Drug Metabolism Reviews.* 24:89-120.

Caines, P.E. 1988. *Linear Stochastic Systems.* New York: Wiley and Sons.

DiStefano, J.J., and E.M. Landaw. 1984. Multiexponential, multicompartmental, and non-compartmental modeling. I. Methodological limitations and physiological interpretations. *American Journal of Physiology.* 246:R651-R664.

Gibaldi, M., and D. Perrier. 1982. *Pharmacokinetics,* 2d ed. New York: Marcel Dekker.

Teorell, T. 1937. Kinetics of distribution of substances administered to the body. *Archives International Pharmacodynamics* 57:205-240.

Wagner, J. G. 1975. *Fundamentals of Clinical Pharmacokinetics.* Lancaster, PA: Technomic Publishing Co.

2

Principles of Drug Movement in the Body

Pharmacokinetics is the study of the time course of drug concentrations in the body. It provides a means of quantitating absorption, distribution, metabolism, and elimination (ADME), the four key physiological processes that govern the time course of drug fate. In the premarketing phase of drug development, it is an essential component in establishing effective yet safe dosage forms and regimens. When applied to a clinical situation, pharmacokinetics provides the practitioner with a useful tool to design optimally beneficial drug dosage schedules for each individual patient. Alternatively, an understanding of pharmacokinetic principles allows more rational therapeutic decisions to be made. In food animals, pharmacokinetics provides the conceptual underpinnings for understanding and utilizing the withdrawal time to prevent violative drug residues from persisting in the edible tissues of food-producing animals. Finally, a comprehensive study of this discipline provides the framework upon which many aspects of pharmacology can be integrated into a rational plan for drug usage.

AN OVERVIEW OF DRUG DISPOSITION

In order to fully appreciate the processes governing the fate of drugs in animals, the various steps involved must be defined and ultimately quantitated. The processes relevant to a discussion of the absorption and disposition of a drug administered by the intravenous (IV), intramuscular (IM), subcutaneous (SC), oral (PO), or topical (TOP) route is illustrated in Figure 2.1. The normal reference point for pharmacokinetic analysis is the concentration of free, non–protein-bound drug dissolved in the serum (or plasma) because this is the body fluid that carries the drug throughout the body and from which samples for drug analysis can be readily and repeatedly collected. Additionally, for the majority of drugs used, drug in the systemic circulation is in equilibrium with the extracellular fluid of well-perfused tissues; thus, serum or plasma drug concentrations generally reflect extracellular fluid drug concentrations. A drug must generally be present at its site of action in a tissue at a sufficient concentration for a specific period of time to produce a pharmacologic effect. Since tissue concentrations of drugs are reflected by extracellular fluid and thus serum drug concentrations, a pharmacokinetic analysis of the disposition of drug in the scheme outlined in Figure 2.1 is useful to assess the activity of a drug in the *in vivo* setting.

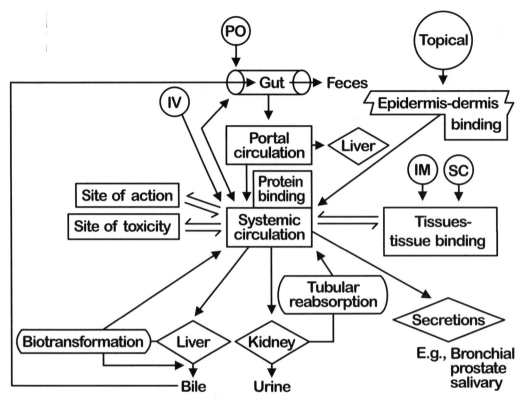

FIGURE 2.1.   Basic schema illustrates how drug is absorbed, distributed, metabolized, and excreted from the body. These processes are those that form the basis for developing pharmacokinetic models.

This conceptualization is especially important in veterinary medicine because species differences in any of these processes may affect the extent and/or time course of drug absorption and disposition in the body. By dividing the overall process of drug fate into specific phases, this relatively complex situation can be more easily handled. It is the purpose of this chapter to present an overview of the physiological basis of absorption, distribution, biotransformation, and excretion. This discussion will then provide a groundwork for the subsequent chapters, which deal with these concepts in more detail.

One should recall that such schemes are created to solve practical problems in pharmacology or therapeutics. The concentration of drug achieved in a tissue can be described using pharmacokinetic techniques. However, the importance of this drug concentration is defined by the user of the data. If a drug is being targeted to a specific tissue (e.g., liver), the liver becomes the site of action. In contrast, if the toxicity of a drug is primarily expressed in the liver, the same organ now becomes the site of toxicity. Finally, the site of action and toxicity may be in different tissues, yet the liver may be the tissue of concern for residues in a food animal. In all three cases, the pharmacokinetic parameters describing the time course of drug concentration in the liver are identical; only the interpretive value associated with the drug concentration is different. This is not a function of the mathematical model describing the drug concentration; rather it is dependent on the use to which the information is put. *Thus, a pharmacokinetic model must be interpreted in the context of the experiment from which it was created.* This relativity will continue to be stressed throughout this book.

Despite the myriad of anatomical and physiological differences among animals, the biology of drug absorption and distribution, and in some cases even elimination, is very

Contain over 100 differeat dissolved solutes.
Plasma - non living fluid natrix (55% of whole blood)
erythrocytes - red blood cells transport origen (45% of whole blood)

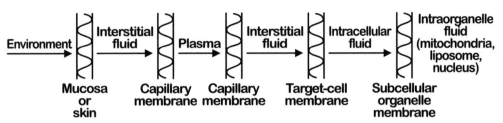

FIGURE 2.2. Illustration of how absorption, distribution, and excretion essentially constitute a journey of drug through various lipoidal membrane barriers.

similar in that it involves drug molecules crossing a series of biological membranes. As illustrated in Figure 2.2, these membranes may be associated with either several layers of cells (tissue) or a single cell, and both living and dead protoplasm may be involved. Despite the different biochemical and morphological attributes of each of these membranes, a unifying concept of biology is the basic similarity of all membranes, whether they be tissue, cell, or organelle. Although the specific biochemical components may vary, the fundamental organization is the same. This fact simplifies the understanding of the major determinants of drug absorption, distribution, and excretion.

These membrane barriers often directly or indirectly define the nature of compartments or other structural units in pharmacokinetic models. Biological spaces are defined by the restrictions of these barriers. The most effective barriers are those that protect the organism from the external environment. These include the skin as well as various segments of the gastrointestinal and respiratory tract, which also protect the internal physiological milieu from the damaging external environment. The interstitial fluid is a common compartment through which any drug must transit either after absorption on route to the blood stream or after delivery by blood to tissue on route to a cellular target. The continuity of this space has recently been taken advantage of in pharmacokinetic studies through the use of implantable microdialysis probes and catheters that allow direct sampling of interstitial fluid. Membranes define homogeneous tissue compartments, and membranes must be traversed in all processes of drug absorption and disposition. The mechanisms by which chemicals cross these ubiquitous membrane barriers often determine the type of pharmacokinetic models appropriate to quantitate the movement of specific drugs.

The basic model of the cellular membrane as originally postulated by Davson and Danielli in 1935 is still the most generally accepted description for the structure of cellular membranes. The major modification is in the increased fluidity of the lipid components, with the resulting fluid mosaic model proposed by Singer and Nicholson depicted in Figure 2.3. A large body of microscopic and biochemical data has now confirmed this insightful model. All cellular membranes appear to be bimolecular lipid leaflets closely associated with globular proteins that may reside on either surface (intracellular or extracellular) or traverse the entire structure. The lipid leaflets are arranged with hydrophilic (polar) head groups on the surface and hydrophobic (nonpolar) tails forming the interior. Several types of lipids are found in biological membranes, with phospholipids and cholesterol predominating. Phosphatidylcholine, phosphatidylserine, and phophatidylethanolamine are the primary phosphatides comprising the charged surfaces with the two fatty acid hydrocarbon chains (typically 16 to 18 but varying from 12 to 22 carbons) comprising the internal nonpolar regions. The specific lipid composition of these membranes varies widely across different tissues and levels of biological organization.

The location of the proteins in the lipid matrix is primarily a consequence of their hydrophobic regions residing in the lipid interior and their hydrophilic and ionic regions

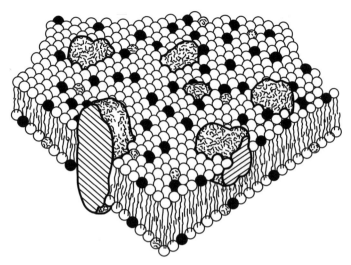

Figure 2.3.   Fluid mosaic model of a bilayer lipid membrane.

occupying the surface. This is the thermodynamically most stable configuration. Some membrane proteins are anchored by microfilaments to the cytoskeleton of the cell. However, the primary force responsible for maintaining structural integrity of both the lipids and proteins are hydrophobic, and to a lesser extent, electrostatic intermolecular interactions. Changes in the fluidity of the lipids alter protein conformations, which then may modulate their activity. In some cases, aqueous channels exist within integral proteins that traverse the membrane. In other cases, these integral proteins may actually be enzymatic transport proteins that function as active or facilitative transport systems. However, the primary pathway for drugs to cross these lipid membranes is by passive diffusion through the lipid environment.

Thus, for a drug to be absorbed or distributed throughout the body, it must be able to pass through a lipid membrane on some part of its sojourn through the body. In some protected sites of the body (e.g., brain, cerebral spinal fluid), additional membranes (e.g., glial cells) may have to be traversed before a drug arrives at its target site. These specialized membranes could be considered a general adaptation to further shelter susceptible tissues from hostile lipophilic chemicals. In this case, drug characteristics that promote transmembrane diffusion would favor drug action and effect (again, unless specific transport systems intervene).

This general phenomenon of the enhanced absorption and distribution of lipophilic compounds is a unifying tenet that runs throughout the study of drug fate. The body's elimination organs can also be viewed as operating according to a somewhat similar principle. The primary mechanism by which a chemical can be excreted from the body is by becoming less lipophilic and more hydrophilic, the latter property being required for excretion in the aqueous fluids of the urinary or biliary system, although amphipathic drugs (having both lipophilic and polar properties) are preferentially excreted in the bile. When a hydrophilic or polar drug is injected into the blood stream, it will be minimally distributed and rapidly excreted by one of these routes. However, if a compound's lipophilicity evades this easy excretion, the liver and other organs may metabolize it to less lipophilic and more hydrophilic metabolites that have a restricted distribution (and thus reduced access to sites for activity) in the body and can be more readily excreted. This basic tenet runs through all aspects of pharmacology.

k_p = permeability coefficient. $k_p = \dfrac{DP}{h}$ (1/time)

D = diffusion coefficient
P = partition coefficient - how well a substance partitions between a lipid and water
h = thickness of path

2 • Principles of Drug Movement in the Body

DRUG PASSAGE ACROSS MEMBRANES

Considerable evidence indicates that lipid-based membranes are permeable to nonpolar lipid-soluble compounds and polar water-soluble compounds with sufficient lipid solubility to diffuse through the hydrophobic regions of the membrane. The rate of diffusion of a compound across a membrane is directly proportional to its concentration gradient across the membrane, lipid:water partition coefficient, and diffusion coefficient. This can be summarized by Fick's law of diffusion in the equation:

$$\text{Rate of diffusion (mg / sec)} = \frac{D \text{ (cm / sec) } P}{h \text{ (cm)}} (X_1 - X_2) \text{ (mg)} \qquad (2.1)$$

where D is the diffusion coefficient for the specific penetrant (nonionized moiety) in the membrane being studied, P is the partition coefficient for the penetrant between the membrane and the external medium, h is the thickness or actual length of the path by which the drug diffuses through the membrane, and $X_1 - X_2$ is the concentration gradient (ΔX) across the membrane. The diffusional coefficient of the drug is a function of its molecular size, molecular conformation and solubility in the membrane milieu. The partition coefficient is the relative solubility of the compound in lipid and water, which reflects the ability of the penetrant to gain access to the lipid membrane. Depending on the membrane, there is a functional molecular size and/or weight cutoff that prevents very large molecules from being passively absorbed across any membrane. As will be demonstrated in Chapter 7, when the rate of a process is dependent upon a rate constant [in this case (DP/h), often referred to as the permeability coefficient k_p] and a concentration gradient, a linear or first-order kinetic process will be operative. In membrane transfer studies, the total flux of drug across a membrane is dependent upon the area of membrane exposed; thus, the rate above is often expressed in terms of cm^2. This relationship holds well *in vitro*, but is only an approximation *in vivo* since in many barriers, penetration is slow, and a long period of time is required to achieve steady-state. When steady-state is not achieved, Fick's second law of diffusion may be used to estimate instantaneous fluxes, a discussion of which is beyond the scope of the present chapter.

If the lipid:water partition coefficient is too great, depending on the specific membrane, the compound may be sequestered in the membrane rather than traverse it. Thus some fraction of X will actually not be available for diffusion through the system. This could be modeled using compartmental schemes similar to that presented in Chapter 7, in which the sequestered portion of the skin is considered to be a separate compartment. However, in general, passage through membranes correlate with various lipid:water partition coefficients. The fluid phase most often used for its determination are octanol:water and olive oil:water. In some cases in which the specific lipid composition of the membrane is known, a slurry of the actual lipids may be employed. This is becoming more sophisticated with the advent of advanced organ culture techniques in which, for example in skin, lipid membranes very similar in composition, structure and function to those *in vivo* can be routinely prepared in culture and used to study drug transport.

Evidence also indicates that membranes are more permeable to the nonionized than the ionized form of weak organic acids and bases. If the nonionized moiety has a lipid:water partition coefficient favorable for membrane penetration, then it will ultimately reach equilibrium on both sides of the membrane. The ionized form of the drug is completely prevented from crossing the membrane because of its low lipid solubility. The amount of the drug in the ionized or nonionized form depends upon the *pKa* (negative logarithm of the acidic dissociation constant) of the drug and the pH of the medium on either side of the membrane (e.g., intracellular versus extracellular fluid;

pKa - negative logarithm of the acidic dissociation constant
'dissociation constant.'

gastrointestinal versus extracellular fluid). Protonated weak acids are nonionized (e.g., COOH), while protonated weak bases are ionized (e.g., NH_3+). If the drug has a fixed charge at all *pH* levels encountered inside and outside of the body (e.g., quaternary amines, aminoglycoside antibiotics), they will never cross lipid membranes by diffusion. This would restrict both their absorption and their distribution and generally lead to an enhanced rate of elimination. It is the unionized form of the drug that is governed by Fick's law of diffusion and described by equation 2.1. For this equation to predict the movement of a drug across membrane systems *in vivo*, the relevant *pH* level of each compartment must be considered relative to the compound's *pKa*, otherwise erroneous predictions will be made.

When the *pH* of the medium is equal to the *pKa* of the dissolved drug, 50% of the drug exists in the ionized state and 50% in the nonionized, lipid-soluble state. The ratio of nonionized to ionized drug is given by the Henderson-Hasselbalch equation.

For acids:

$$pKa - pH = \log\ [(H\ Acid)^0\ /\ (Acid)^-] \qquad (2.2)$$

For bases:

$$pKa - pH = \log\ [(H\ Base)^+\ /\ (Base)^0] \qquad (2.3)$$

These equations are identical as they involve the ratio of protonated (*H*) to nonprotonated moieties. The only difference is that for an acid, the protonated form (*H Acid*)^0 is neutral, and for a base, the protonated form (*H Base*)$^+$ is ionized.

As can be seen by these equations, when the *pH* is one unit less or one unit more than the *pKa* for weak bases or acids, respectively, the ratio of ionized to nonionized form is 10. Thus each unit of *pH* away from the *pKa* results in a tenfold change in this ratio. This phenomenon allows for a drug to be differentially distributed across a membrane in the presence of a *pH* gradient. The side of the membrane with the *pH* favoring ionized drug (high *pH* for an acidic drug; low *pH* for an alkaline drug) will tend to have higher total (ionized plus nonionized) drug concentrations. This *pH* partitioning results in so-called ion-trapping in the area where ionized drug predominates. Figure 2.4 illustrates this concept with an organic acid of *pKa* = 3.4 partitioning between gastric contents of *pH* = 1.4 and plasma of *pH* = 7.4. Assuming that the nonionized form of the drug (*U*) is in equilibrium across the membrane, then according to equation 2.2, there will be a 100-fold (log 2; 3.4 − 1.4) difference on the gastric side and a 10,000-fold (log 4; 7.4 − 3.4) difference on the plasma side of the membrane, for a transmembrane concentration gradient of total drug (*U* + *I*) equal to 10,001 / 1.01 where *I* is the ionized form of the drug. Note that the unionized concentration on both sides of the membrane are in equilibrium. It is the total drug concentrations that are different. In this case, the gradient is generated by the difference in *pH* across an ion-impermeable barrier generated by the local milieu.

Such a gradient would greatly favor the absorption of this weak acid across the gastrointestinal tract into plasma. This is the situation that exists for weak acids, such as penicillin, aspirin, and phenylbutazone. In contrast, a weak base would tend to be trapped in this environment and thus minimal absorption would occur. Examples of such weak bases are morphine, phenothiazine, and ketamine. This is toxicologically significant with the weakly basic strychnine. If strychnine were placed into the strongly acidic stomach, no systemic toxicity would be observed. However, if the stomach was then infused with alkali, most of this base would become nonionized, readily absorbed, and lethal. In summary, weak acids are readily absorbed from an acid environment and sequestered in

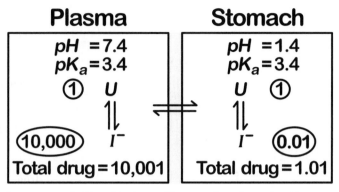

FIGURE 2.4.   The phenomenon of *pH* partitioning and ion-trapping of a weak acid.

an alkaline medium. In contrast, weak bases are absorbed in an alkaline environment and trapped in an acidic environment.

This *pH* partitioning phenomenon is important not only for understanding absorption (as illustrated above) but also in any situation in which the *pH* values of fluid compartments across a biological membrane are different (see Figure 2.2). It will occur for a drug distributing from plasma (*pH* = 7.4) to milk (*pH* = 6.5 – 6.8), to cerebrospinal fluid (*pH* = 7.3), to the rumen (*pH* = 5.5 – 6.5), or to intracellular sites (*pH* = 7.0). Thus, weakly acidic drugs will tend not to distribute into the milk after systemic distribution (e.g., penicillin), while weakly basic drugs (e.g., erythromycin) will. If a disease process alters the *pH* of one compartment (e.g., mastitis), the normal equilibrium ratio will also be perturbed. In mastitis, in which the *pH* level may increase almost one unit, this preferential distribution of basic antibiotics will be lost. The relatively acidic *pH* of cells relative to plasma is responsible for the relatively large tissue distribution seen with many weakly basic drugs (e.g., morphine, amphetamine). Similarly, in the ruminant, many basic drugs tend to distribute into the rumen, resulting in distribution volumes much larger than those in monogastric animals. In fact, a drug that distributes into this organ may then undergo microbial degradation, resulting in its elimination from the body.

There are a number of mathematical transformations that can be made to these basic equations to facilitate the calculation of concentration gradients. For example, to calculate the equilibrium ratio (*R*) of two compounds across a membrane, the following equations could be used. For two acids (*a* and *b*):

$$R\ (a\,/\,b) = \frac{1 + 10^{(pH(a) - pKa)}}{1 + 10^{(pH(b) - pKa)}} \tag{2.4}$$

For two bases (*a* and *b*):

$$R\ (a\,/\,b) = \frac{1 + 10^{(pKa - pH(a))}}{1 + 10^{(pKa - pH(b))}} \tag{2.5}$$

This phenomenon is also very important for the passive tubular reabsorption of weak acids and bases being excreted by the kidney. For carnivores with acidic urine relative to plasma, weak acids tend to be reabsorbed from the tubules into the plasma, while weak bases tend to be preferentially excreted. This principle has been applied to the treatment of salicylate (weak acid) intoxication in dogs in which alkaline diuresis promotes ion-trapping of the drug in the urine and hence its more rapid excretion. Disease-induced changes in urine *pH* will likewise alter the disposition of drugs sensitive to this phenomenon.

In summary, one can appreciate that many of the principles that govern diffusion of a drug across biological membranes are applicable to many phases of drug disposition. However, there are several specialized membranes that possess specific transport systems. In these cases, the laws of diffusion and *pH* partitioning do not govern transmembrane flux of drugs. These specializations in transport can best be appreciated as mechanisms by which the body can exert control and selectivity over the chemicals that are allowed to enter the protected domain of specific organs, cells, or organelles. Such transport systems can be rather nonspecific as are those of the kidney and liver, which excrete charged waste products.

A similar situation occurs in the gastrointestinal tract, where relatively nonspecific transport systems allow for the absorption, and thus entrance to the body, of essential nutrients that do not have sufficient lipophilicity to cross membranes by diffusion. In specific tissues, they allow for select molecules to enter cells depending upon cellular needs, or allow compounds that circulate throughout the body to only have a biological response in a tissue possessing the correct transport receptor.

The primary example is the protein carrier-mediated processes of active transport or facilitated diffusion. These systems are characterized by specificity and saturability. In the case of active transport, biological energy is utilized to move drug against its concentration gradient. In facilitated diffusion, the carrier protein binds to the drug and carries it across the membrane down its concentration gradient. The drugs transported by these systems normally cannot cross the membrane by passive diffusion because they are not lipophilic. These systems are important for the gastrointestinal absorption of many essential nutrients, for cellular uptake of many compounds (e.g., glucose), for the removal of drugs from the cerebral spinal fluid through the choroid plexus, and for the biliary and renal excretion of numerous drugs.

The precise molecular mechanisms behind facilitated and active transport systems are beyond the scope of a pharmacokinetic book such as this. Texts in biochemistry or cellular physiology should be consulted for more detail. For most drugs, the principle of passive diffusion suffices for constructing pharmacokinetic models. Active transport systems are primarily encountered in processes of elimination, which will be dealt with in Chapters 5 and 6.

Active transport processes may dramatically alter the pharmacokinetics of a compound when the process is saturated at concentrations attainable in the body. At this point, unlike with diffusion, drug flux across a membrane is no longer directly proportional to concentration as was described by equation 2.1. This scenario is depicted in Figure 2.5. In pharmacokinetic terminology, concentration dependence is termed linear or first-order and is an assumption made in most generally applicable pharmacokinetic models, be they compartmental, noncompartmental, physiological, or population based. When the telltale plateauing of a saturable process is detected, so called nonlinear or zero-order processes are involved, and specific models must be employed to handle them. The development of such models, which are also encountered in drug protein binding and biotransformation, will be introduced in the chapters discussing these concepts. The incorporation of these processes into pharmacokinetic models will be formally presented in Chapter 9 on nonlinear models.

There are other transport processes important for certain drugs. Some membranes have pores or fenestrae, which allow filtration to occur. In these cases, relatively small molecules (molecular weights < 1000) can pass through independent of their lipid solubility, but larger molecules are excluded. This phenomenon is very important in excretory

flux - rate of transfer of fluid, particles, or energy across given surface.

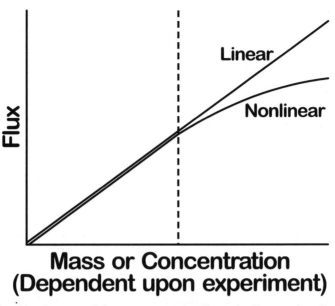

**Mass or Concentration
(Dependent upon experiment)**

FIGURE 2.5.   Relationship of compound flux to concentration illustrating linear and nonlinear kinetics.

processes. The primary route of excretion for most compounds is the kidney, which possesses just such a porous endothelium in its glomerular basement membrane. Thus hydrophilic drugs in solution in the aqueous plasma are readily excreted into the glomerular filtrate. In addition, most capillaries in the body have "leaky" junctions, which allow compounds in solution in the plasma to enter the extracellular fluids. However, unless inflammation is present, which increases capillary permeability, proteins are excluded.

In all of these scenarios, drugs move through these tissues as a solute dissolved in water and essentially are transported wherever the water goes. This process is termed bulk-flow and is dependent upon the concentration of drug dissolved in the plasma or tissue fluid. This is a linear process and thus is easily modeled by most pharmacokinetic systems. Exceptions are few (e.g., Donnan exclusion principle in glomerular filtration) and will be dealt with where appropriate. The only general exception that may affect the structure of some models is limitation of molecular size, which is generally encountered only in disposition of proteins, oligonucleotides, or synthetic polymers.

In some tissues, cells may absorb drugs by endocytosis or pinocytosis, processes in which a compound binds to the surface of the membrane, which then invaginates and interiorizes the compound. This is not a primary mechanism of transmembrane passage for most therapeutic drugs. Finally, most inorganic ions, such as sodium and chloride, are sufficiently small that they easily can cross aqueous membrane pores and channels. The movement of these charged substances is generally governed by the transmembrane electrical potential maintained by active ion pumps. Again, drugs and chemicals commonly modeled in pharmacokinetic studies do not have these properties and thus are not relevant to the scope of this text.

The principles governing the translocation of drugs across membranes and distribution throughout the body are based on the physical-chemical properties of the drug, which affects its interactions with the molecular components of the body. From the perspective of pharmacokinetics, the major processes that determine drug absorption and disposition, and the ones that are quantitated using mathematical models, are related to mass movement of drug across biological barriers. Energy is required to move any chemical across these barriers. This energy is usually related to a physical-chemical concept called thermodynamic activity, which reflects the energy ultimately responsible for moving a compound across membranes. This holds for most processes (except those mediated by active biological pumps) encountered in pharmacokinetics that are responsible for movement of drug into, through, and out of the body.

The best way to increase or create diffusion-driven transport is to create a concentration gradient, or increase the potential energy by creating a large driving force on only one side of a membrane. This can be accomplished by increasing dose or by asymmetrical mechanisms such as ion-trapping, which cause the same result. Whatever the source, most linear pharmacokinetic processes are driven by concentration gradients ultimately related to the administered dose.

It is the nature and relative rate of drug movements across these membranes, and drug distribution in the spaces defined by these multiple barriers, that provide for the subtle changes in drug concentration that allow pharmacokinetic models to be constructed. As will be developed in later chapters, differences in the rate and extent of drug movement across different barriers (natural or synthetic as in the case of slow-release drug delivery formulations) allow models to be constructed that provide mathematical links to these events and thus give one the ability to predict the concentration achieved over time after administering specific doses.

In conclusion, an understanding of the processes that govern the movement of drugs across lipid-based biological membranes is important to the study of drug absorption, distribution, and excretion. Lipid-soluble drugs are easily absorbed into the body and well distributed throughout the tissues. In contrast, hydrophilic drugs are not well absorbed but are easily eliminated. If membranes separate areas of different *pH* levels, concentration gradients may form due to *pH* partitioning or ion-trapping. All of these principles will be repeatedly encountered in the study of drug disposition presented in the remaining chapters of this text.

SELECTED READINGS

Alberts, B., D. Bray, J. Lewis, M. Raff, K. Roberts, and J.D. Watson. 1989. *Molecular Biology of the Cell*, 2ed. New York: Garland Publishing Co.

Brodie, B.B., J.R. Gillette, and H.S. Ackerman. 1971. *Handbook of Experimental Pharmacology, Vol. 28, Part I, Concepts in Biochemical Pharmacology.* Berlin: Springer.

Davson, H., and J.F. Danielli. 1952. *Permeability of Natural Membranes,* 2ed. London: Cambridge University Press.

Pratt, W.B. and P. Taylor. 1990. *Principles of Drug Action,* 3ed. New York: Churchill Livingstone.

Singer, S.J., and G.L. Nicholson. 1972. The fluid mosaic model of the structure of cell membranes. *Science.* 175:720-731.

3

Absorption

Absorption is the movement of drug from the site of administration into the blood. There are a number of methods available for administering drugs to animals. The primary routes of drug absorption from environmental exposure in mammals are gastrointestinal, dermal, and respiratory. The first two are also used as routes of drug administration for systemic effects, with additional routes including intramuscular, subcutaneous, or intraperitoneal injection and intravenous administration. Other variations on gastrointestinal absorption include intrarumenal, sublingual, and rectal drug delivery. Many techniques are also used for localized therapy, which may result in systemic drug absorption as a side effect. Among others, these include topical, intramammary, intra-articular, subconjunctival, and spinal fluid injections.

GASTROINTESTINAL ABSORPTION

One of the primary routes of drug administration is oral ingestion of a pill or tablet that is designed for drug delivery to cross the gastrointestinal mucosa. The common factor in all forms of oral drug administration is the delivery of a drug such that it gets into solution in the gastrointestinal fluids, from which it can then be absorbed across the mucosa and ultimately reach the submucosal capillaries and the systemic circulation. Examples of oral drug delivery systems include solutions (aqueous solutions, elixirs) and suspensions, pills, tablets, boluses for food animals, capsules, pellets, and sustained-release mechanical devices for ruminants. The major obstacle encountered in comparative and veterinary medicine is the enormous interspecies diversity in comparative gastrointestinal anatomy and physiology, which results in major species differences in strategies for and efficiency of oral drug administration. This is often appreciated but overlooked when laboratory animal data are extrapolated to humans. Rats and rabbits are widely utilized in preclinical disposition and toxicology studies, although many investigators fail to appreciate that these animals' gastrointestinal tracts are very different from one another and from those of humans.

From a pharmacologist's perspective, the gastrointestinal tract of all species can be simply presented as diagrammed in Figure 3.1. As discussed in Chapter 2, the gastrointestinal tract is best conceptualized as actually being part of the external environment, which, in contrast to the skin, is protected and whose microenvironment is closely regulated by epithelium – an animal tissue that forms the covering or lining of all free body surfaces, both external and internal

epi – upon, onto.

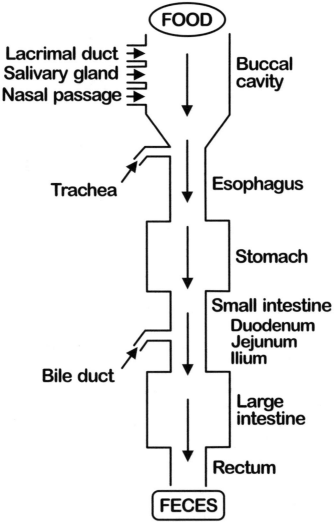

FIGURE 3.1.   Functional structure of the gastrointestinal tract.

mucosa – inner layer of the stomach wall

– any membrane that secretes mucus (a slimy protective substance) eg) membrane lining the stomach and intestine

glands of the stomach lining secrete mucus

the organism. Because of its central role in digestion and nutrient absorption, there are many evolutionary adaptations to this basically simple mucosa structure that allow for physical, chemical, enzymatic, and microbial breakdown of potential food for liberation and ultimate absorption of nutrients. This tract is further adapted such that these digestive processes do not harm the organism's own tissues, which in carnivores may be identical to the food being eaten.

The gastrointestinal tract presents a significant degree of heterogeneity relative to morphology and physiology, which translates to great regional variations in drug absorption. In the oral cavity, where food is masticated, some absorption may occur in sublingual areas. In fact, this site is actually utilized as a route for systemic drug (e.g., nitroglycerin) and nicotine (e.g., oral tobacco) delivery. The esophagus and cranial portion of the stomach is lined by cornified epithelium, which provides an effective barrier and often decreases the chance of absorption for drugs formulated for intestinal drug delivery. The structure and function of this cornified epithelium is actually very similar to that of skin

epithelium –

[handwritten annotations at top:]
villi — small fingerlike growth
microvilli — epithelial cells covering the folds and villi have a brush border, consisting of closely packed cylindrical process

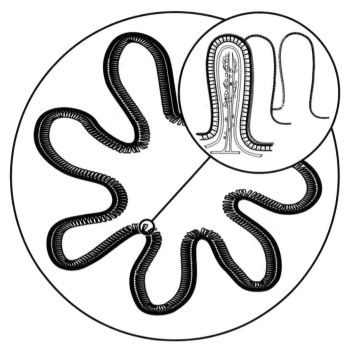

FIGURE 3.2.   Cross-section of the small intestine showing villi adaptations, which increase surface area available for absorption.

described later, except for the presence of mucosal glands. A great deal of recent research has been focused on developing new transbuccal drug delivery systems. As mentioned, the prototype example was sublingual nitroglycerin tablets. Newer systems use novel adhesive technology, which allows actual polymer patches to adhere to the buccal mucosa. This route is a comparatively more permeable barrier than skin. Additionally, compared to oral gastrointestinal absorption, it bypasses the portal vein and thus eliminates the potential for first-pass hepatic biotransformation. *[handwritten: liver]* *[handwritten: blood from capillaries of intestine and stomach is collected, which goes to liver]*

The simple mucosal lining of the stomach allows absorption; however, the presence of surface mucus, which protects the epithelium from self-digestion secondary to acid and enzyme secretion, may be a barrier for some drugs. The acidity and motility of the stomach also creates a hostile environment for drugs and even influences the absorption of drugs farther down the tract. For oral drug absorption to be successful, the drug must be capable of surviving this relatively harsh environment. For some drugs (e.g., penicillin G) susceptible to acid hydrolysis, minimal absorption by the oral route will occur unless they are administered in a formulation that protects them in an acid environment but liberates them in the more alkaline environment of the intestines.

The primary site for most drug absorption is the small intestine. In this region of the gastrointestinal tract, the pH of the contents are more alkaline, and the epithelial lining is conducive to drug absorption. The blood flow to this region is also much greater than to the stomach. The small intestine is lined by simple columnar epithelium resting on a basement membrane and a submucosal tissue bed that is very well perfused by an extensive capillary and lymphatic network. This capillary bed drains into the hepatic portal vein. One of the major anatomical adaptations for absorption in this region is the presence of microvilli that increase the surface area of the small intestine some 600-fold over that of a simple tube. The second anatomical adaptation is that of the villi of the intestine, which can be easily appreciated by examining a cross-section (Figure 3.2). Since diffusion is the primary mechanism for drug absorption, the increase in area due to these two anatomical configurations significantly increases absorption, as can be seen by realizing that equation 2.1 is expressed per unit surface area.

The viable epithelial cells of the intestines are also endowed with the necessary enzymes for drug metabolism, which contributes to a second first-pass effect. Recent research has also indicated that the mechanism and extent of absorption, and the magnitude of local intestinal metabolism, vary between the tips and crypts of the villi. The final determinant of a drug's tortuous journey through the gastrointestinal tract is the resident microbial population that inhabits the intestinal contents. Many bacteria are capable of metabolizing specific drugs, resulting in a third component of the first-pass effect. This epithelial and bacterial biotransformation is generally categorized as "presystemic" metabolism to differentiate it from that which occurs following portal vein delivery of drug to the liver. However, from the perspective of pharmacokinetic analysis of plasma drug concentrations following oral drug administration, all three components are indistinguishable and become combined in the aggregate process of oral absorption assessed as K_a.

Disintegration, Dissolution, Diffusion, and Other Transport Phenomena.   In order for a drug to be absorbed across the intestinal mucosa, the drug must first be dissolved in the aqueous intestinal fluid. Two steps—disintegration and dissolution—may be required for this to occur. Disintegration is the process whereby a solid dosage form (e.g., tablet) physically disperses so that its constituent particles can be exposed to the gastrointestinal fluid. Dissolution occurs when the drug molecules then enter into solution. This component of the process is technically termed the *pharmaceutical phase* and is controlled by the interaction of the formulation with the intestinal contents. Some dosage forms, such as capsules and lozenges, may not be designed to disintegrate, but rather to allow drug to slowly elute from their surface. Dissolution is often the rate-limiting step controlling the absorption process and can be enhanced by formulating the drug in salt form (e.g., sodium or hydrochloride salts), buffering the preparation (e.g., buffered aspirin), or decreasing dispersed particle size (micronization) so as to maximize exposed surface area. Alternatively, disintegration and dissolution can be decreased so as to deliberately provide slow release of drug. This strategy is used in so-called extended-release or slow-release dosage forms and involves complex pharmaceutical formulations that produce differential rates of dissolution. This may be accomplished by dispersing the dosage form into particles with different rates of dissolution or by using multilaminated dosage forms, which delays release of the drug until its layer is exposed. All of these strategies decrease the overall rate of absorption. Similar strategies can also be used to target drugs to the distal segments of the gastrointestinal tract by using delayed-release enteric coatings, which dissolve only at specific pH ranges, thereby preventing dissolution until the drug is in the region targeted. This strategy has been applied for colonic delivery of drugs in humans for treatment of Crohn's disease.

In extended-release formulations, the end result is that absorption becomes slower than all other distribution and elimination processes, making the pharmaceutical phase the rate-limiting or rate-controlling step in the subsequent absorption and disposition of the drug. When this occurs, as will be seen in the pharmacokinetic modeling chapters that follow, the rate of absorption controls the rate of apparent drug elimination from the body, and a so-called *flip-flop* scenario becomes operative.

After the drug is in solution, it must still be in a nonionized, relatively lipid soluble form to be absorbed across the lipid membranes that make up the intestinal mucosa. For orally administered products, the pH of the gastrointestinal contents becomes very important, as is evident from the earlier discussion on pH partitioning in Chapter 2. Specifically, a weak acid would tend to be preferentially absorbed in the more acidic environment of the stomach since a larger fraction would be in the nonionized form. However, the much larger surface area and blood flow available for absorption in the more alkaline intestine may, coupled with a relatively acidic pH ($\simeq 5.5$) at the apical membrane's mucous layer, override this effect. It is important to mention why a weak acid such as aspirin is better absorbed in a bicarbonate buffered form, which would tend to increase the ionized fraction and thus decrease membrane passage. The paradox is that dissolution, a process favored by the ionized form of the drug, must first occur. Only the dissolved ionized aspirin is available to the partitioning phenomenon described in Chapter 2. Thus, when more aspirin is dissolved in the buffered microenvironment, more is available for partitioning and diffusion across the mucosa. It is a misconception that the very small amount of buffering activity in the tablet actually increases gastric pH. In contrast to the situation of a weak acid, a weak base tends to be better absorbed in the more alkaline environment. However, it must be repeated that the very large surface area available in the intestines, coupled with high blood flow and a pH of approximately 5.3 in the immediate area of the mucosal surface, makes it the primary site of absorption for most drugs (weak acids with pKa > 3 and weak bases with pKa < 7.8). An obstacle to absorption is that the compound must also be structurally stable against chemical or enzymatic attack. Finally, compounds with a fixed charge and/or very low (or very high) lipid solubility for the uncharged moiety may not be significantly absorbed after oral administration. Examples include the polar aminoglycoside antibiotics, the so-called enteric sulfonamides, and quaternary ammonium drugs.

There are also specific active transport systems present within the intestinal mucosa of the microvilli that are responsible for nutrient absorption. However, these systems have a very high capacity, and if a specific drug or toxicant has the proper molecular configuration to be transported, saturation is unlikely. There is some evidence that select therapeutic drugs (e.g, ampicillin) may be absorbed by active transport systems in the small intestine. These drugs behave as if their absorption were linear and, from a pharmacokinetic perspective, they can be modeled using the same first-order rate constants as passively absorbed drugs unless nonlinear behavior is clearly evident. These modeling techniques will be presented in much greater detail in later chapters.

Enterohepatic Recycling.   The gastrointestinal tract has also evolved into an excretory organ for elimination of nonabsorbed solid wastes and other metabolic by-products excreted in the bile. The bile duct drains into the upper small intestine. For some drugs, this results in a phenomenon called *enterohepatic recycling,* whereby a drug from the systemic circulation is excreted into the bile and is reabsorbed from the small intestine back into the blood stream. In many cases, drugs that are metabolized by phase II conjugation reactions are "unconjugated" by resident bacterial flora, which generates free drug for reabsorption. Thus compounds that are excreted into the bile may have a prolonged sojourn in the body because of the continuous opportunity for intestinal reabsorption. The cardinal sign of this process is a "hump" in the plasma drug concentration-time profile after administration (Figure 3.3). Bile also serves to emulsify fatty substances that are not capable of solubilizing in the primarily aqueous environment of the intestines. The result of this detergent-like action of bile is the formation of large surface area micelles that have a hydrophilic surface and hydrophobic interior. These act as transport vehicles to deliver fat-soluble drugs to the intestinal brush border surface for diffusion across the lipid membrane into the cell. Without the interaction of bile acids, fatty substances would not be available for absorption because they could not traverse this "dissolution" barrier. Thus, unlike most drugs, compounds that are absorbed by this route often must be administered with a meal to promote bile acid secretion and associated micelle formation. Chapter 6 should be consulted for an in-depth discussion of biliary secretory processes.

ruminant - chew again what has been chewed slightly and swallowed
rumen - large first compartment of stomach of ruminant in which cellulose
          is broken down

26 *Comparative Pharmacokinetics: Principles, Techniques, and Applications*

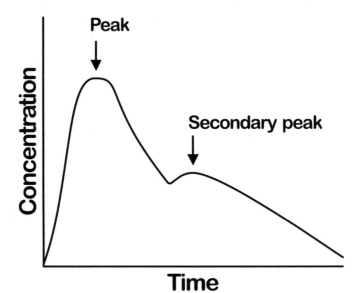

FIGURE 3.3. Profile of concentration versus time demonstrates a secondary peak that could result from enterohepatic recycling.

Species Effects on Gastrointestinal Transit Time and Food Interactions. Food may also interact with other aspects of oral drug absorption and have opposite effects for more-hydrophilic drugs. Depending on the physicochemical properties of the specific drug, administration with food may significantly decrease absorption. Such effects are not only drug-dependent, but also are species-dependent due to the continuous foraging behavior of ruminants and some other omnivores compared to the periodic feeding habits of predatory carnivores. These variables are difficult to incorporate into formal pharmacokinetic models, yet they add to the variability in parameters derived from these studies.

The first potential interaction relates to the rate of drug delivery to the small intestine, which is governed by the rate of drug release from the stomach, the so-called gastric emptying time. This process is dependent upon the eating habits of the species. Continuous foraging animals (e.g., herbivores such as horses and ruminants) have a steady input of drug and a relatively stable gastric pH compared to periodic eaters (e.g., carnivores such as dogs and cats and omnivores such as pigs), which have more variable eating patterns and large swings in gastric pH depending on the presence or absence of food. In addition, the drug may directly interact with the ingested food, as is the case of chelation of tetracyclines with divalent cations such as Mg^{++} in antacids or Ca^{++} in milk products. Thus the decision to administer a compound with or without food is species- and drug-dependent and may significantly alter the bioavailability (rate and extent of absorption) of the drug.

The unique physiology of the equine and ruminant gastrointestinal tract deserves further discussion. Both species have significant anatomical adaptations to allow for microbial digestion of polysaccharides. An obvious problem could arise from the use of microcellulose-based, sustained-release tablet formulations designed for humans. Administered to a herbivore, such tablets would be digested and the drug quickly absorbed rather than the tablet remaining intact as they do in a monogastric animal. Absorption would be dramatically decreased if the drug were metabolized by endogenous microbes. In contrast, if the drug is an antimicrobial, it may disturb this microflora and alter digestive processes.

The forestomachs of a ruminant provide a major obstacle to the delivery of an oral dosage form to the true stomach (abomasum) for ultimate release to the intestines, although a significant amount of drug absorption may occur from this site. The rumen is essentially a large fermentation vat (> 50 L in cattle, 5 L in sheep) lined by stratified squamous epithelium, buffered at a pH of approximately 6 by extensive input of saliva, which maintains it in a fluid to soft consistency designed primarily for the absorption of volatile fatty acids. If drugs dissolve in this medium and remain intact, they undergo tremendous dilution, which decreases their rate of absorption. They then are pumped from the rumen and reticulum through the omasum for a rather steady input of drug into the true stomach. An understanding of ruminant physiology has allowed for the development of some unique and innovative mechanical drug-delivery technologies termed *rumen retention systems*. These essentially are encapsulated pumps that "sink" to the bottom of the rumen and become trapped, as do many unwanted objects (e.g., nails and wire in hardware disease) when ingested by a ruminant. These submarine-like devices then slowly release drug into the ruminal fluid for a true sustained-release preparation. In preruminant calves, drug may bypass the rumen entirely through the rumen-reticulo groove and essentially behave as if administered to a monogastric animal. In contrast, fermentation in the horse occurs after drug absorption by the small intestine and thus has less impact than in ruminants. However, nonabsorbed drug that reaches the equine large intestines and cecum, the site of fermentation, may have disastrous effects (e.g., colic) if digestive flora or function is perturbed. As alluded to earlier, a similar strategy is used to target drugs to the human colon. In addition to extended-release or delayed-release enteric coatings, pro-drug approaches have been used that inhibit drug absorption until specific enzymes are encountered in the distal gastrointestinal tract. These enzymes liberate the active moiety from the pro-drug (e.g., azo reduction).

First-Pass Metabolism.   Another unique aspect of oral drug absorption is the fate of the absorbed drug once it enters the submucosal capillaries. Drug absorbed distal to the oral cavity and proximal to the rectum enters the portal circulation and is transported directly to the liver, where biotransformation may occur. This can be appreciated in Figures 2.1 and 3.1 and is the major cause for differences in a drug's ultimate disposition compared to all other routes of administration. This may result in a significant "first-pass" biotransformation of the absorbed compound. Some of the more complex pharmacokinetic models are needed to quantitate drugs with a significant first-pass effect. Finally, some drugs that are too polar to be absorbed across the gastrointestinal wall are formulated as ester conjugates to increase lipid solubility and enhance absorption. Once the drug crosses the gastrointestinal epithelium in this form, subsequent first-pass hepatic biotransformation enzymes and circulating blood and mucosal esterases cleave off the ester moiety, releasing free drug into the systemic circulation. Chapter 6 on biotransformation should be consulted for more details on drug metabolism by the liver.

As discussed earlier, for some drugs there is also a significant loss secondary to gastric acid hydrolysis or metabolism by enzymes in the brush border of intestinal mucosal cells. This severely restricts the absorption of protein, peptide, and oligonucleotide (e.g., antisense) drugs administered orally. This presystemic intestinal breakdown of peptides deserves further comment. Peptidases are located in the microvilli epithelium, which is present to digest protein and peptides into their constituent amino acids. Proteases from the pancreas complete the process of digestion of proteins that were not completely hydrolyzed by stomach acids. Protein digests and peptides are then efficiently broken down into amino acids to allow for absorption. Despite substantial pharmaceutical research efforts over the past decade to overcome this obstacle to the delivery of these products of the modern biotechnology industry, little progress has been made, and administering peptide drugs orally only contributes to the extent of the caloric value of the amino acid constituents.

The use of selected drug administration sites prevents first-pass hepatic metabolism by allowing absorption through gastrointestinal tract segments *not* drained by the portal vein. These include the oral cavity buccal and rectal routes of drug administration. As discussed earlier, the keratinized buccal mucosa is very similar to skin. Rectal drug administration is accomplished with suppositories and formulations (e.g., diazepam), which allow retention and adhesion of drug to the distal rectum. Drug absorption by this route is by passive diffusion and obeys the diffusion principles discussed previously.

Absorption Models.   It must be stressed that the de facto standard for assessing oral absorption is based upon the use of intact animals. The design of these studies is often driven by regulatory guidelines. However, there are also a number of *in vitro* methodologies available. The simplest, classic technique is the use of *in vitro* diffusion cells (water-jacketed to control temperature), whereby a piece of gastrointestinal mucosa is clamped between two chambers (Figure 3.4). An intestinal membrane may be grown using cell culture techniques. The most widely used system is the Caco model derived from a human intestinal carcinoma cell line. However, its use has recently been challenged on the grounds that metabolism in these transformed cells may be different from that in normal human intestinal cells. Depending upon the purpose of the study, drug is placed in solution in the donor chamber, and the appearance of drug is monitored in the receptor chamber. This technique has also been extensively used to study the biophysics and bioenergetics of active transport processes. More sophisticated models acknowledge the complexity of the *in vivo* setting and study drugs by using *in situ* intestinal flap preparations or isolated perfused intestinal segments, a technique facilitated by the arcuate vascular distribution to discrete intestinal segments. In these situations, drugs are placed in the intestinal contents, and the appearance of drug is monitored in the venous drainage or perfusate. Finally, the most sophisticated techniques available are conducted in conscious, nonmedicated animals or humans and use remote-controlled microprocessor-embedded drug devices administered orally. The passage of these submarine-like devices is monitored by fluoroscopy, and when the capsule reaches a specific segment of the gastrointestinal tract, the device is activated and drug released. Drug absorption is then monitored by assaying blood samples. In all of these cases, the pharmacokinetic models

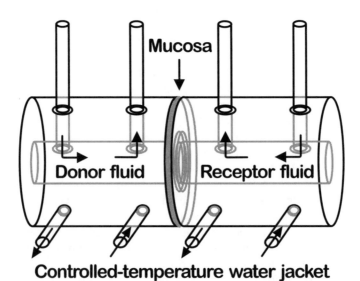

FIGURE 3.4.   *In vitro* chamber used to assess absorption across gastrointestinal membranes.

discussed in subsequent chapters are then used to derive parameters to quantitate absorption.

In conclusion, oral drug administration is the most convenient but most species-specific and variable method for drug administration by the veterinarian. The quantitative estimate of the rate and extent of drug absorption, termed *bioavailability*, will be discussed at the end of this chapter.

Formulation Factors. The pharmaceutical literature is replete with formulation factors that may influence the dissolution and absorption of a drug preparation, assuming in the first place that one has an active component of known purity and potency. The issue then becomes,what are the potential interactions that can occur between the active ingredients and the excipients that make up the formulation? Additionally, what are the effects of the practitioner's compounding techniques (materials used, mixing efficacy, etc.) on the amount of active ingredients ultimately appearing in the formulation? Although this discussion is the focus of a biopharmaceutics text, the strategies are often encountered in pharmacokinetics as they may affect the parameters estimated after oral administration.

Table 3.1 lists the pharmaceutical processes involved in absorption that may be affected by formulation. Following oral administration of tablets, disintegration must first occur. The speed and efficacy of this process will determine how much drug is actually available for subsequent steps. The resulting particle size (and hence surface area) is an important determinant for the next dissolution phase, in which the drug enters solution, an absolute prerequisite for diffusion across the mucosal barrier. Dissolution also involves diffusion across the liquid boundary layers, which are an interface between the particles and the absorption milieu. Many pharmaceutical factors may affect the efficiency of the disintegration and dissolution processes. For tablets, the nature and homogeneity of the excipients become important considerations. As previously discussed using the aspirin example, buffers must be included to ensure that all of the drug particles adequately and rapidly dissolve. These factors are the primary determinants of differences in efficacy between so-called pioneer and generic drug products. Once the drug is in solution, then binding or complexation to inert filler ingredients may occur. It is important to remember that all of this is happening while the particles are in transit through the gastrointestinal tract. Thus, if the formulation results in a decreased rate of disintegration or dissolution, the rate and extent of absorption may be decreased. These processes are competing kinetic events and thus are sensitive to all of the rate processes involved.

TABLE 3.1. Pharmaceutical Factors Affecting Absorption

Disintegration
    Excipients
    Compaction pressure
    Enteric coatings, capsules
    Homogeneity

Dissolution
    Particle size/surface area
    Binding
    Local pH, buffers
    Boundary layers

Barrier Diffusion
    Solubility
    Transit time

Similar factors are involved with oral capsules and even liquid dosage forms, in which case the drug may interact with the vehicle. In fact, these scenarios are probably most pertinent to practitioner compounding. For capsules, the breakdown of the capsule replaces tablet disintegration as the initial rate-determining step. After release of the capsule contents, all of the above factors come into play. It cannot be overstated that such pharmaceutical factors are critical determinants of the extent and rate of subsequent drug absorption.

TOPICAL AND PERCUTANEOUS ABSORPTION *through the skin*

The skin is a complex, multilayered tissue comprising 18,000 cm² of surface in an average human male. The quantitative prediction of the rate and extent of percutaneous penetration (into skin) and absorption (through skin) of topically applied chemicals is complicated by the biological variability inherent in skin. Mammalian skin is a dynamic organ with a myriad of biological functions. The most obvious is its barrier property, which is of primary concern in the absorption problem. Another major function is thermoregulation, which is achieved and regulated by three mechanisms in skin: thermal insulation provided by pelage and hair, sweating, and alteration of cutaneous blood flow. Other functions of skin include mechanical support, neurosensory reception, endocrinology, immunology, and glandular secretion. These additional biological roles lead to functional and structural adaptations that affect the skin's barrier properties and thus the rate and extent of percutaneous absorption.

The skin is generally considered to be an efficient barrier, preventing absorption (and thus systemic exposure) of most topically administered compounds. It is a membrane that is relatively impermeable to aqueous solutions and most ions. It is, however, permeable in varying degrees to a large number of solid, liquid, and gaseous xenobiotics. Although one tends to think of most cases of poisoning as occurring through the oral or, less frequently, the respiratory route, the widespread use of organic chemicals has enhanced exposure to many toxicants that can penetrate the dermal barrier. An example is the large number of agricultural workers who have experienced acute dermal poisoning from direct exposure to parathion (dermal LD50 = 20 mg/kg) during application or from more casual exposure, such as contact with vegetation previously treated with such insecticides. Similar situations often occur in veterinary species.

The gross features of mammalian skin are illustrated in Figure 3.5. Compared to most routes of drug absorption, the skin is by far the most diverse across species (e.g., sheep versus pig) and body sites (e.g., human forearm versus scalp). Three distinct layers and a number of associated appendages make up this nonhomogenous organ. The epidermis is a multilayered tissue varying in thickness in humans from 0.15 mm (eyelids) to 0.8 mm (palms). The primary cell type found in the epidermis is the keratinocyte. Proliferative layers of the basal keratinocyte (stratum germinativum) differentiate and gradually replace the surface cells as they deteriorate and are sloughed from the epidermis. A number of other cell types are also found interspersed in the epidermis, including the pigmented melanocytes; Merkel cells, which may play a sensory role; and Langerhans cells, which probably play a role in cutaneous immunology. These cells are not important contributors to the skin's barrier properties. The basal keratinocyte layer consists of nucleated cuboidal to columnar cells. As these cells move toward the surface, they lose their shape, becoming rounded and ultimately flattened. Three loosely defined layers—the stratum spinosum, stratum granulosum, and stratum lucidum—are areas of considerable morphological and biochemical change, and although variable, their width is several times that of the final surface layer.

The primary morphological changes that occur as the keratinocytes progressively die are that they become greatly flattened, and the nuclei become progressively less obvious. In respect to penetration, the primary biochemical change is the production of fibrous,

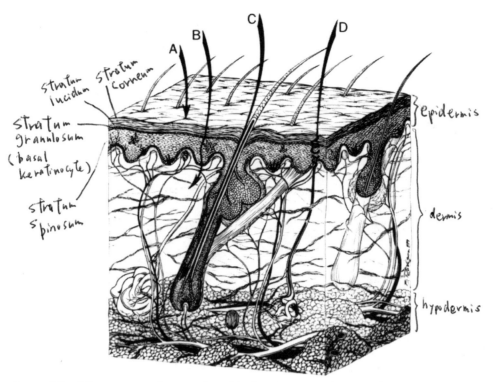

FIGURE 3.5. Microstructure of mammalian skin showing potential routes of penetration. A, intercellular; B, transcellular; C, intrafollicular; D, via sweat ducts. (Reproduced with permission. Riviere, J.E., and N.A. Monteiro-Riviere. 1991. The isolated perfused porcine skin flap as an *in vitro* model for percutaneous absorption and cutaneous toxicology. Critical Reviews in Toxicology. 21:329-344.)

insoluble keratin that fills the cells, and a sulfur-rich amorphous protein that comprises the cell matrix and thickened cell membrane. In addition, the keratinocytes synthesize a variety of lipids that form the distinguishing granules in the stratum granulosum and release their contents into the intercellular spaces. The result in the stratum corneum is dead proteinaceous keratinocytes embedded in an extracellular lipid matrix, a structure referred to by Elias as the "brick and mortar" model depicted in Figure 3.6. The intercellular lipid composition is not homogenous in all layers of the epidermis, making the lipid topography complex. Species differences (lipid composition) also occur.

The Stratum Corneum Barrier. It is the final layer, the stratum corneum, that provides the primary barrier to the penetration of foreign compounds. This barrier consists of eight to 16 layers of flattened, stratified, highly keratinized cells embedded in a lipid matrix composed primarily of sterols, other neutral lipids, and ceramides. These cells are approximately 25 to 40 μm wide, lie tangential to the skin surface, and are oriented as relatively impermeable shingles to form a layer approximately 10 μm thick. The sequence of events from basal cell to stratum corneum formation requires about 4 weeks. Although highly water retarding, the dead, keratinized cells are highly water absorbent (hydrophilic), a property that keeps the skin supple and soft. A natural oil covering the skin, the sebum, appears to maintain the water-holding capacity of the epidermis but has no appreciable role in retarding the penetration of xenobiotics.

Disruption of the stratum corneum removes all but a superficial deterrent to penetration. One line of evidence utilizes "stripping" experiments, in which an adhesive (cellophane tape) is placed on the skin repeatedly, removing progressive sections of the

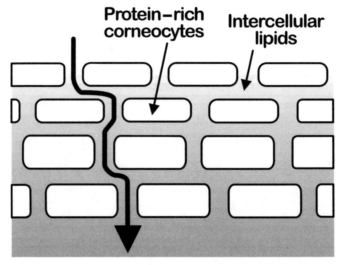

Figure 3.6.   Conceptual "brick and mortar" model of the stratum corneum demonstrating predominant intercellular pathway for topically applied compounds.

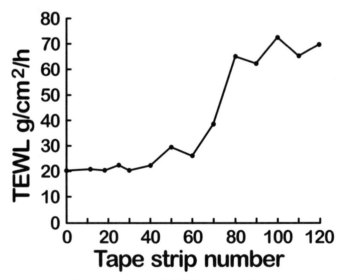

FIGURE 3.7.   Increase in transepidermal water loss (TEWL) in porcine skin as a function of stratum corneum barrier removal with cellophane tape stripping.

corneum. The skin continuously loses its ability to retard penetration, and compound flux increases greatly. This can be noninvasively assessed by measuring the skin's ability to prevent insensible water loss from the body to the environment by using water as a marker of molecular transport across the cutaneous barrier. This is performed by measuring transepidermal water loss (TEWL). This value increases greatly when the stratum corneum is either stripped away using adhesive tape (Figure 3.7) or removed by extracting the intercellular barrier lipids.

For many compounds, the stratum corneum has been calculated to afford 1000 times the resistance to penetration as the layers beneath it. Exceptions to this rule are extremely lipid-soluble compounds with tissue:water partition coefficients greater than 400. As in most other epithelial tissues, the two deeper layers of the skin (dermis and subcutaneous tissue) generally offer little resistance to penetration, and once a substance has penetrated the outer epithelium, these tissues are rapidly traversed. For the highly lipid-soluble compounds, this may not be true, and the dermis may function as a barrier preventing a chemical that has penetrated the epidermis from being absorbed into the blood.

Dermis and Appendages.   The dermis is a highly vascular area, providing ready access for drug distribution once the epithelial barrier has been passed. The blood supply in the dermis is under complex, interacting neural and local humoral influences whose temperature-regulating function can have an effect on distribution by altering blood supply to this area. This function of mammalian skin is different from that of the other epithelial tissues discussed and offers another variable for predicting transdermal drug delivery. The absorption of a chemical possessing vasoactive properties would be affected through its action on the dermal vasculature; vasoconstriction would retard absorption and increase the size of a dermal depot, while vasodilation may enhance absorption and minimize any local dermal depot formation.

The appendages of the skin are found in the dermis and extend through the epidermis, as can readily be appreciated from examining Figure 3.5. The primary appendages are the sweat glands (eccrine and apocrine), hair, and sebaceous glands. Since these structures extend to the outer surface, they play a role in the penetration of certain compounds.

Topical Drug Delivery and the Definition of Dose.   From the perspective of pharmacokinetic models of transdermal and topical drug delivery systems, there are significant differences from other routes of administration (e.g., oral, injection) as to what constitutes a dose. Dermatological preparations target drugs to the skin (penetration is important), whereas transdermal preparations target drugs to the systemic circulation (absorption is important). In veterinary medicine, many pour-on pesticides are in fact transdermal delivery systems. For most exposures, the concentration applied to the surface of the skin exceeds the absorption capacity. Thus, application of higher doses results in a decreased fraction of dose absorbed but an increase in actual drug flux (Table 3.2). However, for therapeutic transdermal patches with a fixed concentration of drug and rate-controlled release properties (much like the oral extended-release formulations discussed earlier), it is the contact surface area that more accurately reflects dose, and thus dose is expressed not in mg/kg, but mg/cm^2 of dosing area. This surface area dependence also holds for any topical application even if absorption capacity is superseded. Yet another source of nonlinearity results secondary to the effects of occlusive (water impermeable) drug vehicle or patches. As the skin hydrates, a threshold is reached at which transdermal flux dramatically increases (approximately 80% relative humidity), as with the topical parathion studies in Figure 3.8. When the skin becomes completely hydrated under occlusive conditions, flux can be dramatically increased. Therefore, dose alone is often not a sufficient metric to describe topical doses, and application method and surface area become controlling factors. Hydration can also markedly affect the pH of the skin, which varies between 4.2 and

TABLE 3.2.   Percutaneous Absorption of Parathion, Paraoxon, and p-Nitrophenol (Flux in µg/cm^2/8 h Using *in vitro* Porcine Skin; Second Row is % Dose)

Dose	4 µg/cm^2	40 µg/cm^2	400 µg/cm^2
Parathion	0.32 ± 0.02	0.77 ± 0.11	1.86 ± 0.14
	7.91 ± 0.38%	1.91 ± 0.28%	0.46 ± 0.04%
Paraoxon	0.61 ± 0.18	3.93 ± 1.16	10.12 ± 1.71
	15.52 ± 4.42%	9.38 ± 2.90%	2.53 ± 0.43%
p-Nitrophenol	0.45 ± 0.09	5.34 ± 0.71	82.99 ± 20.03
	11.21 ± 2.28%	13.35 ± 1.77%	20.75 ± 6.00%

Adapted from: Chang, Dauterman, and Riviere. 1994. *Pesticide Biochemistry and Physiology.* 48:56-62.

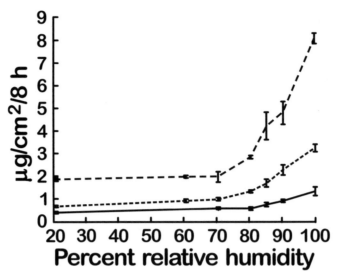

FIGURE 3.8.   Increase in parathion percutaneous absorption as a function of increasing relative humidity. Applied doses: — , 4; - - - -, 40; – – – –, 400 μg/cm².

7.3. For drugs or chemicals with pKa levels in this range, the principles embedded in the Henderson-Hasselbalch equations 2.2 and 2.3 become important. The unionized fraction may change as a function of skin pH, thereby further modulating percutaneous absorption.

Pathways for Dermal Absorption.   Anatomically, percutaneous absorption might occur through several routes. The current consensus is that the majority of nonionized, lipid-soluble toxicants appear to move through the intercellular lipid pathway between the cells of the stratum corneum, the rate-limiting barrier of the skin. It was previously thought that the primary route was transcellular (through the cells), but recent work has discredited this view. A third possible route is through the appendages, such as hair follicles or sweat ducts. Very small and/or polar molecules appear to have more favorable penetration through appendages or other diffusion shunts, but only a small fraction of drugs are represented by these molecules. Initial penetration particularly may be aided by appendages. In addition, the epidermal surface area is 100 to 1000 times the surface area of the skin appendages. Passage through the skin is passive, there being no evidence for active transport. Simple diffusion seems to account for penetration through the skin, whether by gases, ions, or nonelectrolytes.

Polar substances, in addition to movement through shunts, may diffuse through the outer surface of the protein filaments of the hydrated stratum corneum, while nonpolar molecules dissolve in and diffuse through the nonaqueous lipid matrix between the protein filaments. The rate of percutaneous absorption through this intercellular lipid pathway is correlated to the partition coefficient of the penetrant. This has resulted in numerous studies correlating the extent of percutaneous absorption with a drug's lipid:water partition coefficient, typified by Figure 3.9. Some workers further correlated skin penetration to molecular size and other indices of potential interaction between the penetrating molecule and the skin which are not reflected in the partition coefficient. For most purposes, however, dermal penetration is often correlated to partition coefficient. If lipid solubility is too great, then compounds which penetrate the stratum corneum may remain there and form a reservoir, evidenced by a plateauing in extent of absorption versus partition coefficient plots (Figure 3.9). Alternatively, penetrated compounds may also form a reservoir in the dermis. For such compounds, slow release from these depots may result in

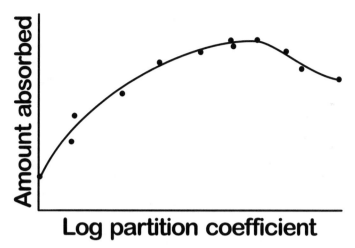

FIGURE 3.9.   Relation between log partition coefficient and amount absorbed.

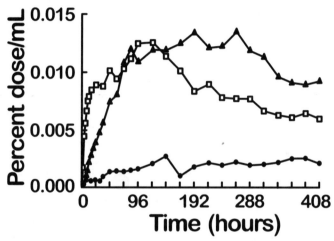

FIGURE 3.10.   Application vehicle effects on the percutaneous absorption of topically dosed pentachlorophenol (40 µg/cm²) on *in vivo* pigs. •••, nonoccluded soil; □, occluded soil; ▲▲▲, occluded soil with antimicrobials.

a prolonged absorption half-life. Conditions that alter the composition of the lipid (harsh delipidizing solvents, dietary lipid restrictions, disease) may alter the rate of compound penetration by changing its partitioning behavior.

Recent studies have demonstrated that the skin may also be responsible for metabolizing topically applied compounds. Both phase I and phase II metabolic pathways have been identified. For some compounds, the extent of cutaneous metabolism influences the overall fraction of a topically applied compound that is absorbed, making this process function as an alternative absorption pathway. Cutaneous biotransformation is used to promote the absorption of some topical drugs that normally would not penetrate the skin. Pro-drugs, consisting of the more lipid-soluble ester analogues, penetrate the stratum corneum, and then the active drugs are liberated through the action of cutaneous or blood esterases. Cutaneous metabolism may also be important for certain aspects of skin toxicology when nontoxic parent compounds are bioactivated within the epidermis, such as benzo[*a*]pyrene to an epoxide. Finally, resident bacteria on the surface of the skin may also metabolize topical drugs, as we recently demonstrated with pentachlorophenol absorption in pig skin dosed in soil with and without antibiotics (Figure 3.10). This effect is potentiated under warm and wet occlusive dosing conditions, which both promote bacterial growth and reduce skin barrier properties.

Variations in Species and Body Region.   Penetration of drugs through different body regions varies. In humans, the rate of penetration of most nonionized toxicants is generally in the following order: scrotal > forehead > axilla = scalp > back = abdomen > palm and plantar. The palmar and plantar regions are highly cornified, producing a much greater thickness (100 to 400 times that of other regions) that introduces an overall lag time in diffusion. In addition to thickness, the actual size of corneocytes may be important. Differences in hair-follicle density may affect absorption of more polar molecules. The scalp should thus be considered in a different light than the rest of the body. Finally, differences in cutaneous blood flow that have been documented in different body regions may be an additional variable to consider in predicting the rate of percutaneous absorption. These factors are also important in animals.

Although generalizations are tenuous at best, human skin appears to be more impermeable, or at least as impermeable, as the skin of the cat, dog, rat, mouse, or guinea pig. The skin of pigs and some primates serve as useful approximation to human skin, but only after a comparison has been made for each specific substance. The major determinants of species differences are thickness, hair density, lipid composition, and cutaneous blood flow.

Factors That Modulate Absorption.   Soaps and detergents are perhaps the most damaging substances routinely applied to skin. Whereas organic solvents must be applied in high concentrations to damage the skin and increase the penetration of solute through human epidermis, only 1% aqueous solutions of detergents are required to achieve the same effect. Alteration of the stratum corneum appears to be the cause of increased penetration. Organic solvents can be divided into damaging and nondamaging categories relative to their effects on the barrier properties of skin. The damaging category includes methanol, acetone, ether, hexane, and mixed solvents such as chloroform:methanol or ether:ethanol. These solvents and mixtures are able to extract lipids and proteolipids from tissues and thereby alter drug permeability. Another mechanism for this solvent effect is that the solvents themselves may partition into the intercellular lipid pathway, changing its lipophilicity and barrier property. Use of more polar or amphoteric solvents may enhance the penetration of polar molecules. In contrast, solvents such as higher alcohols, esters, and olive oil do not appear to damage skin appreciably. However, the penetration rate of solutes dissolved in these solvents is often reduced. This is best explained by partitioning of the penetrant into the nonabsorbed solvent, preventing release of the chemical into the stratum corneum. This is very similar to the strategies used to formulate injectable depot preparations.

For a specific chemical, rate of penetration can be drastically modified by the solvent system used. In transdermal patches, specific chemical enhancers (e.g., solvents such as ethanol; other lipid-interacting moieties) are included in the formulation to reversibly increase skin permeability and enhance drug delivery. Alternatively, drug release is formulated to be rate-limiting from the patch system (membranes, microencapsulation, etc.) so that a constant (zero-order) release from the patch occurs, thereby providing controlled drug delivery. In environmental exposures, the chemical may come into contact with the skin as a mixture or in contaminated soil. In mixtures, other components may function as solvents and modulate the rate of absorption. Other components may retard absorption through surface chemical interactions. In soil, a large fraction of the toxicant may remain bound to soil constituents, thereby reducing the fraction absorbed. Similarly, metabolism by soil bacteria may further modify absorption profiles. These vehicles and medium effects can be seen in the studies conducted in our laboratory (Figure 3.10) after topical application of pentachlorophenol in pigs. All of these phenomena are currently under investigation. Not surprisingly, lipid-soluble toxicants may be markedly resistant to removal by washing within a short time after application due to depot formation. For example, 15 minutes after application, a substantial portion of parathion cannot be removed from exposed skin by soap and water.

Another strategy for transdermal delivery is to overcome the cutaneous barrier by using electrical (iontophoresis) or ultrasonic (phonophoresis) energy, rather than the concentration gradient in diffusion, to drive drug through the skin. These techniques hold the most promise for delivering peptides and oligonucleotide drugs that now can be administered only by injection. In these cases, dose is based on the surface area of application and the amount of energy required to actively deliver the drug across skin. In iontophoresis, this amounts to a dose being expressed in $\mu A/cm^2$. Formulation factors are also very different since many of the excipients used are also delivered by the applied electrical current in molar proportion to the active drug. Finally, a recent but related strategy is to use very short-duration high-voltage electrical pulses (electroporation) to reversibly break down the stratum corneum barrier, allowing larger peptides and possibly even small proteins to be systemically delivered. From the perspective of pharmacokinetic modeling, the classic models to be presented in subsequent chapters are then used to quantitate disposition. The only difference is that the dose is now expressed in terms of applied electrical current rather than drug mass, which is used when a chemical gradient provides the driving force.

Experimental Models.   Before leaving the subject of dermal penetration, it is important to consider briefly the experimental techniques used to assess percutaneous absorption. Whole-animal *in vivo* studies generally assess the fraction of the applied dose that is absorbed using techniques to be discussed later. There are many *in vitro* approaches to assess topical penetration. Most employ diffusion cell systems, which sandwich skin of various thicknesses between a donor and a receiver reservoir, the same systems used to assess gastrointestinal transport (Figure 3.4). The chemical is placed in the donor side (epidermis), and appearance of compound in the receiver (dermal) is monitored over time. This system can use a variety of "skin" sources ranging from full-thickness specimens (epidermis and dermis), to epidermis alone, to various "artificial" membranes such as lipid layers. In most skin studies, unlike other mucosa, the donor reservoir is usually left open to the ambient environment. This basic diffusion cell (Figure 3.11) in which the receiver solution is a fixed volume is called a static cell. If, instead, the receiver solution is continuously pumped through the dermal reservoir of the cell, a "flow-through" system results that mimics the *in vivo* setting in which blood continuously removes absorbed compound. Various cell and organ culture approaches have also been developed that assess absorption across cultured epidermal and/or dermal membranes. All of these systems have also been used to assess cutaneous metabolism.

The next level of complexity in an *in vitro* system is the use of isolated perfused skinflap preparations that employ surgically prepared vascularized skin flaps harvested from animals and then transferred to an isolated organ perfusion chamber. This model, developed in the author's laboratory, allows absorption to be assessed in skin that is viable, is anatomically intact, and has a functional microcirculation.

RESPIRATORY ABSORPTION

The third major route for systemic exposure to drugs and toxicants is the respiratory system. Since this system's primary function is gas exchange (O_2, CO_2), it is always in direct contact with environmental air as an unavoidable part of breathing. A number of

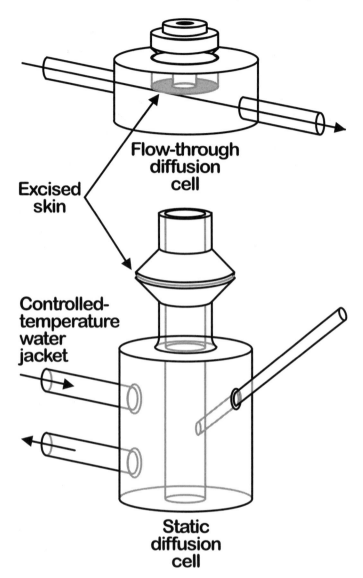

Flow-through diffusion cell

Excised skin

Controlled-temperature water jacket

Static diffusion cell

FIGURE 3.11.   Flow-through and static diffusion cells used to assess *in vitro* percutaneous absorption.

alveolus - actual site of gas exchange, a small cavity

toxicants are in gaseous (CO, NO_2, formaldehyde), vapor (benzene, CCl_4), or aerosol (lead from automobile exhaust, silica, asbestos) forms and are potential candidates for entry via the respiratory system. Each of these modes of inhalational exposure results in a different mechanism of compound absorption and, for the purposes of this text, a different definition of dose. A textbook of anesthesiology should be consulted for more details on disposition and absorption of gases in humans and animals.

Opportunities for systemic absorption are excellent through the respiratory route since the cells lining the alveoli are very thin and profusely bathed by capillaries. The surface area of the lung is large (50 to 100 m²), some 50 times the area of the skin. Based on these properties and the diffusion equation presented earlier (equation 2.1), the large surface area, the small diffusion distance, and high level of blood perfusion maximize the rate and extent of passive absorption driven by gaseous diffusion.

At the alveoli (site of gas exchange), the epithelial membranes are exceedingly thin and

pulmonary circulation - blood enter right side of heart, to lungs, to left side of heart
systemic circulation - from left side of heart, capillaries, veins, to right side of heart.
pulmonary veins - from lung to heart

3 • *Absorption*   **39**

have an intimate association with the capillary walls of the vascular system. There is minimal interstitial space for an absorbed chemical to traverse. During each passage through the lung, blood cells must pass single file in immediate proximity to the site of gas exchange. The distance from the vasculature to the "outside" membrane is only about 1.5 μm for the alveoli. This enables an exceedingly rapidly exchange of gases, approximately 5 seconds in the case of CO_2 and 1/5 second for O_2. A thin film of fluid wetting the alveolar membrane aids in the initial absorption of toxicants from the alveolar air by providing an easy mechanism for entry into solution. However, in some cases the phospholipids of the surfactant monolayer may interact with more lipophilic compounds to retard uptake.

The process of respiration involves the movement and exchange of air through several interrelated passages, including the nose, mouth, pharynx, trachea, bronchi, and successive smaller airways terminating in the alveoli, where gaseous exchange occurs. All of these anatomical modifications protect the internal environment of the air passages from the harsh outside environment by warming and humidifying the inspired air. The passages also provide numerous obstacles and baffles to prevent the inhalation of particulate and aerosol droplets. Thus the absorption of particulate and aerosolized liquids is fundamentally different from that of gases. As will be developed, the absorption of such impacted solids and liquids along the respiratory tract has much more in common with oral and topical absorption, with the critical caveat that the precise dose of compound finally available for absorption is very difficult to determine.

The volume of the respiratory tree where gaseous exchange does not occur results in a residual volume, which is the amount of air retained by the lung despite maximal expiratory effort. Toxicants in the respiratory air may not be cleared immediately because of slow release from this volume. Although the dynamics of air exchange that occurs during inhalation and expiration cycles is beyond the scope of this chapter, this must be considered should a precise estimate of inhalational exposure be desired.

Another unique aspect of respiratory exposure is the fact that the pulmonary blood circulation is in series with the systemic circulation. Thus, in contrast to cutaneous or oral exposure, compounds absorbed in the lung will enter the oxygenated pulmonary veins, which drain to the systemic arterial circulation. Compared to oral administration, this reduces first-pass hepatic metabolism.

Vapors and Gases.   Since the rate of entry of vapor-phase toxicants is controlled by the alveolar ventilation rate, the toxicant is presented to the alveoli in an interrupted manner, whose frequency is equal to the rate of breathing; about 20 times per minute. The diffusion coefficient of a gaseous toxicant in the fluids of, and associated with, pulmonary membranes is an important consideration, but doses are more appropriately discussed in terms of the partial pressure of the gas in the inspired air. Upon inhalation of a constant tension of a toxic gas, arterial plasma tension of the gas approaches its tension in the expired air. The rate of entry is then determined by the blood solubility of the toxicant. If there is a high blood:gas partition coefficient, a larger amount must be dissolved in the blood to raise the partial pressure. Gases with a high blood:gas partition coefficient require a longer period to approach the same tension in the blood as in inspired air than it takes for less soluble gases. Similarly, a longer period of time is required for blood concentrations of such a gas to be eliminated, thus prolonging detoxification. Simple diffusion accounts for the somewhat complex series of events in the lung regarding gas absorption.

Another important point to consider in determining how much of an inhaled gas is absorbed into the systemic circulation is the relation of the fraction of lung ventilated to the fraction perfused. Increased perfusion of the lung will favor a more rapid achievement of blood-gas equilibrium. Decreased perfusion will decrease the absorption of toxicants, even those that reach the alveoli. Various ventilation-perfusion "mismatches" may alter the amount of an inhaled gas that is systemically absorbed. Similarly, pulmonary diseases that thicken the alveoli or obstruct the airways may also affect overall absorption.

Aerosols and Particulates.   The absorption of aerosols and particulates is affected by a number of physiological factors specifically designed to preclude access to the alveoli. The upper respiratory tract, beginning with the nose and continuing down its tubular elements, is a very efficient filtering system for excluding particulate matter (solids, liquid droplets). A coal miner is subject to an inhalation of 6000 g of coal-dust particles during the occupational lifetime, but only 100 g are found postmortem; it is therefore obvious that the protective filtering mechanism is an effective one. The parameters of air velocity and directional air changes favor impaction of particles in the upper respiratory system. Particle characteristics such as size, coagulation, sedimentation, electrical charge, and diffusion are important to retention, absorption, or expulsion of airborne particles. In addition to these characteristics, a mucous blanket propelled by ciliary action clears the tract of particles by directing them to the gastrointestinal system (via the glottis) or to the mouth for expectoration. This system is responsible for 80% of toxicant lung clearance. The deposition of various particle sizes in different respiratory regions is summarized in Table 3.3; particles larger than 6 μm do not reach the alveolus. In addition to this mechanism, phagocytosis is very active in the respiratory tract, both coupled to the directed mucosal route and via penetration through interstitial tissues of the lung and migration to the lymph, where phagocytes may remain stored for long periods in lymph nodes. Ninety percent of material deposited in the respiratory tract may be cleared in less than 1 hour. Compared to absorption in the alveoli, absorption through the upper respiratory tract is quantitatively of less importance. However, inhaled toxicants that become deposited on the mucous layer can be absorbed into the myriad of cells lining the respiratory tract and exert a direct toxicologic response. This route of exposure is often used to deliver pharmaceutics by aerosol. If a compound is extremely potent, systemic effects may occur.

The end result of this extremely efficient filtering mechanism is that most inhaled drugs deposited in nasal or buccal mucus ultimately enter the gastrointestinal tract. This can best be appreciated by examining the respiratory drainages depicted in Figure 3.1. There-

TABLE 3.3.   Percent Retention of Inhaled Aerosol Particles in Various Regions of the Human Respiratory Tract (450 cm² Tidal Air)

Region	Percent retention of indicated particle sizes				
	20 μm	6 μm	2 μm	0.6 μm	0.2 μm
Mouth	15	0	0	0	0
Pharynx	8	0	0	0	0
Trachea	10	1	0	0	0
Pulmonary bronchi	12	2	0	0	0
Secondary bronchi	19	4	1	0	0
Tertiary bronchi	17	9	2	0	0
Quaternary bronchi	6	7	2	1	1
Terminal bronchioles	6	19	6	4	6
Respiratory bronchioles	0	11	5	3	4
Alveolar ducts	0	25	25	8	11
Alveolar sacs	0	5	0	0	0
Total	93	83	41	16	22

Adapted from: Hatch and Gross. 1964. *Pulmonary Deposition and Retention of Inhaled Aerosols.* New York: Academic Press.

pinocytosis (cellular drinking) - ingest extracellular fluid or to transport it across a cellular barrier.
endocytosis - a cell encloses the substance in a membrane-bounded vesicle that is pinched off from the cell membrane.

fore, the disposition of aerosols and particulates largely mirrors that of orally administered drugs. This is an important consideration when interpreting inhalational exposures in which the endpoints are metabolism, pharmacokinetics, or systemic toxicity. Except for drug that is locally absorbed into the epithelium underlying this ubiquitous mucous blanket, or for that small fraction of drug that actually penetrates into the alveoli, most drug is ultimately presented to the gastrointestinal tract for absorption. This fraction of drug undergoes first-pass hepatic biotransformation and thus shares a metabolic fate with drug orally administered. The disposition patterns are thus often mixed and must be compared to both parenteral and oral routes for the complete process to be understood.

Nasal administration is a preferred route for many inhalant medications. In these cases, great care is made to deliver aerosols of the specific size for deposition on the nasal mucosa and upper respiratory tract. The bioavailability of these compounds is assessed using the techniques developed for other routes, although a local effect is often desired. The problems with this strategy are the attainment of an accurately delivered dose and the inactivation and binding of administered drug by the thick mucous blanket. A great deal of effort has been focused on using metered nasal delivery for peptide drugs such as insulin; however, the inherent variability makes the delivery of a precise dose very difficult. Drugs delivered by this route usually have a wide therapeutic window and large safety index.

The direct penetration of airborne toxicants at alveolar surfaces or in the upper respiratory tract is not the only action of toxicological importance. Both vapors and particulates may accumulate in upper respiratory passages to produce irritant effects. Despite the effectiveness of ciliary movement and phagocytosis, the cumulative effects of silica, asbestos, or coal dust ultimately cause important chronic fibrosis even though direct absorption is of minor importance. Thus, phagocytosis prevents acute damage but may contribute to chronic toxicity.

There is little evidence for active transport in the respiratory system (phenol red and disodium chromoglycate are notable exceptions), although pinocytosis may be of importance for penetration. The lung is an area of extensive metabolic activity, although detoxification mechanisms do not appear to be of major importance. Perhaps less well appreciated is the fact that the lung is also an excretory route for ethanol, forming the scientific basis for the breath analyzer test for alcohol intoxication.

The final point to consider relates to some specific peculiarities of nasal absorption. In the region of the olfactory epithelium, there exists a direct path for inhaled compounds to be absorbed directly into the olfactory neural tissue and central nervous system, thereby bypassing both the systemic circulation and the blood-brain barrier. The mass of drugs involved in this uptake process is very small and thus would not affect a pharmacokinetic analysis. However, this route has obvious toxicological significance and is being explored as a potential biological mechanism for some aspects of the putative multiple chemical sensitivity syndrome.

OTHER ROUTES OF ADMINISTRATION

In order to make this discussion of absorption complete, it is important to realize that other extravascular drug administration routes are often encountered. Relative to pharmacokinetic analysis, these are dealt with in the same fashion as the primary routes discussed above. The important difference is that in all cases, the barrier to absorption is less than that encountered in oral or topical delivery. Secondly, all of these routes involve an invasive procedure to inject drug into an internal body tissue, thereby bypassing the epithelial barriers of the skin and gastrointestinal tract. They are relevant to therapeutic drug administration, but not to toxicology, since they are an invasive technique.

The primary therapeutic routes of drug administration are subcutaneous (SC or SQ) and

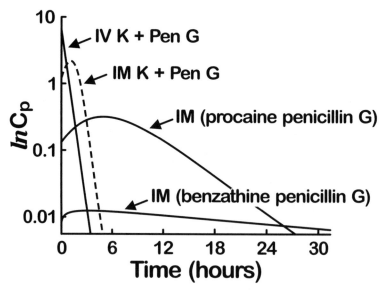

FIGURE 3.12.   Effects of formulation and route of administration on the plasma concentration-versus-time profiles of penicillin G.

(IM) intramuscular. In these cases, the total dose of drug is known and is injected into tissue that is well perfused by systemic capillaries that drain into the central venous circulation. Both of these routes as well as intravenous administration are termed *parenteral* to contrast primarily with oral (*enteral*) and topical dosing, which are classified as *nonparenteral* routes of drug administration. A primary difference between these two classes is that parenteral routes bypass all of the body's defensive mechanisms. Parenteral dosage forms are manufactured under strict guidelines that eliminate microbial and particulate contamination, resulting in sterile preparations that must be administered using aseptic techniques. This restriction does not apply to oral or topical dosage forms. As with all methods of drug administration, there are numerous variables associated with SC and IM dosing, which can be conveniently classified into pharmaceutical and biological categories.

By far, the dosing form has the greatest influence on the rate and extent of absorption of parenteral drugs. The classic examples are potassium, procaine, and benzathine penicillin G (Figure 3.12). The formulation strategy is to complex the active drug (e.g., penicillin G) with a moiety that delays its release to the surrounding capillary beds by modulating the drug's solubility. A pharmaceutics text should be consulted for the chemistry of these processes. The result is that the rate of release of the compound from the dosing formulation becomes slower than that of the drug's elimination and, as with the slow-release oral and transdermal patches discussed earlier, this release becomes rate limiting.

The potential problems with these strategies are two-fold. If one considers antimicrobial therapy, for bacteria with very high therapeutic thresholds (e.g., minimum inhibitory concentrations [MICs]), the prolonged release formulations may never provide therapeutic drug concentrations. In fact, prolonged subtherapeutic concentrations may select for antimicrobial resistance. Secondly, such so-called depot preparations in food animals may result in persistent drug concentrations in tissues, thereby prolonging the withdrawal time (see Chapter 17). Furthermore, drug depots at injection sites may persist much longer than effective blood concentrations do and be easily detected at slaughter. One must exhibit care to differentiate drug tissue concentrations at injection sites from those achieved after absorption and systemic distribution. This scenario also nicely illustrates the reason that knowledge of both the extent and rate of drug absorption are needed to

peritoneal- the smooth transparent serous membrane that lines the cavity of
the abdomen and folded inward over the abdominal viscera.

3 • *Absorption*   **43**

adequately describe the absorption of a drug.

The development of depot preparations has received a lot of attention from pharmaceutical companies. Some contraceptives in humans achieve monthly dosing intervals through injection in the subcutaneous tissue of insoluble tablets that result in very slow drug release, the best example being the use of levonorgestrel implanted capsules (Norplant®). Similar strategies have been employed in veterinary medicine for the administration of growth promotants. These include estradiol formulated in rubber implants (Compudose®), progesterone and estradiol pellets (Implant-C®) and zeranol (Ralgro®). These formulations stress the necessity of knowing the dosage form used when conducting any pharmacokinetic analysis as it is the rate-controlling factor in drug disposition. These considerations will be discussed in more detail in Chapter 7 when the required pharmacokinetic techniques will be presented.

The second major variable concerning parenteral injections relates to the physiology of the injection site. For a drug to be adequately absorbed from a depot preparation, there must be access to the perfusing capillaries and an adequate rate of tissue perfusion. A major source of variability is the muscle into which IM injections are made. Studies have elegantly demonstrated in horses that if the injection is made in between the fascial tissue bundles of a muscle group, less systemic absorption will occur than if the injection is made in the muscle mass. Similarly, if the muscle group or, more likely, the SC injection site, has poor blood perfusion, then less absorption may occur. If the injection results in a local tissue reaction, subsequent inflammation and fibrosis may "wall off" the drug formulation, preventing absorption. Changes in ambient temperature, with compensatory changes in skin blood perfusion, may modulate absorption rate. There are numerous variables in these processes, and it is often only through the use of careful pharmacokinetic analyses that their influence on drug absorption can be ascertained.

Finally, other routes of drug administration are occasionally employed that require absorption for activity. Administration of drugs by intraperitoneal injection is often used in toxicology studies in rodents since larger volumes can be administered. Peritoneal absorption is very efficient, provided adequate "mixing" of the injection with the peritoneal fluid is achieved. Most of the drug absorbed after interperitoneal administration enters the portal vein and thus may undergo first-pass hepatic metabolism. The disposition of intraperitoneal drug thus mirrors that of oral administration.

Some drugs are administered by conjunctival, intravaginal, or intramammary routes. In these cases, achievement of effective systemic concentrations is often not required for what is an essentially local therapeutic effect. Prolonged absorption from these sites may result in persistent tissue residues in food-producing animals if the analytical sensitivity of the monitoring assay is sufficiently low. The systemic absorption of these dosage forms is quantitated using procedures identical to those employed for other routes of administration.

BIOAVAILABILITY

The final topic to consider is the assessment of the extent and rate of absorption after oral, topical, or inhalational drug administration. The extent of drug absorption is defined as absolute systemic availability and is denoted in pharmacokinetic equations as the fraction of an applied dose absorbed into the body (F). Although this topic will also be discussed extensively in the subsequent modeling chapters of this text when distribution and elimination principles and quantitating techniques have been presented, it is important and convenient at this juncture to introduce the basic concepts so as to complete the discussion of drug absorption.

If one is estimating the extent of drug absorption by measuring the resultant concentrations in either blood or excreta, one must have an estimate of how much drug normally would be found if the entire dose were absorbed. To estimate this, an intravenous dose is required since this is the only route of administration that guarantees that 100% of the dose is systemically available (F = 1.0) and the pattern of disposition and metabolism can be quantitated. Parameters used to measure systemic availability are thus calculated as a ratio relative to the intravenous dose. The only problems encountered using intravenous data as a benchmark for extent of absorption arise if precipitation occurs after dosing and, paradoxically, the intravenous dose is not completely available.

For most therapeutic drug studies, systemic absorption is assessed by measuring blood concentrations. In contrast, for pesticides and other toxicants that may be very lipophilic and thus produce very low blood concentrations, urine and feces are often collected to reflect systemic exposure. In both cases, the amount of drug collected after administration by the route under study is divided by that collected after intravenous administration. When drug concentrations in blood (or serum or plasma) are assayed, total absorption is assessed by measuring the area under the (concentration-time) curve (AUC), as shown in Figure 3.13 using the trapezoidal method presented in Chapter 8. This is a geometrical technique that breaks the AUC into corresponding trapezoids based on the number of samples assayed. The terminal area beyond the last data point (a triangle) is estimated and added together with the previous trapezoidal areas. Absolute systemic availability then is calculated as

$$F\,(\%) = \frac{[\text{Urine} + \text{Feces}]_{\text{route}}\ \text{Dose}_{\text{iv}}}{[\text{Urine} + \text{Feces}]_{\text{iv}}\ \text{Dose}_{\text{route}}} \tag{3.1}$$

$$F\,(\%) = \frac{\text{AUC}_{\text{route}}\ \text{Dose}_{\text{iv}}}{\text{AUC}_{\text{iv}}\ \text{Dose}_{\text{route}}} \tag{3.2}$$

The selection of which technique to use is dependent upon the nature of the compound studied. There are further mathematical limitations to these techniques (e.g., best method to extrapolate the terminal triangle, problems with slow-release dosage formulations), which can be overcome using some of the pharmacokinetic techniques presented in subsequent chapters. Additionally, calculation of F only provides an estimate of the extent, and not rate, of drug absorption. To calculate rate, pharmacokinetic techniques are required; these are presented in Chapter 7. Finally, so-called relative systemic availability may be calculated for two nonintravenous formulations in which the data for the reference product are in the denominator, and the test formulation is in the numerator. In many instances, for environmental chemicals and pesticides, urine is more readily accessible and analytically preferred for assessing exposure, although complete urine collections are required. Collection of random urine voids can be independently assessed by simultaneously measuring creatinine concentrations in urine since creatinine is produced at a relatively constant rate and will normalize the data to compensate for incomplete collections.

In summary, knowledge of the biological principles involved in drug absorption by any route is important to the proper application of pharmacokinetics to therapeutic and toxicological problems. The unique biology associated with any specific route must often be taken into consideration when constructing models and sampling strategies, especially when data from such studies are extrapolated to the real world. Assumptions used in building models must be based on the relevant biology of the animal being studied.

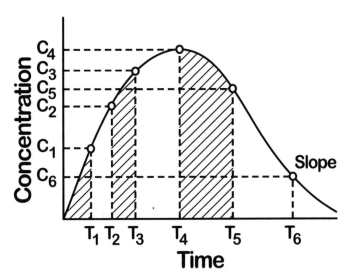

Figure 3.13. Breakdown of a plasma concentration-versus-time curve into trapezoids used to calculate the area under the curve.

SELECTED READINGS

Barry, B.W. 1983. *Percutaneous Absorption.* New York: Marcel Dekker.

Borchardt, R.T., P.L. Smith, and G. Wilson. 1996. *Models for Assessing Drug Absorption and Metabolism.* New York: Plenum Press.

Bronaugh, R.L., and H. I. Maibach. 1989. *Percutaneous Absorption,* 2ed. New York: Marcel Dekker.

Bronaugh, R.L., and H. I. Maibach. 1991. *In Vitro Percutaneous Absorption-Principles, Fundamentals and Applications.* Boca Raton, FL: CRC Press.

Csáky, T.Z. 1984. *Handbook of Experimental Pharmacology, Vol. 70, Parts I and II, Pharmacology of Intestinal Permeation.* Berlin: Springer-Verlag.

Edman, P., and E. Björk. 1992. Routes of delivery: Case studies. (1) Nasal delivery of peptide drugs. *Advanced Drug Delivery Reviews.* 8:165-177.

Firth, E.C., J.F.M. Nouws, F. Driessenss, P. Schmaetz, K. Peperkamp, and W.R. Klein. 1986. Effect of injection site on the pharmacokinetics of procaine penicillin G in horses. *American Journal of Veterinary Research.* 47:2380-2384.

Gizurarson, S. 1990. Animal models for intranasal drug delivery studies. *Acta Pharmacology Nord.* 2:105-122.

Hardee, G.E., and J.D. Baggot. 1998. *Development and Formulation of Veterinary Dosage Forms,* 2 ed. New York: Marcel Dekker.

Hatch, T.F., and P. Gross. 1964. *Pulmonary Deposition and Retention of Inhaled Aerosols.* New York: Academic Press.

Hayes, A.W. 1994. *Principles and Methods of Toxicology,* 3ed. New York: Raven Press.

Klaasen, C.D. 1996. *Casarett and Doull's Toxicology: The Basic Science of Poisons,* 5ed. New York: McGraw-Hill.

Lee, V.H.L., and A. Yamamoto. 1990. Penetration and enzymatic barriers to peptide and protein absorption. *Advanced Drug Delivery Reviews.* 4:171-207.

Martinez, M.N., and J.E. Riviere. 1994. Review of the 1993 Veterinary Drug Bioequivalence Workshop. *Journal of Veterinary Pharmacology and Therapeutics.* 17:85-119.

Patton, J.S., and R.M. Platz. 1992. Routes of delivery: Case studies. (2) Pulmonary delivery of peptides and proteins for systemic action. *Advanced Drug Delivery Reviews.* 8:179-196.

Qiao, G.L., and J.E. Riviere. 1997. Pentachlorophenol dermal absorption and disposition from soil in swine: Effects of occlusion and skin microorganism inhibition. *Toxicology and Applied Pharmacology.* 147:234-246.

Read, N.W., and K. Sugden. 1987. Gastrointestinal dynamics and pharmacology for the optimum design of controlled release oral dosage forms. *Critical Reviews of Therapeutic Drug Carrier Systems.* 3:221-262.

Riviere, J.E. 1994. Influence of compounding on bioavailability. *Journal of the American Veterinary Medical Association.* 205:226-231.

Riviere, J.E., and M.C. Heit. 1997. Electrically assisted transdermal drug delivery. *Pharmaceutical Research.* 14:691-701.

Riviere, J.E., and N.A. Monteiro-Riviere. 1991. The isolated perfused porcine skin flap as an *in vitro* model for percutaneous absorption and cutaneous toxicology. *Critical Reviews in Toxicology* 21(5):330.

Riviere, J.E., N. A. Monteiro-Riviere, and P.L. Williams. 1995. Isolated perfused porcine skin flap as an *in vitro* model for predicting transdermal pharmacokinetics. *European Journal of Pharmacy and Biopharmaceutics.* 41:152-162.

Roth, W.L., R.A. Freeman, and A.G.E. Wilson. 1993. A physiological based model for gastrointestinal absorption and excretion of chemicals carried by lipids. *Risk Analysis.* 13:531-543.

Toutain, P.L. and G.D. Koritz. 1997. Veterinary drug bioequivalence determination. *Journal of Veterinary Pharmacology and Therapeutics.* 20:79-90.

Traver, D.S., and J.E. Riviere. 1981. Penicillin and ampicillin therapy in horses. *Journal of the American Veterinary Medical Association.* 178:1186-1189.

Traver, D.S., and J.E. Riviere. 1982. Ampicillin in mares: A comparison of intramuscular sodium ampicillin or sodium ampicillin-ampicillin trihydrate injection. *American Journal of Veterinary Research.* 43:402-404.

United States Pharmacopeia 23rd Edition / National Formulary 18th Edition. 1995. Rockville: United States Pharmacopeial Convention, Inc.

Wang, R.G.M., J.B. Knaak, and H.I. Maibach. 1993. *Health Risk Assessment: Dermal and Inhalational Exposure and Absorption of Toxicants.* Boca Raton, FL: CRC Press.

4

Distribution

A toxicant absorbed into the systemic circulation following any route of administration must reach its site of action at a high enough concentration for a sufficient period of time to elicit a biological response. Distribution processes determine this outcome. Figure 2.1 (see Chapter 2) should be consulted to assess how distribution processes need to be understood in the context of predicting drug disposition. There are numerous tissues to which a chemical may be distributed, some of them capable of eliciting a pharmacological or toxicological (intended versus unintended) response, while others serve only as a "sink" or "depot" for the chemical. Sinks may also be formed as a result of chemical binding to tissue or plasma proteins. The toxicologic significance of such sinks is that chemicals will be distributed to, and in some cases stored in, these tissues and only slowly be released back into the systemic circulation for ultimate elimination. Such tissue binding may actually protect against acute adverse effects by providing an "inert" site for toxicant localization.

Storage may, however, prolong the overall residence time of a compound in the body and promote accumulation during chronic exposure—two processes that would potentiate chronic toxicity. Thus, when a toxicant is stored in a depot removed from the site of action (such as polychlorinated biphenyls in fat or lead in bone), no adverse effect may be manifested immediately, although the potential for toxicity exists. For example, lead stored in bone is not thought to cause harm, but it has the potential for mobilization into soft tissues, whereupon toxic symptoms may appear. As the toxicant in storage depots is in equilibrium with the free toxicant in plasma, mobilization is constant, and exposure to the target organ is constant (although at a low level). Thus, the opportunity for chronic effects is always present. In fact, it is possible that the mechanism of toxicity for a compound may be solely related to its ability to mobilize a second bound toxicant from its site of storage and thereby elicit a toxicologic effect not directly associated with the compound itself. Finally, this phenomenon may be used to therapeutic advantage by administering compounds that can redistribute harmful chemicals from storage sites and promote elimination. This is the rationale for using systemic chelation therapy to mobilize stored metals.

If the animal is a food-producing species, such tissue storage may result in residues in the edible meat products. Tissue concentrations thus become an endpoint in themselves, devoid of a biological or toxicological relevance in the tissue in which they are found.

Their relevance is set by regulations that legally establish safe tissue tolerances or maximum residue levels for specific tissues and species. These are based upon extrapolations of safety to the consuming human population and food consumption patterns. Phenomenological confusion often results when tissue concentration data are presented independent of the context of their use. Tissue depletion data collected in the very low concentration ranges appropriate for tissue residue studies are not appropriate to be used to estimate therapeutic efficacy against a tissue-residing bacterium or as an indicator of tissue distribution. As will be seen, the pharmacokinetic techniques used to describe these two different scenarios may be similar, although the resulting parameters may be very different.

Distribution of chemicals to peripheral tissues is dependent on four factors: (1) the physiochemical properties of the compound, (2) the concentration gradient established between the blood and tissue, (3) the ratio of blood flow to tissue mass, and (4) the affinity of the chemical for tissue constituents. The physiochemical properties of the chemical (pKa, lipid solubility, molecular weight) are most important in determining its propensity to distribute to a specific tissue. For most molecules, distribution out of the blood into tissue is by simple diffusion down a concentration gradient, hence distribution is generally described by first-order rate constants. The principles discussed in Chapter 2 for movement of compounds across diffusion barriers also apply here, as one could consider distribution as absorption into the tissues from the blood. The complicating factors are that the driving concentration is now dependent upon blood flow, the surface area for absorption into tissues is dependent upon tissue mass, the relevant partition coefficient is the blood-tissue ratio, and plasma/tissue protein binding complicates the picture. An understanding of distribution is a prerequisite to predicting pharmacological response.

endocrine - produce and release hormones

PHYSIOLOGICAL DETERMINANTS OF DISTRIBUTION

extracellular

Body fluids are distributed among three primary compartments, only one of which, vascular fluid, is thought to have an important role in the distribution of most compounds throughout the body. Human plasma amounts to about 4% of the total body weight and 53% of the total blood volume. By comparison, the interstitial tissue fluids account for 13% and intracellular fluids 41% of body weight. Use of recently developed microdialysis probes and catheters allows the concentration of drug to be directly monitored in the interstitial fluid and thus further opens the window for pharmacokinetic analysis. The concentration that a compound may achieve in the blood following exposure depends in part upon its apparent volume of distribution. If it is distributed only in the plasma, a high concentration could be achieved in the vascular system. In contrast, the concentration would be markedly lower if the same quantity of toxicant were distributed to a larger pool, including the interstitial water and/or cellular fluids.

The next major consideration is the relative blood flow to different tissues. Two factors will potentiate chemical accumulation into a tissue: high blood flow per unit mass of tissue and a large tissue mass. Tissues with a *high blood flow-mass ratio* include the *brain, heart, liver, kidney,* and *endocrine glands*. Tissues with an *intermediate ratio* include *muscle* and *skin*, while tissues with a *low ratio* (indicative of poor systemic perfusion) include *adipose tissue* and *bone*. These ratios are generalizations, and some tissues may actually be categorized in two disparate groups. An excellent example is the kidney, where the renal cortex receives some 25% of cardiac output and thus has a very high blood flow-mass ratio. However, the renal medulla receives only a small fraction of this blood flow and thus could be categorized in the intermediate to low group.

If the affinity of the chemical for the tissue is high, then it will still accumulate in poorly perfused tissues (such as fat), although it will take a long period of time to "load" or "de-

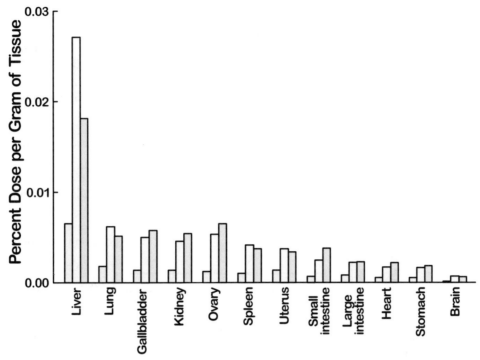

FIGURE 4.1. Comparative tissue distribution at 17 days after topical pentachlorophenol dosing (300 mg) in soil on pigs. Histograms represent [nonoccluded/occluded/occluded with antimicrobials] dosing conditions. Note the predominant distribution to liver. *exposed to air* *block air.*

plete" these tissues. A relatively low blood flow-mass ratio is a major physiological explanation for depot formation.

Differences in perfusion and affinity have therapeutic and toxicological implications, as will now be illustrated. Figure 4.1 depicts the relative tissue concentrations in pigs of the environmental contaminant pentachlorophenol (PCP) dosed topically in soil (relevant environmental exposure conditions) for three weeks with the skin either occluded or exposed to air. Two trends can be immediately noted. Higher accumulation of PCP occurred in well-perfused tissues such as liver, lung, kidney, and ovary. Also, as discussed in Chapter 3, occlusion of the dosing site increased the absorbed dose and thus tissue concentrations (recall Chapter 3, Figure 3.10). Many antibiotics used in comparative medicine show preferential distribution to liver and kidney over muscle and other tissues. This is shown in Figure 4.2, which depicts the tissue depletion for intravenous gentamicin in pigs relative to simultaneous serum concentrations. Numerous examples of similar relative tissue distributions can be seen throughout the literature for many classes of drugs and toxicants, reinforcing the general principle of organ flow-dependent diffusion. This topic will be revisited in Chapter 17 in which the pharmacokinetics of tissue residue depletion is presented.

The data above required no pharmacokinetic analysis as only comparative tissue concentrations were employed. However, in some cases, performing very simple manipulations of the data, using the concept of the area under the (concentration-time) curve (AUC) presented in Chapter 3, may shed more light on the problem at hand and simplify interpretation of the data. Our laboratory has performed studies designed to induce changes in the distribution of systemic blood flow by using systemic hyperthermia. Previous studies had demonstrated such blood flow shunting using imaging and microsphere techniques. The strategy was to target peripheral tissues with the chemotherapeutic drug

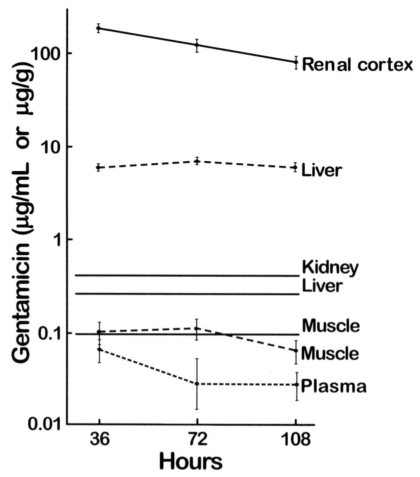

FIGURE 4.2.   Mean (± SEM, standard error of the mean) gentamicin concentrations in pigs after a multiple-doseage regimen shows predominant distribution to kidney and liver. Horizontal lines are legal tissue tolerances. Renal cortex (—); liver (– – –); muscle (- - -); plasma (---).

cisplatin while simultaneously shunting flow away from the kidney, where drug toxicity may occur. Cisplatin covalently binds to tissue sites, and thus tissue concentrations largely reflect total exposure. Experimental dogs were given three different doses of cisplatin by intravenous infusion. Blood and tissue concentrations were determined by atomic absorption spectroscopy. The observed blood AUCs were linearly related to infusion dose, indicating that saturation of any disposition process did not occur. Because of this linearity, observed tissue concentrations were also dose-dependent, and thus tissue concentration should be normalized to AUC, a metric representing blood-tissue partitioning, as an indicator of systemic exposure. When the ratio of these normalized tissue concentrations in hyperthermic animals (42°C) were compared to those of normal dogs (37°C), statistically significant differences in tissue ratios were observed. A ratio of 1.0 would indicate no preferential tissue accumulation with hyperthermia. The liver, lung, and several gastrointestinal tissues tended to accumulate drugs, while the renal medulla, lymph nodes, and skin had lower ratios, indicating restricted distribution (Table 4.1). These differences are significant for a drug such as cisplatin with a low therapeutic index, as doses may be reduced to avoid nephrotoxicity while still maintaining effective concentrations in target tissues such as the lung.

glial cell - provide neurons with nutrients, help maintain a homogeneous environment.
epithelial cell - external and internal tissue that forms the covering or lining of all free body surfaces.

4 • *Distribution*   **51**

TABLE 4.1.   Comparison of Hyperthermic and Normothermic Tissue Distribution of Cisplatin Administered in Three 1-Hour Infusions (20, 50, and 80 mg/m^2)

Tissue	Ratio*
Lung	2.3 ± 0.4
Ileum	2.0 ± 0.2
Adrenal	1.8 ± 0.1
Pyloric stomach	1.7 ± 0.2
Colon	1.6 ± 0.2
Duodenum	1.6 ± 0.1
Spleen	1.5 ± 0.2
Pancreas	1.5 ± 0.2
Outer renal cortex	1.5 ± 0.1
Rectum	1.4 ± 0.2
Jejunum	1.4 ± 0.2
Heart	1.4 ± 0.3
Esophagus	1.3 ± 0.1
Ovary	1.2 ± 0.2
Thyroid	1.2 ± 0.2
Cardiac stomach	1.2 ± 0.1
Inner renal cortex	1.2 ± 0.1
Uterus	1.2 ± 0.1
Muscle	1.1 ± 0.3
Fat	1.0 ± 0.3
Bone marrow	0.96 ± 0.32
Renal medulla	0.79 ± 0.08
Skin	0.79 ± 0.13
Cervical lymph node	0.64 ± 0.11

$$*Ratio\ (\pm SEM) = \frac{[Platinum]_{42°C} / AUC}{[Platinum]_{37°C} / AUC}$$

TISSUE BARRIERS TO DISTRIBUTION

Some organs have unique anatomical barriers to xenobiotic penetration. The classic and most studied example is the blood-brain barrier, which has a glial cell layer interposed between the capillary endothelium and the nervous tissue. In the membrane scheme depicted in Figure 2.2 (see Chapter 2), this amounts to an additional lipid membrane between the capillary and target tissue. Only nonionized lipid-soluble compounds can penetrate this barrier. Similar considerations apply to ocular, prostatic, testicular, synovial, mammary gland, and placental drug or toxicant distribution. In addition, the pH partitioning phenomenon discussed in Chapter 2 also may occur since the protected tissue (e.g., cerebrospinal fluid) may have a lower pH level than the circulating blood plasma. Chemicals may also distribute into transcellular fluid compartments, which are also demarcated by an epithelial cell layer. These include cerebrospinal, intraocular, synovial, pericardial, pleural, peritoneal, and cochlear perilymph fluid compartments.

A few tissues possess selective transport mechanisms that accumulate specific chemicals against concentration gradients. For example, the blood-brain barrier possesses glucose, L-amino acid, and transferrin transporters. If the toxicant resembles an endogenous transport substrate, then it may preferentially concentrate in a particular tissue. Recent work with the blood-brain barrier has demonstrated that some of these tissues also employ drug efflux transport processes that remove drug from the protected sites. Two such

ligand— a group, ion, or molecule coordinated to a central atom in a complex

processes are p-glycoprotein associated with multidrug resistance and the weak organic acid cell-to-blood efflux systems. P-glycoprotein is a member of the so-called ATP-binding cassette proteins, which include the cystic fibrosis transmembrane regulator and the sulfonylurea-sensitive ATP-dependent potassium channel. Drugs such as vinblastine, vincristine, and cyclosporine, which have the proper physiochemical characteristics (high lipophilicity) to enter the brain, do not achieve effective concentrations because of this active efflux mechanism. Similar processes and transport systems for peptides and other compounds are also found in other organs (e.g., the liver).

PLASMA PROTEIN BINDING

Following entry into the circulatory system, a chemical is distributed throughout the body and may accumulate at the site of toxic action, be transferred to a storage depot, or be transported to organs that will detoxify, activate, or eliminate the compound. Although many toxicants have sufficient solubility in the aqueous component of blood to account for simple solution as a means of distribution, the primary distribution mechanism for insoluble toxicants appears to be in association with plasma proteins. Although cellular components (e.g., red blood cells) may also be responsible for transport of drugs, such transport is seldom the major route. The transport of compounds by lymph is usually of little quantitative importance. It must be recognized, however, that both erythrocytes and lymph can play roles in the transport of some lipophilic drugs and toxins, in some instances to an important extent.

Studies of plasma proteins have shown albumin to be particularly important in the binding of drugs. This is especially true for weak acids, with weak bases often binding to acid glycoproteins. For certain hormones, specific high-affinity transport proteins are present. Studies of toxicant binding have been more limited, but there is evidence of a significant binding/partitioning role for lipoproteins in carrying very lipophilic chemicals in the blood.

Ligand-Protein Interactions.   An interesting aspect of disposition is the apparent contradiction that, although many toxicants are "unreactive" in a strictly chemical sense, they can be reversibly bound to a variety of biological constituents. In the case of most ligand-protein interactions, reversible binding is established that follows the law of mass action and provides a remarkably efficient means whereby toxicants can be transported to various tissues. The toxicant-protein interaction may be simply described according to the law of mass action as

$$[T]_F + [Free\ sites] \underset{k_2}{\overset{k_1}{\rightleftharpoons}} [T]_B \tag{4.1}$$

where $[T]_F$ and $[T]_B$ are free (ultrafilterable) and bound toxicant molecules, respectively, and k_1 and k_2 are the specific rate constants for association and dissociation. It is important to stress that k_2 dictates the rate of toxicant release to a site of action, inaction, or storage. The ratio k_2 / k_1 is identical to the dissociation constant, K_{diss}. Among a group of binding sites on proteins, those with the smallest K_{diss} value for a given toxicant will bind it most tightly. In contrast to reversible binding seen with most therapeutic drugs, agents like cisplatin and some potentially carcinogenic metabolites that are formed from chlorinated hydrocarbons (such as CCl_4) are covalently bound to tissue proteins. In this case, there is no true distribution of the ligand, as k_2 is nonexistent; thus there is no opportunity for dissociation.

Once a molecule binds to a plasma protein, it moves throughout the circulation until it

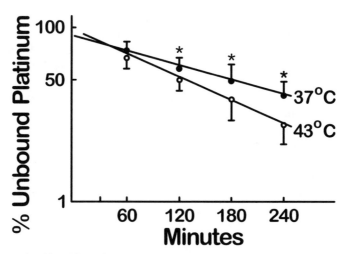

FIGURE 4.3.   Percent ultrafilterable (unbound) cisplatin in canine serum incubated at 37°C and 43°C demonstrating increased rate of covalent binding at elevated temperatures.

dissociates, usually for attachment to another large molecule. Dissociation occurs when the affinity for another biomolecule or tissue component is greater than that for the plasma protein to which the toxicant was originally bound. Thus, forces of association must be strong enough to establish an initial interaction, and they must also be weak enough such that a change in the physical or chemical environment can lead to dissociation. Dissociation could occur by binding to proteins of greater affinity (lower K_{diss} values); binding with a higher concentration of proteins of lower affinity; or changes in K_{diss} with changes in ionic strength, pH, temperature, or conformational changes in the binding site induced by binding of other molecules. As long as binding is reversible, redistribution will occur whenever the concentration of one pool (i.e., blood or tissue) is diminished. Redistribution must occur when the concentration is diminished in order to reestablish equilibrium.

Covalent Binding.   Proteins complex with ligands by a variety of mechanisms. Covalent binding may have a profound direct effect on an organism due to modification of an essential molecule, but it usually accounts for a minor portion of the total dose and is of no importance in further distribution of toxicants since such compounds cannot dissociate. As previously mentioned, when metabolites of some compounds are covalently bound to proteins, there may be no opportunity for subsequent release of the ligand apart from release upon breakdown of the protein itself. The cancer chemotherapeutic drug cisplatin covalently binds to albumin through an aquation reaction. In incubation studies, "aging" occurs after a short period of time independent of drug concentration, and the majority of circulating cisplatin is covalently bound (Figure 4.3). Hyperthermia thermodynamically accelerates this process and thus reduces effective filterable (and thus diffusible) drug concentrations even sooner. However, cisplatin may also bind to lower molecular weight nucleophiles (e.g., peptides, amino acids) and be distributed to tissues in association with these more mobile molecules. Once in the cell, the free cisplatin is regenerated, which can exert a toxicologic effect. Similar scenarios may occur with other covalently bound toxicants.

Noncovalent Binding.   Noncovalent binding is of primary importance with respect to distribution because of the opportunities to dissociate after transport. In rare cases, the noncovalent bond may be so tight (K_{diss} extremely small) that a compound remains in the blood for very lengthy periods. For example, 3-hydroxy-2,4,4-triiodo-α-ethyl hydrocinnamic acid has a half-life of about 1 year with respect to its binding to plasma albumin. Types of interactions that lead to noncovalent binding include the following:

Ionic Binding. Charged drugs may be bound to plasma proteins by ionic interactions. Electrostatic attraction occurs between two oppositely charged ions on a drug and a protein. Proteins are thereby capable of binding charged metal ions. The degree of binding varies with the chemical nature of each compound and the net charge. Dissociation of ionic bonds usually occurs readily, but some members of the transition group of metals exhibit high association constants (low K_{diss} values), and exchange is slow. Ionic interactions may also contribute to binding of alkaloids with ionizable nitrogenous groups and other ionizable toxicants.

Hydrogen Binding. Hydrogen bonds arise when a hydrogen atom, covalently bound to one electronegative atom, is "shared" to a significant degree with a second electronegative atom. As a rule, only the most electronegative atoms (O, N, and E) form stable hydrogen bonds. Protein side chains containing hydroxyl, amino, carboxyl, imidazole, and carbamyl groups can form hydrogen bonds, as can the N and O atoms of peptide bonds themselves. Hydrogen bonding plays an important role in the structural configuration of proteins and nucleic acids.

Weak Interactions. Van der Waals forces produce weak interactions that act between the nucleus of one atom and the electrons of another atom; i.e., between dipoles and induced dipoles. The attractive forces arise from slight distortions induced in the electron clouds surrounding each nucleus as two atoms are brought close together. The binding force is critically dependent upon the proximity of interacting atoms and diminishes rapidly with distance. However, when these forces are summed over a large number of interacting atoms that "fit" together spatially, they can play a significant role in determining specificity of toxicant-protein interactions.

A final mechanism of binding is based on hydrophobic interactions. When two nonpolar groups come together, they exclude the water between them, and this mutual repulsion of water results in a hydrophobic interaction. In the aggregate, they present the least possible disruption of interactions among polar water molecules and thus can lead to thermodynamically stable complexes. Some authorities consider this a special case involving van der Waals forces. The minimization of thermodynamically unfavorable contact of a polar grouping with water molecules provides the major stabilizing effect in hydrophobic interactions.

Methods for Assessing Protein Binding. A number of *in vitro* methods have been employed to study ligand-protein interactions, including ultrafiltration, electrophoresis, equilibrium dialysis, solvent extraction, solvent partition, ultracentrifugation, spectrophotometry, and gel filtration. The most widely used techniques are ultrafiltration and equilibrium dialysis. The basic concept is that a semipermeable membrane is used that restricts passage of protein but allows unbound drug to cross the barrier, according the diffusion. Bound drug is placed on one side of the membrane, and samples are collected from the protein-free side. Ultrafiltration allows rapid protein-drug separation, while equilibrium dialysis requires time for the separation to occur. The fraction of free drug is then calculated based on the amount of total drug used. For some membranes and cationic basic drugs, binding to the membrane may occur, which would confound the analysis. This must be ruled out, otherwise erroneous results may occur. The mathematical methods presented below are then used to characterize the nature of the drug-protein interaction.

A characteristic of ligand-protein interactions is the great number of binding possibilities for attachment of a small molecule (drug or toxicant) to a large molecule (protein). Although highly specific (high-affinity, low-capacity) binding is known to occur with a number of drugs, examples of specific binding for toxicants are limited. In most cases, low-affinity, high-capacity binding describes the interactions, and often the number of binding sites cannot be accurately determined because of the nonspecific nature of the interactions.

To understand the physiochemical and biological significance of toxicant binding to a protein, several factors must be considered. The number of ligand molecules bound per protein molecule, v, and the maximum number of binding sites, n, are important considerations as they comprise the definitive binding capacity of the protein. Another consideration is the binding affinity, $K_{binding}$ (or $1 / K_{diss}$). If the protein has but one binding site for the toxicant, a single value of K_{diss} (or $K_{binding}$) describes the strength of the interaction. More usually, the value of the binding constant will vary when more than one binding site is present, each site having its intrinsic association constant, $K_1, K_2, \ldots$ This is especially true in the case of those toxicants for which van der Waals forces and hydrophobic binding appear to contribute to binding of a nonspecific, low-affinity nature. Of course, the chemical nature of the binding site is of critical importance in determining the binding characteristics. The environment of the protein, the three-dimensional molecular structure of the binding site, the general location in the overall protein molecule, cooperativity, and allosteric effects are all factors that influence binding. Studies have not generally provided an adequate elucidation of these factors; i.e., binding is usually too complex to be accurately described by any one set of equations.

Methods for analyzing binding phenomena are legion, and all possess unique terminology depending upon the roots of their disciplines (e.g., biochemistry versus physiology versus pharmacology). The examples presented will be less complex. Many of the classic techniques utilized have been challenged on mathematical and statistical grounds, and thus this presentation is only intended to illustrate basic principles. This section also serves as an introduction to the techniques used to describe saturable processes, since many of these essentially nonlinear pharmacokinetic interactions will be dealt with more extensively in Chapter 9 using a terminology consistent with pharmacokinetic models.

Chemical-protein complexes that are held together by relatively weak bonds (energies of the order of hydrogen bonds or less) readily associate and dissociate at physiological temperature, and a state of thermodynamic equilibrium can be readily attained. The law of mass action can be applied as follows:

$$K_{binding} = \frac{[TP]}{[T][P]} = \frac{1}{K_{diss}} \qquad (4.2)$$

where $K_{binding}$ is the equilibrium constant for association, $[TP]$ is the concentration of chemical-protein complex, $[T]$ is the concentration of free chemical, and $[P]$ is the concentration of total protein. This equation does not describe the binding sites or binding affinity. To incorporate these parameters and estimate the extent of binding, double reciprocal plots may be utilized to test the specificity of binding. This is illustrated in Figure 4.4 with binding of the lipophilic antibiotic doxycycline with albumin in cats. Regression lines passing through the origin imply infinite binding. In the case of infinite binding, calculation of an affinity constant becomes of questionable value.

Toxicant-protein binding may be defined as (1) specific, high-affinity, low-capacity, and (2) nonspecific, low-affinity, high-capacity. The term high-affinity implies an affinity

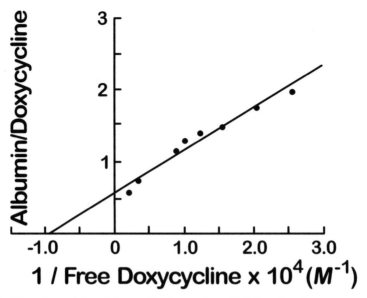

FIGURE 4.4.   Double reciprocal plot of doxycycline interaction with feline albumin.

constant ($K_{binding}$) of the order of 10^8 M^{-1} or greater, while low affinity implies a $K_{binding}$ of the order of 10^4 M^{-1} or less. Nonspecific, low-affinity binding appears to be most characteristic of nonpolar compounds.

Where high-affinity binding is manifest, the method of Scatchard is preferable for describing the action in which the equation

$$v = \frac{nk[A]}{1 + k[A]}$$
(4.3)

is rearranged for purposes of graphic solution to

$$\frac{v}{[A]} = k(n - v)$$
(4.4)

where v is the moles of ligand bound per mole of protein, $[A]$ is the concentration of free ligand, k is the intrinsic affinity constant, and n is the number of sites exhibiting such affinity. When $v[A]$ is plotted against v, a straight line is obtained (provided the protein has only one class of binding sites), the slope being $-k$ and the intercept on the v axis being n. With more than one class of sites, a curve is obtained from which the constants may be derived. This is illustrated for binding of doxycycline to feline albumin in Figure 4.5. Computer programs usually solve such data by determining one line for the specific binding and one line for nonspecific binding, the latter being an average of many possible solutions. In the case of doxycycline, one high-affinity specific and one very low-affinity nonspecific binding site were identified. Significant differences were also detected when the analysis was performed from albumin obtained from different species.

Hydrophobic binding of highly lipid toxicants (many environmental contaminants) is probably not limited to a single plasma protein. The binding of DDT to five human plasma proteins was strongest for albumin and lipoprotein fractions, although binding to any of three other proteins could adequately explain transport of DDT in the blood. Similar results have been reported for dieldrin, parathion, and carbaryl.

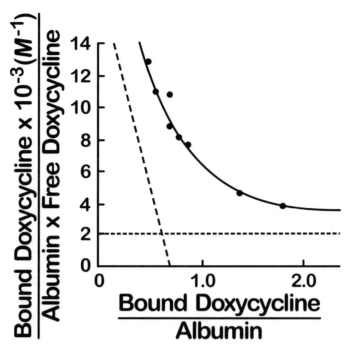

Figure 4.5.   Scatchard plot of doxycycline interaction with feline albumin demonstrating one high-affinity binding site (–––) and one nonspecific binding site (---).

Protein-binding data are frequently expressed in terms of percent of ligand bound. Although useful, the limitations should be recognized, for as ligand concentration is lowered, the percentage of binding increases. When a compound has a high affinity for a protein (e.g., albumin), percent binding falls sharply when the total ligand concentration exceeds a certain value that saturates the binding sites available. This topic will be revisited in greater detail when nonlinear pharmacokinetic models are developed in Chapter 9. A basic text in biochemistry should be consulted for more details on the analysis of ligand-protein interactions.

Displacement.   If a toxicant or drug is administered after binding sites on a protein are occupied by another chemical, competition for the site occurs, and toxic effects or enhanced activity may be noted due to a higher concentration of free toxicant. A number of fatty acids and derivatives, as well as the drug phenylbutazone, bind to the same site as the anticoagulant warfarin. Figure 4.6 illustrates the situation in which phenylbutazone displaces warfarin from its binding site of albumin. The increased anticoagulant effect observed *in vivo* when the compounds are administered concurrently may be attributable to an increase of free warfarin at its cell receptor site. To further illustrate, Hg^{2+} has a greater affinity for metallothionein than has Cd^{2+} and displaces Cd from the protein *in vitro*. The displacing substance may also be an endogenous ligand. In renal disease, accumulation of so-called uremic toxins may occur, which displaces administered drugs and results in enhanced toxicity, as is discussed in Chapter 15. This disease-induced increase in a compound's free fraction may be responsible for disease-induced increases in a toxicant's distribution volume.

Competition for the same site on plasma proteins may have especially important consequences when one of the potentially toxic ligands has a very high affinity. If compound A has low fractional binding (for example, 30%), and compound B displaces 10% of A

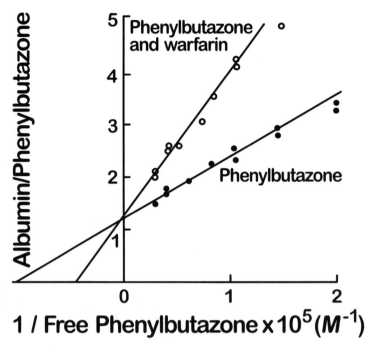

FIGURE 4.6. Double-reciprocal plot of phenylbutazone demonstrating competitive binding.

from the protein, the net increase of free A is from 70% to 73%, a negligible increase. However, if A is 98% bound and 10% is displaced, the amount of free A increases from 2% to 12%, a sixfold increase in free toxicant, which could result in a severe toxicological reaction. Competitive binding for very nonpolar compounds with infinite binding sites would be unlikely to occur at physiological concentrations. A change in binding may also occur when a second ligand produces an allosteric effect resulting in altered affinity of the protein for the originally bound compound (noncompetitive binding).

Most pharmacokinetic models in the human and comparative medical literature only assess total drug concentrations. When the extent of protein binding differs dramatically among species, inappropriate extrapolations often occur, as will be seen with doxycycline in Chapter 16. Similarly, interpretation of the extent of tissue distribution when the extent of protein binding is not known may be misleading. The most precise predictions can often be made when the free fraction of drug is known over the concentration ranges of the study being conducted.

OTHER FACTORS AFFECTING DISTRIBUTION

Among the factors that affect distribution, apart from binding to blood macromolecules per se, are the route of administration, molecular weight, rate of metabolism, polarity and stereochemistry of the parent compound or metabolic products, and rate of excretion. Molecular weight, charge, and/or polarity have been discussed. Stereoselectivity in the disposition of a drug is an often ignored phenomenon that could influence many studies. Its impact on metabolism is obvious; however, any receptor-mediated binding or transport process, including high-specificity protein binding, could be affected. Propranolol and ibuprofen have been shown to demonstrate stereoselective distribution.

A major factor determining distribution is the extent of tissue binding, a process identical to that of serum protein binding except that the results on drug disposition are opposite. Tissue binding is governed by the same mechanisms as discussed above and tends to increase a drug's distribution, although not necessarily activity, if the drug is sequestered away from active drug receptors or target microorganisms. Covalent binding also occurs and is relevant to toxicology and tissue residue depletion. Depending on the pharmacokinetic model employed, irreversible covalent tissue binding may actually be mathematically detected as an increase in the drug's elimination if only blood samples are used in the analysis since there is no redistribution of drug back into the blood. For distribution to be quantitated, the basic assumption in most modeling systems is that the process is reversible, and thus an equilibrium will ultimately be achieved between drug movement into and out of tissue. When irreversible binding occurs, compound is extracted from blood, and when excretory output (e.g., urine, feces, expired air) is not monitored, this is interpreted in many models as elimination. These model assumptions are often ignored. The quantitation of tissue binding and its effects on pharmacokinetic model development will be covered in Chapter 9.

Route of administration may affect the extent of absorption. Gastrointestinal and intraperitoneal absorption provide immediate passage of a compound to the liver via the portal system, whereas the dermal and respiratory routes provide at least one passage through the systemic circulation prior to reaching the liver. The metabolism of most toxicants results in products that are more polar and thus more readily excreted (than the parent molecule). Therefore, the rate of metabolism is a critical determinant in the distribution of a compound since those compounds that are readily metabolized are usually readily excreted, but their reduced hydrophobicity makes them proportionally less prone to distribute to and accumulate in the tissues. This effect would be seen if the analytical method used could not distinguish metabolites from parent compound. The same principle holds for polarity, since the greater the polarity, the more readily a xenobiotic may be excreted but be less able to cross membrane barriers and distribute to tissues.

As can be appreciated from this discussion, there are numerous factors that could affect distribution of a compound to tissues. Another factor is the methodology used to assess tissue distribution. Autoradiography is an excellent technique to anatomically localize distributed drug to the level of organs, cells, and even subcellular components. However, most pharmacokinetic studies rely on analytical techniques. When a tissue sample is collected from an animal, the sample is actually a homogenate of cells, extracellular fluid, and blood. The concentration measured cannot be uniquely assigned to any specific tissue or body fluid compartment. The use of microdialysis provides a direct estimate of extracellular fluid concentrations. There are many techniques available to separate tissue from fluid components; however, the investigator must be sure that drug diffusion doesn't occur during the procedures and again confound results.

All of these factors are important considerations when selecting the proper pharmacokinetic model. Many of these factors are implicit, especially when physiological pharmacokinetic models are employed. However, they strongly affect the interpretation of the primary parameter that quantitates distribution, the volume of distribution (Vd). As will be seen throughout the text, Vd is a proportionality factor that relates the mass of drug in a compartment (or dose) to the volume into which it is diluted, yielding a concentration:

$$Vd \text{ (mL)} = Mass \text{ (mg)} / Concentration \text{ (mg/mL)} \qquad (4.5)$$

Vd appears in equations that relate drug concentration to pharmacokinetic or physiological variables. The calculation of its value will be dependent upon the modeling scheme adopted. It is the physiological and protein-binding properties discussed above that change the nature of the concentration profile being modeled and thus will change the value of Vd obtained. As will be repeatedly stressed, Vd is a primary pharmacokinetic parameter whose precise estimation is central to any model used.

SELECTED READINGS

Ariens, E.J., W. Soudijn, and P.B.M.W.M. Timmermans. 1983. *Stereochemistry and Biological Activity of Drugs.* Oxford: Blackwell Scientific Press.

Artursson, P., R.H. Guy, D. Scherman, and P. Wils. 1996. *Passage of Drugs Across Physiological Barriers.* Table Ronde Roussel Uclaf nº 85: Paris.

Bai, S.A., U.K. Walle, M.J. Wilson, and T. Walle. 1983. Stereoselective binding of the (−) enantiomer of propranolol to plasma and extravascular binding sites in the dog. *Drug Metabolism and Disposition.*11:394-395.

Barza, M. 1981. Principles of tissue penetration of antibiotics. *Journal of Antimicrobial Chemotherapy, Supplement C.* 8:7-28.

Elmquist, W.F., and R.J. Sawchuck. 1997. Application of microdialysis in pharmacokinetic studies. *Pharmaceutical Research.* 14:267-288.

Kenakin, T.P. 1987. *Pharmacologic Analysis of Drug Receptor Interaction.* New York: Raven Press.

Khan, A.Z., and L. Aarons. 1989. Design and analysis of protein binding experiments. *Journal of Theoretical Biology.* 140:145-166.

Koch-Weser, J., and E.M. Sellers. 1976. Binding of drugs to serum albumin. *New England Journal of Medicine.* 294:311-316, 526-531.

LeBlanc, P.P. 1988. Drug distribution in the body. *General Pharmacology.* 3:357-360.

Mammarlund-Udenaes, M., L.K. Paalzow, and E.C.M. deLange. 1997. Drug equilibration across the blood-brain barrier: Pharmacokinetic considerations based on the microdialysis method. *Pharmaceutical Research.* 14:128-134.

Meijer, D.K.F., and P. van der Sluijs. 1989. Covalent and noncovalent protein binding of drugs: Implications for hepatic clearance, storage, and cell-specific drug delivery. *Pharmaceutical Research.* 6:105-118.

Notarianni, L.J. 1990. Plasma protein binding of drugs in pregnancy and in neonates. *Clinical Pharmacokinetics.* 18:20-36.

Peterson L.R., and D. Gerding. 1980. Influence of protein binding of antibiotics on serum pharmacokinetics and extravascular penetration: Clinically useful concepts. *Reviews of Infectious Diseases.* 2:340-348.

Poulin, P., and K. Krishnan. 1995. A biologically based algorithm for predicting human tissue:blood partition coefficients of organic chemicals. *Human and Experimental Toxicology.* 14:273-280.

Putnam, F.W. 1975. *The Plasma Proteins: Structure, Function and Genetic Control.* New York: Academic Press.

Riond, J.L., and J.E. Riviere. 1988. Multiple intravenous dose pharmacokinetics and residue depletion profile of gentamicin in pigs. *Journal of Veterinary Pharmacology and Therapeutics.* 11:210-214.

Riond, J.L., and J.E. Riviere. 1989. Doxycycline binding to plasma albumin of several species. *Journal of Veterinary Pharmacology and Therapeutics.* 12:253-260.

Riviere, J.E., R.L. Page, M.W. Dewhirst, K. Tyczkowska, and D.E. Thrall. 1986. Effect of hyperthermia on cisplatin pharmacokinetics in normal dogs. *International Journal of Hyperthermia.* 2:351-358.

Riviere, J.E., R.L. Page, R.A. Rogers, S.K. Chang, M.W. Dewhirst, and D.E. Thrall. 1990. Non-uniform alteration of cis-diammine dichloroplatinum (II) tissue distribution in dogs with whole body hyperthermia. *Cancer Research.* 50:2075-2080.

Tozer, T.N. 1981. Concepts basic to pharmacokinetics. *Pharmacology Therapeutics.* 12:109-131.

Upton, R.N. 1990. Regional pharmacokinetics I. Physiological and physiological basis. *Biopharmaceutics and Drug Disposition.* 11:647-662.

Upton, R.N. 1990. Regional pharmacokinetics II. Experimental methods. *Biopharmaceutics and Drug Disposition.* 11:741-752.

Williams, K., R. Day, R. Knihinicki, and A. Duffield. 1986. The stereoselective uptake of ibuprofen enantiomers into adipose tissue. *Biochemical Pharmacology.* 35:3403-3405.

Yamaoka, T., Y. Tabata, and Y. Ikada. 1994. Distribution and tissue uptake of poly(ethylene glycol) with different molecular weights after intravenous administration to mice. *Journal of Pharmaceutical Sciences.* 83:601-606.

5

Renal Elimination

The ultimate route for drug elimination from the body is the kidney. Drugs can also be eliminated in bile, sweat, saliva, tears, milk, and expired air; however, for most therapeutic drugs these routes are generally not quantitatively important as mechanisms for reducing total body burden of drug. The degree of lipid solubility and extent of ionization in blood determines how much of drug will be excreted by the kidney. For drugs that are first biotransformed by the liver, the more water-soluble metabolites are then ultimately excreted through the kidney in the urine. The kidney has also been the most widely studied excretory organ because of the accessibility of urine to collection and analysis. Many of the principles utilized by pharmacologists in quantitating excretory organ function, especially clearance, were originally developed by renal physiologists to noninvasively assess kidney function. Smith's classic reference on renal physiology is still instructive for the determination of renal clearance.

There are two components relevant to any discussion of renal drug excretion: physiology and quantitation. This chapter will introduce the physiology and expand upon the perspective developed earlier. Renal drug excretion can be considered using the same principles of membrane transport, except in this case the movement is from the vascular system to outside the body. Generally, only drugs that are either dissolved in the plasma or bound to circulating blood proteins are available for excretion. Many of the methods routinely used in pharmacokinetics to quantitate drug excretion are dependent upon the specific modeling techniques employed. However, the final parameter estimated by most of these approaches is the renal clearance of the drug. The concept of clearance, deeply rooted in renal physiology, will be extensively developed here and expanded on in the next chapter (on hepatic drug elimination). Precise and practical methods for its experimental determination will be introduced; however, full development must wait until the basic pharmacokinetic models have been presented in later chapters.

RENAL PHYSIOLOGY RELEVANT TO CLEARANCE OF DRUGS

For a perspective of drug excretion from the body, the kidney should be considered as an excretory organ designed to remove foreign compounds (e.g., drugs) and metabolic by-products (e.g., creatinine, urea) from the blood. As will become evident, the major clinical indices of renal function, such as blood urea nitrogen, serum creatinine, and creatinine clearance, are actually pharmacokinetic parameters of creatinine and urea excretion.

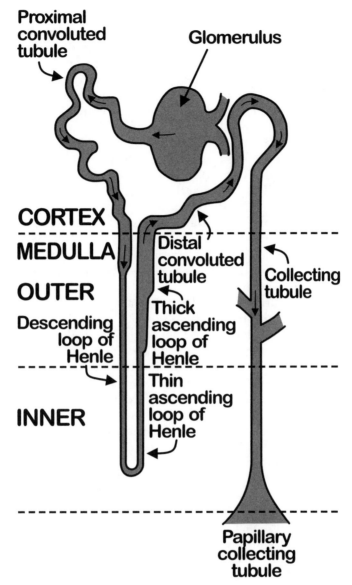

FIGURE 5.1. Structure of a nephron.

As discussed relative to distribution in the last chapter, the kidney receives approximately 25% of the cardiac output and thus processes a prodigious amount of blood. The kidney functions in a two-step manner to accomplish its function. The first step is passage through a filtering unit to retain formed cellular elements (e.g., erythrocytes, white blood cells) and proteins in the blood, only allowing the passage of plasma fluid into the remainder of the kidney. The second step utilizes a system of anatomically and physiologically segmented tubules to further modify the contents of the filtered fluid depending on a host of physiological needs including but not limited to fluid, electrolyte, and acid-base balance and the regulation of systemic blood pressure.

The primary functional unit of the kidney is the nephron depicted in Figure 5.1. Depending on the species, there may be 500,000 nephrons per kidney. The sum of their individual function is the observed organ function. Their specific anatomical arrangement is species-dependent, often determined by the evolutionary adaptation of the animal to its environment relative to the need to conserve body fluids. The filtration unit is the glomerulus, while the remainder of the fluid processing is accomplished by the extensive tubular system, whose segments are named in relation to their relative distance (proximal versus distal) measured *through* the tubules from the glomerulus. The junction between these is a unique anatomical adaptation called the loop of Henle, which is designed to use countercurrent exchangers to efficiently produce a concentrated urine since most of the water that is filtered by the glomerulus must be reabsorbed back into the body. The loop of Henle also forces the distal tubules to return toward the surface of the kidney to inter-act with the glomeruli. Grossly, the region of the kidney containing the glomeruli as well as the proximal and returning distal tubules is on the outside toward the surface and comprises the renal cortex. This region of the kidney is very well perfused by blood and is primarily characterized by oxidative metabolic processes. The interior region is the medulla, which is occupied by the penetrating loops of Henle; it is poorly perfused and is characterized by anaerobic metabolism.

The reabsorption of sodium, chloride, and urea produces osmotic gradients for the subsequent reabsorption of water. This is facilitated by the very low medullary blood flow, which maintains a hyperosmotic (relative to blood) environment characterized by high sodium chloride and urea tonicity. The tubular segments involved in this reabsorp-tion (primarily the proximal tubule and loop of Henle) are the primary targets for di-uretic drugs that function by blocking sodium or chloride reabsorption. As fluid moves from the proximal to distal segments, the fluid contents become more concentrated as water is reabsorbed. Filtrate in the distal tubules from individual nephrons then drains into the collecting ducts for excretion from the body as urine. The distal nephron is the fi-nal control point for the ultimate volume of urine produced. Urine volume is regulated by antidiuretic hormone (ADH, vasopressin), which alters the permeability of the collecting ducts exposed to the hyperosmotic medulla, through which the tubules penetrate. When permeable, water is reabsorbed back into the medulla, the urine is more concentrated, and diuresis is reduced (hence antidiuretic).

The amount of tubular fluid filtered by the glomeruli is thus acted upon by the various nephron segments to reabsorb wanted materials (primarily water and sodium) back into the blood and to let the remainder be excreted into the urine. Most of these processes are regulated by neural and hormonal systems whose function is control of fluid homeostasis and blood pressure. Because of the role of fluid balance in maintaining systemic blood pressure, there are additional anatomical adaptations that allow for this regulation. The primary one is that the distal tubules of nephrons course back up to the glomeruli at the point that the arterial blood supply enters, forming the juxtaglomerular apparatus. Dif-ferent nephron segments may associate with different glomeruli, which results in the gross kidney averaging of individual nephron function, an anatomical arrangement that introduces a certain degree of heterogeneity and thus variability in any renal excretory process. This anatomical adaptation is the major manifestation that allows for the opera-tion of the renin-angiotensin system to regulate blood pressure. Part of the function of this system is modulated by changing nephron blood flow, which secondarily may alter the ability of the kidney to excrete drugs. Finally, the kidney is also the site where acid-base balance is metabolically tuned by controlling acid and base excretion. Some of these processes are coupled to electrolyte secretion (e.g., potassium and sodium) and thus are further modulated by hormones, such as aldosterone. These nephron functions may in-advertently alter the amount of drug eliminated in the tubules by changing tubular fluid pH and consequently the ionized fraction of weak acids and bases according to the Henderson-Hasselbach equation presented in Chapter 2. This modification in tubular fluid may affect the value of renal clearance determined in pharmacokinetic studies.

There are specific tubular transport systems that excrete products directly into the tubular fluid, which are not filterable because of plasma protein binding. Other transport systems reabsorb essential nutrients (e.g., glucose) back into the blood that were filtered into the tubular fluid. Drugs are also processed by these same transport systems, making drug excretion dependent upon the physiological status of the animal. This is especially true when a drug biochemically resembles an endogenous substrate. As is similar to all transport processes, saturation and competition may occur, and as will be developed in subsequent chapters, nonlinear behavior may become detectable.

A full discussion of these varied functions of the kidney would take multiple books to adequately cover, and in fact many multivolume references in renal physiology and nephrology admirably accomplish this task and should be consulted for further details. The purpose of this brief review is to present sufficient anatomy and physiology so that the process of drug excretion is intelligible. Some select aspects of renal physiology in disease states will also be presented in Chapter 15 when the effects of renal disease on drug disposition must be taken into account. Now, effort will be focused on demonstrating how different methods for determining renal function are derived and relate to similar pharmacokinetic parameters.

MECHANISMS OF RENAL DRUG EXCRETION

Drugs are normally excreted by the kidney through the processes of (1) glomerular filtration, (2) active tubular secretion and/or reabsorption, and/or (3) passive, flow-dependent, nonionic back diffusion. These processes can be considered as vectorial quantities, each possessing magnitude and direction relative to transport between tubular fluid and blood. Their sum determines the ultimate elimination of a specific drug by the kidney as illustrated in Figure 5.2. *The total renal excretion of a drug equals its rate of filtration plus secretion minus reabsorption.* If a drug is reabsorbed back from the tubular fluid into the blood, its net renal excretion will be reduced. In contrast, if a drug is secreted from the

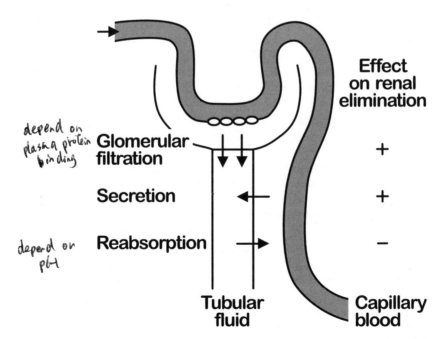

FIGURE 5.2. Vectorial processes of nephron function and their net effect on overall renal drug elimination.

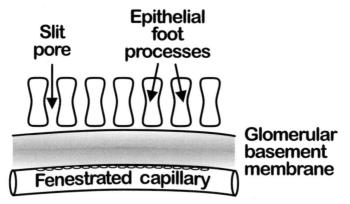

FIGURE 5.3.   The glomerular filtration barrier.

blood into the tubular fluid, its net excretion will be increased. These events will be subsequently quantitated.

Glomerular Filtration.   Excretion by this process is unidirectional with drug removal from the blood by bulk flow. Only non–protein-bound drugs are eliminated by this process, since only neutral molecules with a diameter of less than 75 to 80 angstroms may be filtered (smaller for charged molecules). The rate of drug filtration, therefore, is dependent upon both the extent of drug protein binding and the glomerular filtration rate (*GFR*), whose calculation will be developed below.

Glomerular filtration is essentially ultrafiltration through the relatively permeable glomerular filtration barrier, which consists of the epithelial cells of Bowman's capsule, the glomerular basement membrane, and the slit pores formed from juxtaposing epidothelial foot processes (Figure 5.3). These possess a fixed negative charge that is a major contributor to the rate-limiting aspect of this barrier. When damaged, filtration selectivity is impaired, and proteins may pass into tubular fluid. This is the primary manifestation of glomerular diseases that affects drug excretion. The anionic nature of the glomerular membrane pores also further restricts excretion of cationic molecules due to a Donnan exclusion effect. This factor can generally be ignored when calculating drug clearances, although in very carefully designed studies with drugs such as polyamines and aminoglycosides, its contribution can be quantitated relative to the filtration of similarly sized uncharged molecules.

The rate of glomerular filtration is dependent not only upon the efficiency of the filtration barrier, but also upon the net filtration pressure (approximately 17 mm Hg). Filtration pressure is a function of blood flow and the balance of hydrostatic pressure (primarily arterial blood pressure) promoting filtration, countered by the nonfiltered glomerular oncotic pressure generated by the tendency of nonfiltered albumin to retain water in the glomerular capillaries. This process is not saturable, and thus a constant fraction of drug presented to the glomeruli will be filtered. Because of the dependency on drug concentration in blood, renal drug excretion due to glomerular filtration is a linear first-order kinetic rate process. Each nephron contributes to the overall ability of the kidney to filter drugs, with the total glomerular filtration capacity being the sum of single nephron filtrations. This has a major influence in renal disease processes marked by loss of nephrons and is the prime contributing factor to reduced glomerular filtration in renal disease. Finally, changes in renal blood flow will also decrease glomerular filtration, and thus vasoactive drugs that cause renal arterial constriction may decrease their own clearance. Drugs that alter the modulators of intrarenal blood flow (e.g., inhibitors

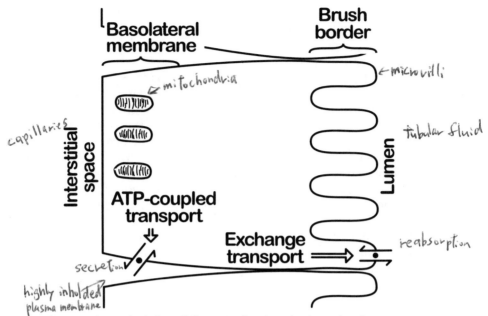

FIGURE 5.4. Schematic of a renal tubular cell illustrating location of active and exchange transport systems.

of prostaglandins, angiotensin, kinins) may also alter their own excretion as a result of changes in the distribution of renal blood flow to the glomeruli. The fraction of plasma that is ultimately filtered through the glomeruli and presented to the tubules for further action is termed the filtered load.

Active Tubular Secretion and Reabsorption. The magnitude of these processes is not affected by the extent of plasma drug protein binding. These saturable, carrier-mediated processes are energy-dependent and described by the laws of Michaelis-Menton enzyme kinetics fully presented in Chapter 9. In order to promote absorption from the tubular filtrate into blood, tubule cells have microvilli, much like the intestinal mucosal cells presented in Chapter 3, that maximize the surface area to cell volume ratio presented to the tubule. For secretion from the interstitial space into the tubule lumen, the basolateral surfaces of these cells (side facing the capillaries) have intensive membrane invaginations that also increase the surface area for interaction with the perfusing capillaries to facilitate active secretion. To provide the energy to drive these processes, proximal tubule cells have high mitochondrial densities to generate adenosine triphosphate (ATP), which fuels the Na+/K+ adenosine triphosphatase (ATPase)–coupled transport systems. This high level of oxidative metabolism is the primary reason for the sensitivity of the kidney to hypoxic or anoxic conditions, which results in renal damage if blood perfusion is interrupted even for short periods of time.

The cellular structure of transport systems across tubule cells involves two separate pairs of transport proteins, which creates an overall "polarity" of tubule cell function relative to the interstitial fluid and tubular lumen (Figure 5.4). One set is located in the brush border of the interface with tubular fluid and the other is located in the basolateral membrane. Energy coupling with ATP generally occurs in the basal portion of the cell (proximity to mitochondria) which, in secretion, builds up intracellular drug concentrations, which are then transported to the tubular fluid by concentration-driven facilitated transport carriers. In reabsorption, the reverse occurs as the basolateral active "pumps" create low intracellular drug concentrations that promote facilitated carrier-mediated reabsorption through the brush-border tubular membrane. Most transport systems are also stoichiometrically coupled to the transport of an electrolyte (e.g., Na+, K+, Cl−, H+), which ensures electrical neutrality and provides a mechanism for modulating the systemic concentrations of these elements.

The primary ion that drives these transporters and regulates overall renal function is sodium. Thus, all drug transport systems are usually coupled to a Na+ ATPase transmembrane system whose structure and polarity will determine the nature and direction of drug movement. The identical motif exists in other organs; thus similar mechanisms will be encountered when we discuss biliary transport systems in Chapter 6. The major difference between renal and hepatic cellular transport mechanisms is that in the kidney, cells are specialized as to the substrates being transported in relation to their location in different nephron segments. In the liver, regional specialization does not occur, and all cells involved in hepatobiliary transport have similar structure and function.

This two-membrane transport process has been studied to explain the mechanism of toxicity of some compounds. The classic example is the antibiotic cephaloridine which, unlike other cephalosporins, is actively transported into proximal tubular cells but does not possess a brush-border transport system to allow drug efflux into the tubular fluid. High concentrations of drug thus accumulate in the tubular cells, which results in nephrotoxicity. A similar phenomenon occurs in some liver cells involved in hepatobiliary secretion.

There are two distinct secretory pathways in the later sections of the proximal renal tubule that are relevant to a discussion of drug and toxicant excretion: one for acidic and one for basic compounds. The primary orientation of this system is from blood to tubular filtrate, removing drugs and/or metabolite conjugates from the blood that were not removed by glomerular filtration. Table 5.1 lists drugs that are actively secreted by the tubules. Active reabsorption systems are also present that act on drug already present in the filtered load. These systems are generally present to recover essential nutrients (e.g., glucose) that have been filtered by the glomerulus. Some drugs reach their target sites by this mechanism, making their tubular fluid concentration more important for predicting activity than their blood concentrations. An excellent example is the diuretic furosemide, which is first secreted by the tubules into the tubular fluid and is then actively reabsorbed back into the tubular cells, gaining access to its receptors for activity. Thus, the best concentration-time profile to predict the diuretic action of furosemide is that of the urine rather than blood.

Drugs (and other endogenous substrates) may compete for tubular transport sites, thereby functioning as reversible, competitive inhibitors. This interaction has been classically studied with the organic acid transport system. Weak acids such as probenecid or phenylbutazone will inhibit secretion of the weak acid penicillin, thereby prolonging penicillin blood concentrations. Thus, when two or more drugs in the same ionic class are administered, their rate and extent of renal excretion will be affected. Many drug metabolites are conjugates (e.g., glucuronides) produced by phase II biotransformation reactions and secreted by the transport system for weak acids, which may further complicate the pattern of drug excretion. In addition, agents secreted by the acid transport system may produce biphasic effects, inhibiting secretion at low doses and reabsorption at high doses. Salicylate inhibition of uric acid secretion follows this pattern. Damage to renal tubules from toxins, interstitial nephritis, and hypercalcemic nephropathy will impair the renal secretion of drugs and conjugates by active tubular processes.

There are direct pharmacokinetic implications to the carrier-mediated mechanism of renal tubular drug secretion. The limited capacity of carrier-mediated processes means that above certain blood drug concentrations, transport will proceed at a maximal rate independent of concentration in blood; that is, so-called nonlinear zero-order kinetics will become controlling, which will have adverse affects on the utility of normal linear

TABLE 5.1.   Renal Tubular Handling of Drugs

Acids	Bases
Acetazolamide (A, P)	Amphetamine (P)
p-Aminohippurate (A)	Chloroquine (P)
Chlorothiazide (A, P)	Diphenhydramine (P)
Chlorpropamide (A)	Dopamine (A)
Cephaloridine (A)	Ephedrine (P)
Dapsone (A)	Fenfluramine (P)
Diodrast (A)	Hexamethonium (A)
Ethacrynic acid (A)	Histamine (A)
Furosemide (A)	Isoproterenol (A, P)
Glucuronides (A)	Morphine (A)
Hippurates (A)	Neostigmine (A)
Indomethacin (A)	Opiates (P)
Mersalyl (A)	Phenothiazine (P)
Methotrexate (A)	Procainamide (A, P)
Nitrofurantoin (P)	Procaine (A)
Penicillin (A, P)	Quinidine (A, P)
Phenolsulfonphthalein (A, P)	Tetraethylammonium (A)
Phenylbutazone (A, P)	Thiamine (A)
Probenecid (A, P)	Trimethoprim (A, P)
Salicylic acid (A, P)	
Spironolactone (A)	
Sulfonamides (A, P)	

A = active tubular secretion or reabsorption; P = passive tubular reabsorption
(nonionic back diffusion).

pharmacokinetic models. These factors may become more important in renal disease states in which renal capacity is already diminished. Under these circumstances, drug renal clearance will approach the glomerular filtration rate, as additional drug concentrations in blood will not now be secreted into the urine. At subsaturation concentrations, renal clearance of an actively secreted substance is dependent on and limited by renal plasma flow. Thus flow-limited mechanisms discussed below, and more extensively in the hepatic elimination chapter, will become important considerations.

Passive Tubular Reabsorption.   The final determinant of a drug's renal disposition is the mechanism of nonionic passive tubular reabsorption, or back diffusion, a process dependent upon urine flow rate, lipid solubility of the nonionized drug moiety, and urine pH. At low urine flow rates, there is greater opportunity for diffusion of drug from the distal tubular fluid back into the blood. Diffusion is facilitated by the high concentration of drug in the tubular fluid. Polar compounds having low lipid solubility, such as many drug metabolites, are not reabsorbed since they cannot cross the lipid membrane. In contrast, lipid-soluble, nonionized drugs are reabsorbed into the blood. This is the identical process discussed for passive drug absorption in Chapters 2 and 3, except in these cases, the outside of the body is now the filtered tubular fluid. The ratio of ionized to nonionized molecules determines the concentration gradient that drives the drug into the fluid. Table 5.1 also lists drugs passively reabsorbed by renal tubules. The extent of reabsorption is again a function of the drug's pKa and the pH of the tubular fluid as described by the Henderson-Hasselbach equations (see Chapter 2, equations 2.3 through 2.5). The pH of the urine can undergo drastic changes as a function of diet and coadministered drugs (e.g., urine acidifiers and alkalizers). Tubular reabsorption of organic acids occurs with pKa values between 3.0 and 7.5 and for basic drugs with pKa values between 7.5 and

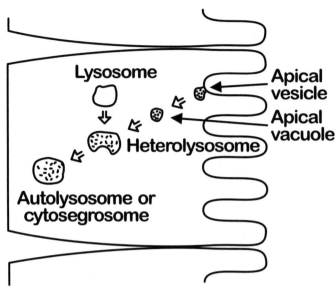

FIGURE 5.5.   Schematic of pinocytotic reabsorption in a tubule cell.

10.5. Weak acids thus are reabsorbed at low urinary pH (acidic), while weak bases are reabsorbed at high urinary pH (alkaline). Therefore, the renal excretion of an acidic drug decreases in acidic urine but increases in alkaline urine.

This principle is employed in treating salicylate intoxication in dogs. A brisk, alkaline diuresis is induced to decrease salicylate reabsorption into the blood and hasten excretion into the urine by trapping the salicylic acid in an ionized form in the alkaline urine. Reabsorption is further decreased by the elevated urinary flow rate. In contrast, induction of an alkaline diuresis will enhance the toxicity of basic drugs by increasing the amount of tubular reabsorption. Drugs often employed in critical care situations, such as procainamide or quinidine, have increased reabsorption and thus systemic activity in this alkaline state.

Species differences in urinary pH can have a major influence on the rate of renal excretion of ionizable drugs. Carnivores tend to have more acidic (pH 5.5 to 7.0) urine than herbivores (pH 7.0 to 8.0). Thus, with all other disposition factors being equal, a weakly acidic drug will have a higher renal excretion in herbivores than in carnivores, and a weakly basic drug will have a greater renal excretion in carnivores than in herbivores. In healthy animals, small changes in urinary pH or urine flow rate do not significantly contribute to altered drug clearance. However, with decreased function in renal disease, there is a decreased tubular load of drug. Altered urinary pH theoretically could further decrease overall drug clearance. Conditions such as renal tubular acidosis and the Fanconi syndrome modify drug elimination by enhancing reabsorption of acidic drugs and decreasing reabsorption of basic drugs.

There are two other peculiarities of renal tubular transport that must be discussed before quantitating these processes. Some drugs are reabsorbed into the tubules by pinocytosis. This occurs by interaction of filtered drug in the tubular fluid with the brush-border membrane (Figure 5.5). This is a very low-capacity and slow process that is easily saturated. Pinocytozed drug is then transferred to lysosomes and generally digested in the cell (e.g., peptides and filtered proteins such as β_2 microglobulin). However, for some compounds, such as the aminoglycosides, enzymatic breakdown does not occur, and the drug is essentially stored in the kidney. Therefore, although the drug is reabsorbed from the tubular fluid, it is not transported through the cell into the blood.

Thus, unlike other tubular reabsorption processes, reabsorption with storage or metabolism does decrease elimination of drug from the body. This is important when considering the meaning of a clearance calculated from pharmacokinetic parameters determined from blood alone. Reabsorption into the renal parenchyma will generally not be detected from blood-centered systemic pharmacokinetic models because any return flux back to the blood is at very low rates. Urine drug concentrations must be included in the analysis for pinocytotic absorption to be detected. However, such reabsorption has toxicologic significance because the drug does accumulate in the tubular cells and could produce an adverse effect. Finally, this phenomenon has a major influence on the prediction of tissue residue profiles in the kidney resulting from drugs with prolonged elimination half-lives (e.g., aminoglycosides).

Renal Drug Metabolism. The final confounding influence on determination of renal drug clearance occurs when drug is metabolized by the kidney. Most of the phase I and phase II enzymatic systems presented in detail in Chapter 6 also exist in the kidney, although different isozymes may be expressed. Oxidative processes generally occur within the proximal tubule cells. Two scenarios may occur. The first is when drug is metabolized solely by the kidney and not the liver, or a combination of both processes occurs. The second is when *relay* metabolism occurs, and the kidney further metabolizes a drug already biotransformed by the liver. A toxicologically relevant example of this is the metabolism of hexachlorobutadiene by the liver to its glutathione conjugate. In the kidney, ß-lyase then cleaves the conjugate with release of free drug into the renal tubule cells. Finally, hepatic metabolites may induce renal enzymes to further metabolize a drug. These interactions are complex and often are of toxicologic significance.

Similar to the discussion above, compound that is metabolized by the kidney is lost to the systemic circulation since parent drug would not be detected, even in the urine. To quantitate this, one must use radiolabeled drug and/or know the specificity of the analytical method relative to separating parent drug and metabolite concentrations. This process contributes to the overall renal elimination of drug from the body and can be easily studied using many of the pharmacokinetic modeling techniques presented in later chapters. Renal drug biotransformation may also occur in the medulla by anaerobic metabolic processes (e.g., prostaglandin endoperoxide synthetase). This process is small relative to reducing overall body burden because only 1% of renal blood flow delivers compounds to this region but has toxicologic significance to the renal medulla where drug and/or metabolite may accumulate. Finally, brush-border enzymes are present that metabolize peptides in the filtered tubular load to amino acids for reabsorption.

A great deal of effort is spent on studying the toxicological significance of renal drug metabolism because lethal synthesis may occur where a nontoxic parent drug is metabolically activated within the renal tubular cells into a toxic metabolite. The classic example of renal cortical drug activation is chloroform to toxic phosgene and carbon tetrachloride to its toxic trichloromethyl free radical. In the medulla, prostaglandin endoperoxide synthetase metabolizes acetaminophen to a toxic free radical that produces interstitial nephritis after chronic treatment and activates benzidine to a carcinogenic metabolite. The biochemical mechanisms of metabolism will be presented in Chapter 6.

Stereoselectivity in both active tubular secretion and metabolism in the kidney may occur with specific drugs (e.g., quinidine). The implications to assessment of renal drug excretion is similar to that of drugs metabolized by the kidney and is usually not taken into account.

This is a limited introduction of the wide range of processes that occur in the kidney and may affect renal drug elimination. A complete assessment of the renal mechanisms requires that both blood and urine data be collected to fully describe these events. If the drug is metabolized, assays must differentiate parent drug from metabolites. Numerous pharmacokinetic strategies will be presented in later chapters to specifically quantitate these processes. When simple blood-based models are used, these mechanisms may be obscured and aberrant predictions made.

THE CONCEPT OF CLEARANCE AND ITS CALCULATION

Urine analysis is required for any detailed study of drug disposition. The problem with simply measuring the concentration of drug in urine as an index of its renal excretion is that the kidney also modulates the volume of urine produced in association with its primary mission of regulating fluid balance. Thus, the concentration of drug alone may be higher or lower depending upon the ultimate urine volume. To accurately assess how much drug is eliminated, the product of volume of urine produced and the concentration of drug in urine (mass/volume) must be determined to provide the amount excreted (mass). If timed urine samples are collected, then an excretion rate (mass/time) is determined. Similarly, to assess how efficient this process is, one must know how much drug is actually presented to the kidney for excretion. This is related to the concentration of drug in the arterial blood. As alluded to above, this is especially important when renal disease lowers the extent of glomerular filtration and reduces the filtered load of drug. The physiological concept of clearance was developed by early workers to generate a parameter that measured the true efficiency of renal excretion processes by assessing the total mass of compound ultimately excreted and relating it to the concentration of drug presented to the kidney for excretion. As will be stressed, the net clearance of a substance is the vectorial sum of glomerular filtration, tubular secretion, tubular reabsorption, and renal metabolism.

Definition of Clearance.   With this background in renal physiology, the task at hand is to establish parameters that are useful to quantitate drug or xenobiotic elimination by the kidney. The parameter that is used throughout physiology and pharmacokinetics to quantitate drug elimination through an organ, and by extension out of the body, is clearance. The relevant equation defining the whole-body clearance (Cl_B) of a drug is the sum of all elimination clearances:

$$Cl_B = Cl_{(renal)} + Cl_{(hepatic)} + Cl_{(other)} \tag{5.1}$$

This equation illustrates the elegance of using Cl_B as the prime estimate of drug elimination since contributory organ function, when expressed as clearances, is simply additive. The only exception to this rule is for a drug eliminated through the lung since the pulmonary circulation is in series with the systemic circulation and receives the total cardiac output. Calculation of Cl_B provides an efficient strategy for estimating how a drug or toxicant is eliminated from the body as it indirectly compares systemic clearance to renal and hepatic clearances. Because of the historical role of renal physiology in defining clearance and the easy accessibility of the kidney's excretory product (urine) for collection and analysis, the concept of clearance and simple methods for its determination will be developed in this chapter. However, Cl_B will be revisited in Chapter 6 when $Cl_{hepatic}$ becomes the parameter of interest.

Renal Clearance.   The first definition of renal clearance is *the volume of blood cleared of a substance by the kidney per unit of time* or, alternatively, the volume of blood required to contain the quantity of drug removed by the kidney during a specific time interval. As will be developed shortly, it is a physiologically based parameter that relates drug excretion directly to a measurable estimate of renal function. This is very important for calculating dosage regimens for patients with renal disease.

Recall from the previous discussion of renal physiology that the actual value for a drug's renal clearance is the vectorial sum of filtration + tubular secretion − tubular reabsorption, making it a parameter that estimates the entire contribution of the kidney to drug elimination. Similarly, any change in renal drug processing will be reflected in renal clearance if it is not compensated for by more distal components of the renal tubules.

Two types of data are needed to calculate clearance: (1) an estimate of blood drug concentration presented to the kidney and (2) the amount of drug removed by the kidney. The latter can be estimated by either measuring the amount of drug excreted by the urine or comparing the difference between the renal arterial and venous drug concentrations to assess how much drug was extracted while passing through the organ.

To begin, we will use the classic approach, which directly measures extraction, based on Fick's law:

$$Cl(mL / min) = (Q)\,(E) = (Q)\frac{(C_{art} - C_{ven})}{(C_{art})} \tag{5.2}$$

where Q is renal arterial blood flow (mL/min), E is the extraction ratio, and C_{art} and C_{ven} are arterial and venous blood concentrations. As will be presented in Chapter 10, this approach is also the basis for many organ specific clearances used in building physiologically based pharmacokinetic models. The obvious difficulty with this approach is that arterial and venous blood samples must be collected. However, renal physiologists realized that this approach could be modified to more easily assess renal function.

The amount of substance removed or extracted by the kidney is equivalent to the amount excreted into the urine. If one makes a timed collection of urine and measures the urine concentration and volume, then the amount (X) of drug extracted by the kidney over a specific time interval, that is, its *rate of renal excretion*, denoted $(\Delta X / \Delta t)$ (the origin of the Δ terminology defined as "change in" will be presented in Chapter 7), is

$$\Delta X / \Delta t \text{ (mg/min)} = [U_x \text{ (mg/mL)}]\, [V \text{ (mL/min)}] \tag{5.3}$$

where U_x is the concentration of drug in urine and V is the urine production. Now the only component needed is the concentration presented to the kidney. Because renal function fluctuates and urine sampling requires relatively long intervals to collect sufficient samples for analysis, blood concentrations should be relatively constant to ensure that the measured values do not change throughout a sampling interval. This is in contrast to using equation 5.2, where short sampling intervals can be employed since simultaneous arterial and venous blood samples may be collected. When urine is collected, fluctuating blood concentrations may bias the results. Thus, workers used constant-rate intravenous infusion of chemicals to ensure that so-called steady-state blood concentrations were achieved. With this experimental design, the renal clearance of substance X is calculated as

$$Cl_{(renal)} \text{ (mL/min)} = (\Delta X / \Delta t) / C_{art} = U_x V / C_{art} \tag{5.4}$$

This expression also provides the second widely used definition for clearance, which is *the rate of drug excretion relative to its plasma concentration*. This expression will serve as the basis for many of the pharmacokinetic techniques to be developed in subsequent chapters.

Some minor discrepancies may result when drug clearances are calculated by use of blood or plasma data alone versus techniques such as this, which employ urine collection. As discussed earlier in this chapter, even for a drug that is excreted solely by the kidney,

TABLE 5.2.   Glomerular Filtration Rates (mL/min/kg) in
Select Species as Assessed by Inulin Clearance (Cl_{inulin})

Cow	1.8
Horse	1.7
Human	1.8
Goat	2.2
Sheep	2.0
Dog	4.0
Rat	10.0

tubular reabsorption with storage (e.g., aminoglycoside antibiotics) will result in a lower $Cl_{(renal)}$ calculated from urine data rather than blood-based methods since, as can be seen from equation 5.2, tubular reabsorption would not be reflected in the venous blood concentrations since the substance is now trapped in the tubular cells. A similar discrepancy may occur with intrarenal drug metabolism since, like renal storage, this process does not return parent drug to venous blood. In a research setting, the difference is often used as conclusive evidence that either of these two phenomena actually occur. This issue will be revisited in Chapter 7.

Estimates of Glomerular Filtration Rate.   The original perspective of the renal physiologists was to develop an estimate of renal *GFR*. In order for $Cl_{(renal)}$ to accurately measure *GFR*, a chemical that is solely cleared by glomerular filtration is required so that the kinetics are linear and thus do not change with varying blood concentrations; i.e., the more variable processes of tubular reabsorption and secretion will not confound the estimate. The classic *GFR* marker, the biologically inert polysaccharide inulin, is not bound to plasma proteins and is only filtered by the glomerulus. Thus the clearance of inulin (Cl_{inulin}) reflects the maximum amount of a compound that could be excreted by filtration alone since all of the inulin presented is free and available for filtration. Finally, in order to provide a reasonably straightforward technique, plasma or serum venous inulin concentrations are used since arterial samples are difficult to obtain. Although this results in a constant overestimation of clearance since C_{ven} is less than C_{art}, it has become a standard practice. Additionally, the inulin concentrations employed are high relative to the amount extracted, and thus the arteriovenous difference is not important as long as the sampling protocols used are the same. *GFR* is thus commonly calculated as

$$GFR(mL/min) = Cl_{inulin} = U_{(inulin)} \, V \, / \, Cp_{(inulin)} \qquad (5.5)$$

where *Cp* is the common nomenclature in pharmacokinetics to denote plasma concentration. *GFR* estimates are commonly normalized to body weight to adjust for different individual body sizes and then expressed in units of mL/(min kg) or mL min^{-1} kg^{-1}. Table 5.2 lists Cl_{inulin} across species ranging from cows to rats. Recently, the radiolabeled *GFR* markers ^{125}I-iothalamate and CrEDTA have been employed to facilitate the assay.

If one compares *GFR* measured as Cl_{inulin} to the renal clearance of a study drug or toxicant, then the ratio of clearances gives some insight into how the kidney excretes this compound relative to the processes of glomerular filtration, tubular secretion, and tubular reabsorption. This ratio, termed the *fractional clearance,* is calculated as

$$Fractional\ clearance\ (X) = \frac{U_{(x)}V / Cp_{(x)}}{U_{(inulin)} \, V \, / \, Cp_{(inulin)}} = \frac{Cl_{(renal)}}{Cl_{(inulin)}} \qquad (5.6)$$

However, applying basic algebra, one notes that V appears in both the numerator and denominator and thus cancel out. Rearrangement yields

$$Fractional\ clearance\ (X) = \frac{U_{(x)}\ Cp_{(inulin)}}{U_{(inulin)}\ Cp_{(x)}} \tag{5.7}$$

Therefore, timed urine collections are not required, and only urine and plasma samples of inulin and the chemical of interest need be assayed in any urine sample. *Fractional clearance* less than 1 implies tubular reabsorption, 1 implies only glomerular filtration, and greater than 1 implies tubular secretion.

Two endogenous substances produced at a constant rate as metabolic products of systemic metabolism have a *fractional clearance* close to unity. The closest, plasma (or serum) creatinine, is produced secondary to muscle metabolism of creatine phosphate. The second, urea, is produced as a by-product of protein metabolism. Creatinine, which is easily assayed in both urine and serum by spectrophotometric techniques, became an excellent surrogate for inulin since the body's metabolic processes provided the constant-rate infusion. Creatinine clearance is the standard clinical test for estimating *GFR* within the method embodied in equation 5.5. It has also been extensively used in pharmacokinetics as an independent estimate of *GFR*. Creatinine clearance is superior to urea clearance because urea is reabsorbed in the distal tubules as part of the countercurrent mechanism to concentrate urine and may vary depending on the hydration status of the animal. Additionally, ruminants metabolically handle urea differently than other species, which confounds its use in certain disease conditions. In some species (e.g., dogs), the *fractional clearance* of creatinine to inulin approaches a value of 1.1, suggesting some tubular secretion of creatinine. However, its ease of measurement and endogenous production overshadows this relatively minor error.

The final estimate of *GFR* is based on monitoring only serum creatinine (*SCR*) or serum urine nitrogen (*SUN*), commonly called blood urea nitrogen (BUN), as a rough estimate of *GFR*. It is instructive to consider how this relationship is derived. When the production of creatinine or urea is constant under normal steady-state conditions, all of the compound produced by the body is excreted by the kidney. A steady state can only be achieved, and in fact is defined, when the rate of input (muscle production of creatinine, protein catabolism to urea) equals its rate of output (excretion), which we defined in equation 5.4 as $\Delta X / \Delta t$. If we rewrite this equation in terms of creatinine,

$$Cl_{cr} \cong GFR = (\Delta CR / \Delta t) / SCR$$

and rearranging, we obtain

$$(SCR)\ (GFR) = \Delta CR / \Delta t \tag{5.8}$$

[handwritten: ← rate of renal excretion]

This suggests that if $\Delta CR / \Delta t$ remains constant, then the product of *SCR* and *GFR* will be constant, or for two different levels of *GFR* (1 and 2),

$$(SCR_1)\ (GFR_1) = (SCR_2)\ (GFR_2) \tag{5.9}$$

[handwritten: $\frac{SCR_1}{SCR_2} = \frac{1}{\frac{GFR_1}{GFR_2}}$]

The ratio of two *SCR*s is therefore inversely proportional to the ratio of the respective *GFR*s. Normal *SCR* is 1 mg/dl when *GFR* is normal, thus $1 / SCR$ reflects the ratio of normal to abnormal *GFR*. If *GFR* is reduced by 50%, *SCR* doubles. If *GFR* is reduced to 75% of normal, *SCR* will increase fourfold, and so on. Because the rate of creatinine production is constant and related to muscle mass, clinicians for humans have developed nomograms to adjust *SCR* to reflect gender differences in muscle mass. This inverse relation (hyperbolic) also explains why, with a decrease in renal function, *SCR* and *SUN* dramatically increase in renal disease, while *GFR* only decreases linearly.

This constant daily excretion of metabolic by-products into the urine allows urine concentrations to be used to normalize the excretion of other chemicals in a manner analogous to *fractional clearance*. In some toxicology and field-monitoring protocols in which drug or chemical excretion into urine is assessed, urine concentrations will often be adjusted by urine creatinine concentrations to correct for differences in urine volumes between study subjects. This provides an internal standard as to the length of the urine collection and ensures that adequate urine volume has been collected. This approach is particularly useful when chemical excretion into the urine is used as a field indicator or *biomarker* of chemical exposure and collection of timed or even complete urine samples cannot be guaranteed. By using urine creatinine concentration as a normalizing factor, urinary toxicant concentrations can be adjusted by creatinine concentrations to compensate for differences in dilution between individuals.

NONLINEARITY OF TUBULAR SECRETION AND REABSORPTION

The discussion thus far has been limited to determining clearances of substances that are primarily eliminated through glomerular filtration. The pharmacokinetics of this process are linear since saturation does not occur, and only non–protein-bound drugs are filtered through the glomerular basement membrane complex. When the renal clearance of a drug eliminated by glomerular filtration is estimated, only the filtration of the free or unbound drug is assessed; thus changes in protein binding will change the net excretion of drug. Drugs and toxicants that undergo passive tubular reabsorption obey Fick's law of diffusion since concentration gradients described again by linear first-order rate constants provide the driving force across the tubular epithelium. In contrast, compounds that are actively secreted from postglomerular capillaries across the renal tubules and into the tubular fluid show saturation at high concentrations, competition with drugs secreted by the same pathways, and dependence on the magnitude of renal blood flow—all hallmarks of nonlinear pharmacokinetic behavior. For such compounds, clearance will not be constant but rather will be dependent upon the concentration of drug presented to the kidney.

As discussed earlier in the physiology section, as tubular secretory pathways become saturated, the ratio of clearance to *GFR* (e.g., the *fractional clearance* of equation 5.6) will decrease. To develop this concept, we will revisit our definition of a drug cleared by *GFR* and acknowledge that only the free or unbound drug concentration (C_f) is eliminated by filtration. Protein-bound drug (C_b) cannot be filtered. Therefore, the rate of renal excretion ($\Delta X / \Delta t$) can be expressed as simply

$$\Delta X / \Delta t = C_f \times GFR \qquad (5.10)$$

As C_f becomes greater, $\Delta X / \Delta t$ will increase in direct proportion (e.g., linearly). However, recalling equation 5.4, its clearance will be $\Delta X / \Delta t$ *divided* by C_{art}. In this case, C_{art} is the total blood concentration presented to the kidney ($C_f + C_b$). Clearance thus equals

$$Cl_{(renal)} = (\Delta X / \Delta t) / C_{art} \qquad (5.11)$$

These relations have two implications. The first is that as total blood concentrations of drug increase, so does $\Delta X / \Delta t$; however, $Cl_{(renal)}$ remains constant since

$$Cl_{(renal)} = (C_f \times GFR) / (C_{art}) \tag{5.12}$$

and C_{art} will increase in direct proportion to $C_f + C_b$ as long as the fraction bound does not change. However, if the extent of protein binding of a drug is increased ($C_f \downarrow$, $C_b \uparrow$), its rate of renal excretion $\Delta X / \Delta t$ will decrease (equation 5.10) as will its clearance since the C_{art} ($C_f + C_b$) will be constant. Therefore, drugs cleared by filtration have constant clearance with changing total drug concentrations but are sensitive to the extent of protein binding. As will be seen in Chapter 6, this is characteristic of low-extraction clearance processes.

For such a drug with high protein binding, only the small fraction presented for filtration can ever be extracted and cleared by the kidney. Since the total renal clearance of a compound is the sum of filtration plus secretion, a drug *solely cleared by filtration* will have a relatively low clearance compared to one that is also actively secreted. If one considers this in terms of the extraction ratio (E) defined in equation 5.2, Cl_B will always be less than the renal blood flow (Q) since the extraction ratio is less than 1 and dependent upon the glomerular filtration fraction. Such drugs are termed *low-extraction* drugs, and their $Cl_{(renal)}$ will be sensitive to the extent of protein binding. Examples of such drugs include inulin, aminoglycosides, antibiotics, tetracyclines, and digoxin.

In contrast, consider a drug that also undergoes active tubular secretion. In this case, even a drug that is protein bound (C_b) or distributed into red blood cells will be secreted into the urine since the affinity for specific tubular transport proteins will be greater than that for the relatively nonspecific protein-binding sites or partitioning in erythrocytes. The extraction ratio will thus approach 1.0, and $Cl_{(renal)}$ will approach the renal blood flow Q. Such drugs are termed *high-extraction* or *perfusion-limited* to acknowledge the relationship of clearance to blood flow. The classic example is para-amino hippurate (PAH) as it is almost completely extracted as it passes through the kidney, making its clearance almost equal to renal plasma flow. In fact, PAH renal clearance was often calculated in clinical situations using equation 5.4 to estimate renal blood flow. Other such drugs include many of the ß-lactam antibiotics (e.g., penicillin) and many sulfate and glucuronide conjugate products of hepatic drug biotransformation. These concepts are developed further in Chapter 6 where low- and high-extraction drugs are discussed (see Table 6.13 and discussion).

The final implication of active tubular secretion is that at sufficiently high concentrations, saturation of the secretory pathways may occur. The point at which this occurs is termed the *maximum tubular transport* (T_m). At concentrations well below saturation, clearance will remain relatively constant since the rate of secretion will be dependent upon the concentration, much as it is with filtered drugs. However, as T_m is approached, the rate of secretion ($\Delta X / \Delta t$) will decrease until it reaches the maximal rate ($Q \times T_m$) and from that point on will be constant and independent of blood concentration. Since $\Delta X / \Delta t$ decreases and C_{art} increases, equation 5.4 suggests that $Cl_{(renal)}$ will also reach a maximal plateau. Since the total renal clearance of a drug is the sum of filtration plus secretion, the rate of secretion for a drug versus its plasma concentration will have a shape characteristic of its elimination pattern, as seen in Figure 5.6. Similarly, if another drug or endogenous compound that competes for tubular secretion is also present (e.g., probenecid coadministered with penicillin), $\Delta X / \Delta t$ and $Cl_{(renal)}$ will decrease.

The final complication occurs when a drug undergoes passive tubular reabsorption. The dependency of this process on urinary pH has already been discussed. In this case, C_{art} will be constant, but $\Delta X / \Delta t$ and thus $Cl_{(renal)}$ will vary depending on the urinary pH. Since this is an equilibrium process, time is required for this diffusion to occur. Thus, if the renal clearance of a drug is dependent upon urine flow, it is presumed to undergo passive tubular reabsorption. When high tubular loads are presented, reabsorption is overloaded as equilibrium cannot be achieved and nonreabsorbed drug is eliminated into the urine.

T_m (mg/min)

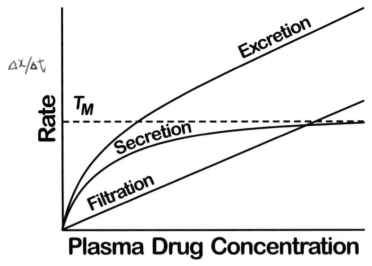

FIGURE 5.6.   Decomposition of the rate of drug excretion into components of glomerular filtration and tubular secretion.

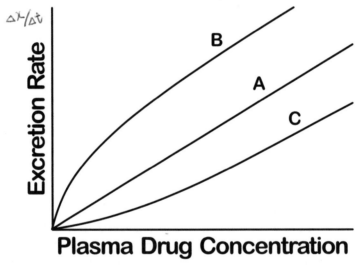

FIGURE 5.7.   Comparison of rate of renal excretion versus plasma drug concentration for a drug handled by (A) glomerular filtration, (B) tubular secretion, or (C) tubular reabsorption.

Using the principles presented in the above paragraphs, one can now examine the dependence of the rate of drug excretion ($\Delta X / \Delta t$) and $Cl_{(renal)}$ on the plasma drug concentration for drugs secreted by these different mechanisms, as shown in Figures 5.7 and 5.8. $\Delta X / \Delta t$ will generally increase with increasing concentrations; however, secretion and reabsorption will make these curves deviate from the linearity seen with solely filtered drugs at high concentrations. In contrast, and more instructive, clearance for a filtered drug is constant and is the value approached by both secreted and reabsorbed drugs at high concentrations.

A final complication arises depending on whether plasma or blood concentrations are measured. As the reader can appreciate from most of the discussions in this text, terms are often used interchangeably in the literature as the difference is usually very small. However, from a theoretical perspective relative to renal clearance, if an exact value of a

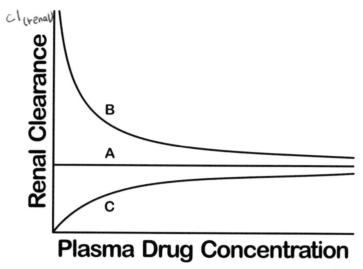

FIGURE 5.8.   Renal clearance versus plasma drug concentration of a drug handled by (A) glomerular filtration, (B) tubular secretion, or (C) tubular reabsorption.

renal extraction ratio is desired, only blood concentrations should be used since concentrations of drug in red blood cells are available for active tubular secretion despite not being filtered at the glomerulus.

SUMMARY

Unfortunately, it is not as easy to assess the function of other organs as it is for the kidney since their excretory fluids are not as experimentally accessible as urine. Techniques used to assess organ clearance require some additional pharmacokinetic techniques that build on the clearance principles developed above. These concepts will be revisited in the pharmacokinetic modeling chapters, in which various strategies for calculating drug clearances will be presented. Many are based on the definitions developed for assessing renal function. For example, the best method for calculating Cl_B is based on using steady-state drug infusions with a formula similar to equation 5.4. Techniques will also be presented to deal with non–steady-state drug concentrations, some of which have been developed into rapid tests for estimating *GFR*.

SELECTED READINGS

Caldwell, J., S.M. Winter, and A.J. Hutt. 1988. The pharmacological and toxicological significance of the stereochemistry of drug disposition. *Xenobiotica.* 18(Supplement 1):59-70.

Garrett, E.R. 1978. Pharmacokinetics and clearances related to renal processes. *International Journal of Clinical Pharmacology.* 16:155-172.

Hayes, A.W. 1994. *Principles and Methods of Toxicology,* 3ed. New York: Raven Press.

Keller, F., and J. Scholle. 1983. Criticism of pharmacokinetic clearance concepts. *International Journal of Clinical Pharmacology, Therapy and Toxicology.* 21:563-568.

Klaasen, C.D. 1996. *Casarett and Doull's Toxicology: The Basic Science of Poisons,* 5ed. New York: McGraw-Hill.

Osborne, C.A., and D.R. Finco. 1995. *Canine and Feline Nephrology and Urology.* Baltimore: Williams & Wilkins.

Riviere, J.E. 1982. Limitation on the physiologic interpretation of aminoglycoside body clearance derived from pharmacokinetic studies. *Research Communications in Chemical Pathology and Pharmacology.* 38:31-42.

Riviere, J.E., K.F. Bowman, and R.A. Rogers. 1985. Decreased fractional renal excretion of gentamicin in subtotal nephrectomized dogs. *Journal of Pharmacology and Experimental Therapeutics.* 234:90-93.

Rowland, M., L.Z. Benet, and G.G. Graham. 1973. Clearance concepts in pharmacokinetics. *Journal of Pharmacokinetics and Biopharmaceutics.* 1:123-136.

Seldin, D.W. ,and G. Giebisch. 1985. *The Kidney: Physiology and Pathophysiology.* New York: Raven Press.

Smith, H.W. 1956. *Principles of Renal Physiology.* New York: Oxford University Press.

Tozer, T.N. 1981. Concepts basic to pharmacokinetics. *Pharmacology and Therapeutics.* 12:109-131.

6

Hepatic Biotransformation and Biliary Excretion

Hepatic disposition is one of the final keys in the absorption, distribution, metabolism, and elimination (ADME) scheme needed to describe the disposition of many drugs and chemicals in the body. The liver is responsible for both biotransformation and biliary excretion as well as enterohepatic recycling. In many ways, the liver should be considered as two separate organs—one encompassing metabolism and the other biliary excretion.

Drug localization and biotransformation in the liver are dependent on many factors associated with both the biological system and drug itself. These factors include the biological properties of the liver (chemical composition, relative activity of major drug metabolism enzymes, hepatic volume/perfusion rate, and drug accessibility to and extraction by hepatic metabolic sites) as well as the physicochemical properties of the drug (pKa, lipid solubility, molecular weight). If single large or multiple doses of a drug are given, hepatic drug binding and metabolic sites may become saturated, which would facilitate drug distribution to other metabolic sites, including the blood, kidney, skin, gastrointestinal tract (including the gut flora), lung, brain, placenta, and other organs. Despite this caveat, in a quantitative sense, the liver is the major drug metabolism organ in the body.

Drug metabolism studies in animals are easier to conduct than in humans due to practical and ethical considerations, including the accessibility of special tissue collection and homogeneity of subject population. However, species differences in drug metabolic rate are, in most cases, the primary source of variation in drug disposition and therefore in drug activity or toxicity, across species. Extrapolation of metabolism data between animal species is an important issue as is the ability to correlate *in vivo* pharmacokinetic and metabolic data with *in vitro* metabolic findings.

Recalling our discussion in Chapter 2 about the phenomenological role of metabolism in drug distribution and excretion, it would be hard to imagine what would happen in biological systems without xenobiotic metabolism. Absorbed compounds would stay in the body for a much longer period of time and have prolonged activity, tissue accumulation and, potentially, toxicity. Metabolism is necessary for the animal or human body to rid itself of lipophilic xenobiotics as an effective defense mechanism against adverse effects. In general, the intensity of drug action is proportional to the concentration of the drug and/or its active metabolite(s) at the target site. On the other hand, drug-associated toxi-

Co-authored by Dr. Gui Lin Qiao

city is also dependent on the chemical form (active or inactive) and concentration at the same or other relevant target site. Therefore, any process or factor that modifies the drug/metabolite concentration at a target site will cause an altered activity or toxicity profile.

Drug metabolism may often result in metabolite(s) with altered chemical structures that change the receptor type affected, drug-receptor affinity, or pharmacological effect. Most parent drugs can be deactivated to inactive metabolites. In contrast, some drugs can also be activated either from an inactive form (pro-drug) to an active drug or from an active form (e.g., meperidine) to an active metabolite (normeperidine) with similar activity/toxicity. Therefore, drug metabolism can either reduce or enhance the parent drug's effect, create another activity, or even elicit toxicity, depending on both the drug and the biological system in question.

Therefore, the pharmacological and pharmacokinetic properties of a drug can be changed by metabolism in one or several of the following ways: pharmacological activation or deactivation, change in disposition kinetics of drug uptake (absorption from application site), distribution, and excretion (e.g., bile excretion, enterohepatic circulation, and renal excretion). For most drugs and toxicants, the liver is the major metabolic organ which, in addition to its role in biliary excretion, makes an understanding of its function central to a knowledge of drug disposition. This chapter will focus on hepatic metabolism and drug hepatobiliary excretion in animal species and introduce some basic biochemical and pharmacokinetic concepts relevant to this role. Although these discussions are focused on the liver, the principles elucidated may also be applicable to extrahepatic sites of drug biotransformation.

PHASE I AND PHASE II REACTIONS

Various metabolic pathways are involved in drug metabolism, including oxidation, reduction, hydrolysis, hydration, and conjunction. These processes can be divided into phase I and phase II reactions (Table 6.1). Some workers have also defined so-called phase III reactions, although this concept has not been well accepted. Phase I includes reactions introducing functional groups to drug molecules necessary for the phase II reactions, which primarily involve conjugation. In other words, phase I products act as substrates for phase II processes, resulting in conjugation with endogenous compounds, which further increases their water solubility and polarity, thus retarding tissue distribution and facilitating drug excretion from the body. The biochemical mechanisms to be presented are also applicable to metabolism in other body sites (e.g., kidney and skin, discussed in earlier chapters). Interested readers should consult standard texts on drug metabolism or biochemical pharmacology/toxicology for specific detailed examples illustrating the chemistry of these processes.

TABLE 6.1.   Drug Metabolism Reactions

Phase I	Phase II
Oxidation	Glucuronidation/glucosidation
-$CytP_{450}$ dependent	Sulfation
-Others	Methylation
Reduction	Acetylation
Hydrolysis	Amino acid conjugation
Hydration	Glutathione conjugation
Dethioacetylation	Fatty acid conjugation
Isomerisation	

In Organic compound

oxidation: increase the number of C-O bonds and/or decreases the number of C-H bonds

reduction: decrease the number of C-O bonds and/or increases the number of C-H bonds

ER= Synthesize new membrane phospholipids, to package proteins into vesicles for transport to other parts of cell, to store calcium ions

6 • *Hepatic Biotransformation and Biliary Excretion* **83**

Our knowledge regarding the molecular mechanisms of drug metabolism has been predominately gained from studies on the liver at different experimental levels, including *in vivo* intact animals, *ex vivo* liver perfusion, and *in vitro* liver slices, hepatocyte cell cultures, isolated/purified subcellular hepatocyte organelles, and isolated enzyme or enzyme components. The later *in vitro* systems are particularly suited for studies with human tissue. Two subcellular organelles are quantitatively the most important: the endoplasmic reticulum (ER) (isolated in the microsome fraction) and the cytosol (isolated in the soluble cell-sap fraction). Phase I oxidation enzymes are almost exclusively localized in the ER, along with the phase II enzyme of glucuronyl transferase. In contrast, other phase II enzymes are mainly present in the cytoplasm. Microsomal fractions of the hepatocyte retain most, if not all, of the enzymatic activity in drug metabolism.

Phase I Metabolism. Phase I metabolism includes four major pathways: oxidation, reduction, hydrolysis, and hydration, of which oxidation is the most important. Some specific phase I reactions with examples are illustrated in Tables 6.2 through 6.4. Special attention will be given to oxidation mediated by the microsomal mixed-function oxidase

TABLE 6.2. Oxidation Reactions Catalyzed by Microsomal Enzymes

Reaction/Enzymes	Example of Substrate
Reaction by MFO Systems	
Alcohol oxidation	Ethanol
Aromatic hydroxylation	Lidocaine
Aliphatic hydroxylation	Pentobarbitone
Dehalogenation	Halothane
N-Dealkylation	Diazepam
O-Dealkylation	Codeine
S-Dealkylation	*S*-Methylthiopurine
Epoxidation	Benzo[*a*]pyrene
Oxidative deamination	Amphetamine
N-Oxidation	3-Methylpyridine, 2-acetylamino-fluorene
S-Oxidation	Chlorpromazine
Phosphothionate oxidation	Parathion
Non-MFO Enzymes	
Alcohol dehydrogenase	Ethanol
Aldehyde dehydrogenase	Acetaldehyde
Alkylhydrazine oxidase	Carbidopa
Amine oxidases	Imipramine
Aromatases	Cyclohexane carboxylic acid CoA
Xanthine oxidase	Theophylline

TABLE 6.3. Hydrolysis Reactions

Substrate	Enzyme
Esters	Plasma: nonspecific acetylcholinesterases, pseudocholinesterases, other esterases
	Liver: specific esterases for particular groups of chemicals
Amides	Liver: amidases
	Plasma: nonspecific esterases
Hydrazides, carbamates	Less common
Peptides, proteins	Enzyme in gut secretions

TABLE 6.4.   Additional Reactions Involved in Drug Metabolism

Reaction	Compound
Hydration	Epoxides (benzo[*a*]pyrene 4,5-epoxide)
Ring cyclisation	Proguanil
N-Carboxylation	Tocainide
Transamidation	Propiram
Isomerisation	α-Methylfluorene-2-acetic acid
Decarboxylation	L-Dopa
Dethioacetylation	Spironolactone

TABLE 6.5.   Phase II Conjugation Reactions

Reaction	Enzyme	Functional group
Glucuronidation	UDP-Glucuronyltransferase	-OH; -COOH; -NH$_2$; -SH
Glycosidation	UPD-Glycosyltransferase	-OH; -COOH; -SH
Sulfation	Sulfotransferase	-NH$_2$; -SO$_2$NH$_2$; -OH
Methylation	Methyltransferase	-OH; -NH$_2$
Acetylation	Acetyltransferase	-NH$_2$; -SO$_2$NH$_2$; -OH
Amino acid conjugation		-COOH
Glutathione conjugation	Glutathione-*S*-transferase	Epoxide, organic halide
Fatty acid conjugation		-OH
Condensation		Various

(MFO) system, for example, cytochrome P$_{450}$ (*CytP*$_{450}$) due to its central role and significance in governing the metabolic disposition of many drugs and xenobiotics. An understanding of this pathway is often critical to making interspecies extrapolations.

The microsomal MFO system responsible for xenobiotic oxidation is present in the ER or microsome fraction of various cell types (especially liver, renal cortex, lung, and intestine). As a general rule, these oxidation reactions require the presence of molecular oxygen (O$_2$), reduced nicotinamide adenine dinucleotide phosphate (*NADPH*), and a complete MFO system (*CytP*$_{450}$, NADPH-*CytP*$_{450}$ reductase, and lipid). The reactions are initiated by insertion of a single oxygen atom into the drug molecule and usually followed by rearrangement and/or decomposition of the product to yield an oxidized metabolite, which may be subject to further metabolism. Compounds undergoing reduction by hepatic microsomes include azo- and nitro-compounds, epoxides, halogenated hydrocarbons, and heterocyclic ring compounds.

Phase II Metabolism.   Phase II conjugating enzymes (Table 6.5) play a very important role in the deactivation of the phase I metabolites of many drugs as well as in direct deactivation of some parent compounds when their specific structure doesn't require phase I modification. For example, the analgesic drug paracetamol can be deactivated directly by phase II reactions using glutathione, glucuronide, and sulfate conjugation mechanisms. Phase II deactivation can be achieved both by gross chemical modification of the drug, thereby decreasing their receptor affinity, and by enhancement of excretion from the body, often via the kidney.

The *CytP*$_{450}$ MFO System.   Among the reactions catalyzed by drug metabolism enzymes in the human hepatic ER, *CytP*$_{450}$-dependent MFO is the most intensively studied. This reaction catalyses the hydroxylation of hundreds of structurally diverse drugs and

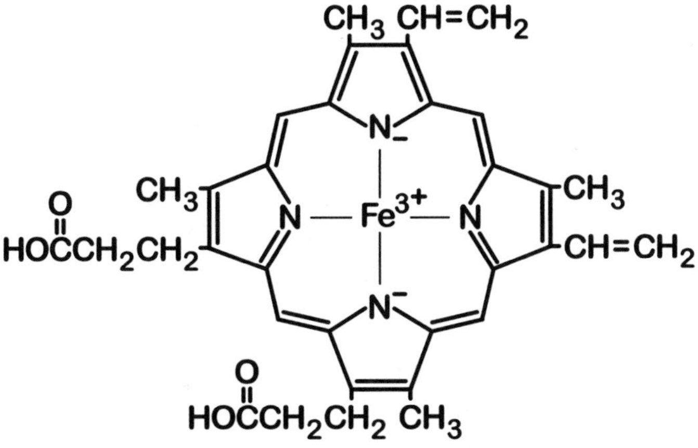

FIGURE 6.1. Structure of ferric protoporphyrin IX, the prosthetic group of *Cyt P$_{450}$*.

compounds, whose only common feature appears to be a relatively high lipophilicity. The MFO reaction conforms to the following stoichiometry:

$$NADPH + H^+ + O_2 + RH \xrightarrow{CytP_{450}} NADP^+ + H_2O + ROH$$

where *RH* represents an oxidizable drug substrate, and *ROH* is the hydroxylated drug metabolite generated as an oxidation product. The overall reaction is catalyzed by the enzyme *CytP$_{450}$*, which also catalyses the *N*-, *O*-, and *S*-dealkylation reactions of many drugs. These heteroatom dealkylation reactions can be considered as a special form of hydroxylation in which the initial event is a carbon hydroxylation (Table 6.2).

Three major components of a complete MFO system have been identified. They are *CytP$_{450}$*, *NADPH-CytP$_{450}$* reductase, and lipid components. *CytP$_{450}$* is the terminal oxidase component of an electron transfer system present in the ER, which is a heme-containing enzyme with iron protoporphyrin IX as the prosthetic group (Figure 6.1). The enzyme consists of a family of closely related isoenzymes embedded in the ER membrane and exists in multiple forms of monomeric molecular weight of 45 to 55 kDa. Its name is based on the fact that the cytochrome is a pigment that exhibits a maximal absorbance wavelength of 450 nm when reduced and complexed with carbon monoxide. The hemoprotein serves as both the oxygen and substrate binding locus for the MFO reaction and, in conjunction with the associated flavoprotein reductase (*NADPH-CytP$_{450}$* reductase), undergoes a cyclic oxidation reduction of the heme iron, which is mandatory for catalytic function of the enzyme.

With the advent of gene cloning and sequencing, and the application of molecular biology techniques to *CytP$_{450}$* structure analysis, tremendous progress was made in the last decade in the isolation and sequencing of the cDNAs encoding multiple forms of the hemoprotein. The rapid determination of full-length *CytP$_{450}$* amino acid sequences enabled the development of a coherent nomenclature system describing about 220 different and unique forms of *CytP$_{450}$*. More details can be found in the related readings.

As mentioned earlier in this chapter, *NADPH-CytP$_{450}$* reductase is another essential component of the MFO system responsible for drug oxidation in that the flavoprotein transfers reducing equivalents from *NADPH + H$^+$* to *CytP$_{450}$* as

$$NADPH + H^+ \rightarrow (FAD - NADPH\text{-}CytP_{450} \text{ reductase} - FMN) \rightarrow CytP_{450}$$

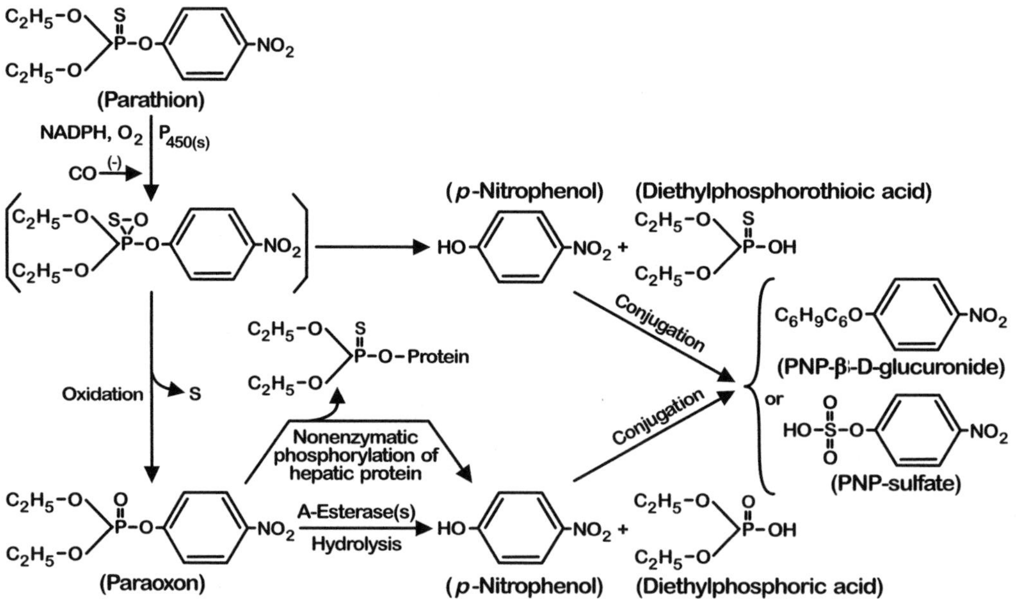

FIGURE 6.2.   Proposed metabolic pathways of parathion in mammals.

$NADPH$-$CytP_{450}$ reductase is a flavin-containing enzyme. This flavoprotein consists of 1 mole of flavin adenine dinucleotide (*FAD*) and 1 mole of flavin mononucleotide (*FMN*) per mole of apoprotein. This is different from other flavoproteins, as usually only one *FAD* or *FMN* can be found as the prosthetic group in the flavoproteins. $NADPH$-$CytP_{450}$ reductase has a monomeric molecular weight of 78 kDa and is closely associated with the $CytP_{450}$ in the ER membrane.

Studies have demonstrated that a heat-stable lipid is essential for MFO activity in drug oxidation. The lipid may function in substrate binding, facilitation of electron transfer, or providing a "template" for the interaction of $CytP_{450}$ and $NADPH$-$CytP_{450}$ reductase.

Impact of Metabolism.   A variety of phase I and phase II reactions can take place simultaneously or sequentially in the body. For example, parathion can be catalyzed by $CytP_{450}$ to an intermediate, which in turn can be either further oxidized to paraoxon or hydrolyzed to *p*-nitrophenol followed by conjugation reactions (Figure 6.2). This complicated metabolic profile has been observed in the pig and will serve as the primary example illustrating a number of topics in this text. As discussed in Chapter 5, a compound metabolized in the liver may be subsequently metabolized in the kidney prior to excretion.

Stereochemistry also plays a major role in drug metabolism since most enzyme systems can be stereoselective. Examples include the enantiomers of amphetamine, cyclophosphamide, pentobarbitone, phenytoin, verapamil, and warfarin.

In summary, phase I metabolism is primarily responsible for drug deactivation, although phase II plays an important role in deactivation of some drugs. Phase I reactions prepare drugs or toxicants for phase II metabolism; i.e., phase I modifies the drug molecule by introducing a chemically reactive group on which the phase II reactions can be carried out for the final deactivation and excretion. Recall in Chapter 2 that generally only lipophilic compounds are capable of crossing biological membranes, including access to drug metabolism enzymes which produce more hydrophilic metabolites. This increased water solubility restricts drug/metabolite distribution to extracellular fluids, thereby enhancing excretion. Since many phase I and phase II reactions can occur on the same drug molecule, there is a possibility of interaction among various metabolic routes in terms of competing reactions for the same substrate (drug, toxicant, or its metabolite). Finally, some species are deficient in phase II conjugation reactions. Cats are poor in their ability to glucuronidate drugs, pigs are deficient in sulfate conjugation, and dogs are relatively poor acetylators.

HEPATIC CLEARANCE

As presented in our discussion on renal excretion (Chapter 5), clearance of a drug by an organ (Cl_{org}) (Chapter 5, equation 5.2) can be ultimately defined as a function of its blood flow (Q_{org}) and its extraction ratio (E_{org}):

$$Cl_{org} = Q_{org} E_{org} \qquad (6.1)$$

The ability of the liver to remove drug from the blood, defined as hepatic clearance, is related to two variables: the intrinsic hepatic clearance (Cl_{int}) and hepatic blood flow rate (Q_h) as defined below:

$$Cl_h = Q_h[Cl_{int} / (Q_h + Cl_{int})] = Q_h E_h \qquad (6.2)$$

where Cl_h is the hepatic clearance, Q_h is the hepatic blood flow, and $Cl_{int} / (Q_h + Cl_{int})$ is the hepatic extraction ratio or E_h. Intrinsic clearance Cl_{int} is conceptualized as the maximal ability of the liver to extract/metabolize drug when hepatic blood flow is not limiting. As indicated in equation 6.2, when $Cl_{int} >> Q_h$, hepatic extraction ratio ≈ 1.0 (*flow-limited or high extraction,* usually seen with $E_h > 0.8$), Cl_h is only dependent on the blood perfusion rate Q_h. In this case, the more blood passing through the liver, the more drug molecules will be extracted by the liver for metabolic elimination. Changes in protein binding will not effect the drug's Cl_h. A hepatic blood perfusion-dependent hepatic clearance will then be seen. In contrast, if $Cl_{int} << Q_h$, the E_h is close to zero, and thus the Cl_h is dependent only on the Cl_{int}; i.e., the liver extracts as many drug molecules as it can from the blood flow presented (*metabolism-limited or low extraction,* usually with $E_h < 0.2$). Protein binding will effect drug clearance in this case. These two extremes occur with propranolol and antipyrine, respectively. Intermediate values of extraction ratio of 0.2 to 0.8 give hepatic clearance rates that can be dependent to varying extents on both hepatic blood perfusion rate and intrinsic clearance. *Therefore, to estimate hepatic drug clearance, one must consider the drug's physicochemical properties, hepatic drug metabolism enzyme activity, and the hepatic blood perfusion rate.* The reader should note the similarity of this discussion to that introduced in Chapter 5 concerning capacity or flow-limited renal tubular secretion. The concepts are identical for both organs; however, they are more often employed when hepatic clearance is modeled.

The intrinsic hepatic clearance has been shown to be related to the following enzymatic and kinetic parameters: maximal velocity of metabolism (V_{max}, nmol min^{-1}g^{-1}), Michaelis-Menten or affinity constant (K_m, μM), and drug concentration (C, μM) following the law of mass action. These concepts will be mathematically developed and fully presented in Chapter 9 (e.g., see Chapter 9, equation 9.4).

In our parathion metabolism modeling studies in swine, we found that parathion can be trapped in the liver as indicated by both a very high liver/blood concentration ratio of 7 and a very high liver/perfusate distribution coefficient of 16 to 20. Therefore, parathion is a high hepatic extraction ratio compound, making its hepatic clearance blood flow limited. In fact, other researchers have found that the perfused liver effectively retains most of the parathion infused into it with little of the oxidation metabolite paraoxon escaping. This indicates that the liver is a very effective sink for both parathion and paraoxon.

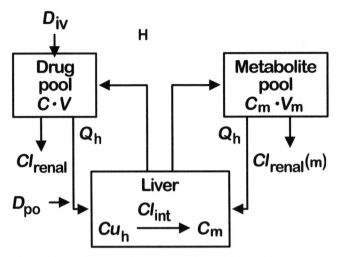

FIGURE 6.3.   A hybrid physiologically based pharmacokinetic model describing hepatic drug metabolism.

In drug metabolism studies, the use of so-called hybrid physiological pharmacokinetic models (see Chapter 10) has gained popularity and received increasing research attention. These models are partially physiological since the organs having metabolic importance are separated out from the other tissues/organs that do not possess significant metabolic capacity for the compound being studied. A hybrid model is illustrated in Figure 6.3, which describes the kinetics of a drug and its metabolite(s) based on their circulating concentrations. Such models apply volume terms to relate circulating drug concentration to the total amount of drug in the system (concepts introduced in Chapter 4, equation 4.5, and Chapter 7, equation 7.14) and use clearance terms to relate the circulating concentration to the elimination processes of drug and metabolites (see Chapter 7, equation 7.17). This model is introduced at this point in order to provide a conceptual framework on which to study hepatic drug metabolism and to introduce the reader to the utility of pharmacokinetic models. Full details of model construction are presented in subsequent chapters.

Within the liver compartment, which is assumed to be the only site in the body possessing considerable metabolic elimination, the unbound drug molecules at a concentration of Cu_h are converted to the metabolite yielding a liver metabolite concentration of C_m according to its intrinsic metabolic clearance (Cl_{int}). The intrinsic clearance of a drug can be further conceptualized as its clearance from liver water. This removal occurs subsequent to dissociation from drug binding sites in the blood, transport into the hepatocyte, and attainment of equilibrium with intracellular binding sites. It is assumed that the final step in this catenating (e.g., sequential) pathway, metabolism, is the rate-limiting process. From an enzymatic viewpoint, the intrinsic clearance of free drug may be regarded as equivalent to the ratio of V_{max} to K_m for the reaction (see Chapter 9 for relevant equations). In this model, as presented in Figure 6.3, the extrahepatic tissues available to the parent drug and metabolite are designated as the drug central pool and metabolite central pool with volume of V and V_m and concentrations of C and C_m, respectively. The compartments are linked by the hepatic blood flow (Q_h) and renal clearances of the drug and metabolite are termed Cl_{renal} and Cl_{renal} (m), respectively. The drug can be administered either intravenously or orally (via portal vein) at a dose of D_{iv} or D_{po}.

The total body clearance of a drug relates the rate of the compound's overall elimination to the blood concentration circulating within the body, as previously defined in Chapter 5, equation 5.1. Therefore, the fraction of the dose metabolized in the liver (f_m) can be used to estimate $Cl_{hepatic}$ from Cl_B as

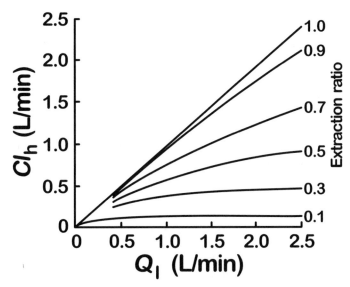

FIGURE 6.4. Relationship between liver blood flow (Q_l) and hepatic clearance (Cl_h) for drugs with different hepatic extraction ratios. Extraction-ratio values are at a blood flow of 1.5 L/min.

$$Cl_{hepatic} = (f_m)\,(CL_B) \tag{6.3}$$

The relationship between hepatic clearance and liver blood perfusion rate for drugs with different extraction ratios can be determined according to equation 6.2 (Figure 6.4) using a logic that parallels the logic of partitioning renal elimination into filtered, absorbed, and secreted components, as presented at the end of Chapter 5. With a lower hepatic extraction drug, the blood perfusion rate is less important to $Cl_{hepatic}$, although for a high hepatic extraction drug, the $Cl_{hepatic}$ is proportional to the blood flow, as discussed earlier.

As two complementary parameters, intrinsic and hepatic clearance can now be used to characterize the rate of elimination of a drug. $Cl_{hepatic}$ is derived from circulating drug blood concentrations, while Cl_{int} reflects the full potential (V_{max} / K_m) of the drug metabolizing or excretory system without any other limitation/restriction and thus has no upper limit of hepatic blood flow.

$$Cl_{int} \approx (liver\ weight)\,(V_{max} / K_m) \qquad zero\ order \tag{6.4}$$
$$Cl_{int} \approx (liver\ weight)\,(V_{max} / K_m + C) \quad first\ order \tag{6.5}$$

Intrinsic clearance may also be expressed in terms of unbound drug fraction (f_u) within the liver (Cl_{int}). Therefore, intrinsic clearance is dependent on neither the drug protein binding nor the rate of hepatic blood perfusion rate, making it an independent measure of hepatocellular "potential" in drug metabolic elimination.

Drug intrinsic clearance can only be assessed directly from blood drug concentration-time data when its hepatic extraction ratio is low (e.g., < 0.3) and its plasma protein binding is low (e.g., < 30%), using equation 6.3. When binding is high but extraction ratio remains low, the relationship can be modified to

$$Cl_{int} = (f_m\ Cl) / f_u \tag{6.6}$$

which clearly shows how these two clearances are related. The most popular model for a drug with medium and high hepatic extraction ratio (e.g., > 0.3) is

$$Cl_{int} = (f_m \, Cl) \, / \, [f_u \, (1 - E_h)] \qquad (6.7)$$

These concepts will be fully developed in subsequent chapters but are presented here only to bridge hepatic physiology to the later development of kinetic models.

Metabolite disposition kinetics can be characterized by analyzing the metabolite concentration-time data generated simultaneously with the parent drug data set. In general, metabolite distribution volume and clearance can be calculated using a similar data processing approach as that used for parent drug. More accurate parameters of metabolite kinetics can be obtained by direct administration of the metabolite to animals. An example of direct administration of metabolite (*p*-nitrophenol) via various dosing routes, to construct and verify its parent (parathion) metabolic disposition model, can be found at the end of Chapter 7.

METABOLISM INDUCTION AND INHIBITION

Drug metabolism is substantially influenced from enzyme induction or inhibition that occurs secondary to the deliberate or passive intake of a number of chemicals that humans and animals are increasingly exposed to in the environment, for medical reasons, or simply as a result of individual lifestyle (smoking, alcohol consumption, etc.). In laboratory animals, contaminants and natural constituents of diet have been shown to affect the pattern of drug metabolism observed. In many cases, the compound itself may alter its own metabolic fate by induction or inhibition.

Induction.   Many currently used drugs, food additives, household chemicals, and environmental contaminants (including pesticides) possessing diverse chemical structure, pharmacology, and toxicology are well known to induce their own metabolism and/or that of other compounds in humans and animals. Some examples are listed in Table 6.6.

In general, there is no structure-activity relationship in the ability of these different inducers to stimulate drug metabolism, and the only common physicochemical property is their lipophilicity. With such a long list of compounds able to alter hepatic metabolism, a great deal of effort has been spent in recent years to understand the mechanisms behind these processes. *This is important from a pharmacokinetic perspective since the intrinsic hepatic clearance of a drug will change if the enzymes responsible for metabolizing it are induced, thereby increasing metabolic capacity.* This is especially important for low-extraction drugs. Similarly, the patterns of phase I and phase II metabolism may be changed if one enzyme component's activity has been modified by inducers. These interactions introduce a significant complexity to pharmacokinetic models, describing the disposition of drugs extensively metabolized by the liver. However, they have also prompted research efforts aimed at elucidating the mechanisms behind these processes which, when understood, should provide a strategy for developing mechanistically meaningful models for simulation of drug metabolic disposition.

Of particular importance to the overall hepatic metabolic clearance of a drug is the activity of the $CytP_{450}$ system. In the mid-1960s, both $CytP_{450}$ and its associated flavoprotein reductase were found to be induced by phenobarbitone pretreatment, which was accompanied by induction of drug metabolism. Induction was generally accompanied by increases in liver microsomal $CytP_{450}$ content. Diverse drug metabolism responses to different inducers, all of which induce hepatic $CytP_{450}$, can be dependent on the substrate of interest (substrate specificity) with stereoselectivity and regioselectivity, suggesting that subpopulations of $CytP_{450}$ (isoenzymes) might be present. This now widely accepted concept has had a profound influence on drug discovery, design of metabolism studies, and the resulting structure of pharmacokinetic models.

TABLE 6.6. Inducers of Drug Metabolism in Humans and Animals

Classification	Example
Drugs	Antipyrine
	Barbiturates
	Carbamazepine
	Chlorimipramine
	Clofibrate
	Griseofulvin
	Helofenate
	Nikethamide
	Phenylbutazone
	Phenytoin
	Pregnenolone-16α-Carbonitrile
	Quinine
	Rifampin
	Spironolactone
	Testosterone
	Triacetyloleandomycin
	Vitamin C
Food additives, nutrients	5,6-Benzoflavone
	Butylated hydroxyanisole/hydroxytoluene
	Ethoxyquin
	Isosafrole
Pesticides	2,3,7,8-Tetrachlorodibenzo-*p*-dioxin (TCDD)
	3,3,4,4-Tetrachlorobiphenyl
	DDT
	Kepone
	Piperonyl butoxide
Contaminants	1-2,Benzanthracene
	Benzo[*a*]pyrene
	Chrysene
	3-Methylcholanthrene
	Phenanthrene
Solvents	Acetone
	Chloroform
	Ethanol
	Toluene
	Xylene

Over 220 individual $CytP_{450}$ isoenzymes have been purified and characterized, although the exact number is not known with certainty and is subject to change as research continues. Different criteria used by different laboratories in defining $CytP_{450}$ heterogeneity, coupled with a lack of standardized techniques in assessing their structure and functional properties, are partially responsible for this large and increasing number of isoenzymes. However, the confusion over the identity of multiple forms of $CytP_{450}$ has been largely clarified by newly accepted gene nomenclature with criteria established to promote a common reference (Table 6.7). One tissue can contain more than one $CytP_{450}$ isoenzyme in a species-dependent way. The human liver contains $CytP_{450}$ isoenzymes similar in terms of structural, functional, and immunological properties to those observed in experimental animals (rats and rabbits). The challenge is to identify which animal species are appropriate for extrapolating to humans (or to one another) as well as to determine how changes in specific isoenzyme activities modify the hepatic clearance of a drug. In many cases, this may be

Catabolism = destructive metabolism involving the release of energy and resulting in the breakdown of complex materials within the organism

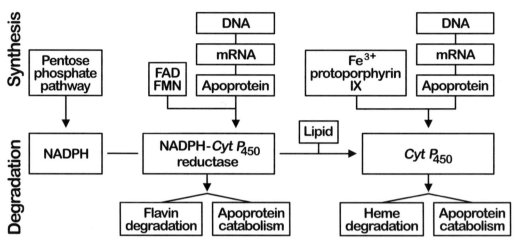

FIGURE 6.5. Synthesis and degradation pathways for components of the hepatic mixed function oxidase (MFO) system.

TABLE 6.7. Assessment of $CytP_{450}$ Heterogeneity in Highly Purified Preparations

Spectral properties of the ferric, ferrous, and carbon monoxyferrous states
Spectral interactions with drug substrates
Monomeric molecular weights, amino acid composition and sequence, peptide fragmentation
  patterns
Substrate specificities in reconstituted enzyme systems
Immunological properties such as lack of antibody cross-reactivity to heterologous $CytP_{450}$
  antigens

TABLE 6.8. Differences in Induction Mechanisms for $CytP_{450}$

P_{450} Isoenzyme	Inducer	Mechanism
1A1	Dioxin	Transcriptional activation by ligand-activated Ah receptor
1A2	3-Methylcholanthrene	mRNA stabilization
2B1/2B2	Phenobarbital	Transcriptional gene activation
2E1	Ethanol, acetone, isoniazid	Protein stabilization (in part)
3A1	Dexamethasone	Transcriptional gene activation
4A6	Clofibrate	Transcriptional activation, mediated by peroxisome proliferator-activated receptor

impossible, and the only solution is to construct pharmacokinetic models capable of using data from experimental studies (*in vitro* and *in vivo*) in one or more species to extrapolate drug disposition in the target species. The liver appears to be a particularly sensitive target organ for the induction of the drug metabolism enzymes in general, and $CytP_{450}$ in particular, whereas the responses of extrahepatic metabolism organs to induction are more variable depending on the inducing agent, drug, organ or tissue, and route of administration.

Induction of metabolism may arise as a consequence of increased synthesis (at different transcriptional/translational levels), decreased degradation, activation of preexisting components, or a combination of these processes (Figure 6.5). Although the precise molecular mechanisms of $CytP_{450}$ induction are not yet fully understood, much research effort (primarily in rats and rabbits) has been expended in trying to rationalize the response

metabolism belong to one of two phases — anabolism & catabolism.
anabolism — complex organic molecules like glucose are assembled
catabolism — living things extract energy from food

Hepatocyte

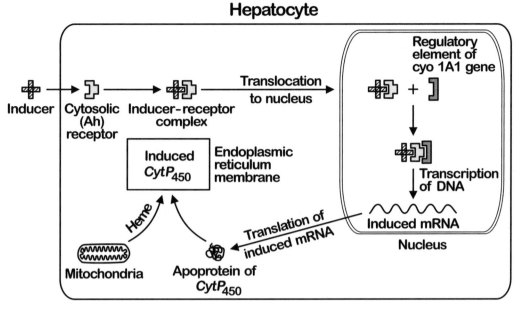

FIGURE 6.6.   Mechanisms of Ah receptor-mediated induction of $CytP_{450}$ by polycyclic aromatic hydrocarbons. (Adapted from Okey AB, 1990, *Pharmacol. Ther.* 45:241-298.)

TABLE 6.9.   Polycyclic Aromatic Hydrocarbon-Related Inducers of $CytP_{450}$

Charcoal-broiled meat
Cigarette smoke
Crude petroleum
Halogenated dibenzo-*p*-dioxins and dibenzofurans
ß-Naphthoflavone and other flavones
Phenothiazines
Plant indoles (e.g., indole-3-acetonitrile, indole-3-carbinol)
Polychlorinated and polybrominated biphenyls
Polycyclic aromatic hydrocarbons (e.g., 3-methoxycholanthrene, benzo[*a*]pyrene, benz[*a*]anthracene, dibenz[*a,h*]anthracene)

of the drug metabolism enzymes to inducers in liver tissue. It has been demonstrated that inducers have a variety of effects on the functional components of the MFO system, particularly on the terminal hemoprotein $CytP_{450}$, as described in Table 6.8. Some examples illustrate this concept.

The major inductive effect of phenobarbitone in rat liver appears to be exerted by increasing specific mRNA levels of CYP2B1 through augmented transcription, rather than stabilizing preexisting levels of protein precursors or increasing translational efficiency. No specific cytoplasmic or nuclear receptor for phenobarbitone has been identified. In contrast, induction by environmental polycyclic aromatic hydrocarbons such as 3MC, benzo[*a*]pyrene, and TCDD (Table 6.9) is recognized to be associated with a specific cytosolic receptor, termed the Ah receptor. The mechanisms are illustrated in Figure 6.6.

The Ah receptor is likely an inducer (e.g., the ligand)-activated transcription factor. The 1A subfamily of the $CytP_{450}$ enzymes is the major induction product for such environmental polycyclic aromatic hydrocarbons. However, ethanol and acetone can induce CYP2E1 by stabilization and inhibition of degradation of the CYP2E1 apoprotein, although multiple mechanisms may be involved depending on the induction stimulus. It is

TABLE 6.10.   Inducers of Non–$CytP_{450}$ Enzymes

Enzyme	Example of Inducers
Epoxide hydrolase	2-Acetylaminofluorene; aldrin; arochlor 1254; dieldrin; isosafrole; 3-methoxycholanthrene; phenobarbitone
Glucuronosyl transferase	Dieldrin; isosafrole; 3-methoxycholanthrene; phenobarbitone; 2,3,7,8-tetrachlorodibenzo-p-dioxin
NADPH-$CytP_{450}$ reductase	2-Acetylaminofluorene; dieldrin; isosafrole; phenobarbitone; polychlorinated biphenyls
Glutathione-S-transferase	2-Acetylaminofluorene; 3-methoxycholanthrene; phenobarbitone; 2,3,7,8-tetrachlorodibenzo-p-dioxin
Cytochrome b_5	2-Acetylaminofluorene; butylated hydroxytoluene; griseofulvin

important to note the potential metabolic changes induced by ethanol and acetone since these two chemicals are often used as administration vehicles in a variety of toxicological and pharmacological studies. The impact of induction on the testing systems and resultant effects may be dramatic when multiple doses are applied in a long-term chronic experiment. Ethanol is also a substance of abuse in humans, making drug activity in alcoholics often significantly different than the normal population.

Non–$CytP_{450}$ enzyme induction may also be relevant to altered drug metabolism. The inducers of the non–$CytP_{450}$ enzyme induction are relatively nonspecific and thus cause a general proliferation of the hepatic endoplasmic reticulum or the enzymes themselves. Enzymes other than $CytP_{450}$ involved in phase I and phase II reactions can be induced by various inducers, as summarized in Table 6.10. This imposes another level of control on the overall metabolic fate of drugs and other relevant chemicals and adds extra complexity to metabolic modeling.

Although much progress has been made in drug metabolism induction studies, a major problem is how to assess the extent of induction of hepatic drug metabolism. The existing methods include assessing increased drug clearance, shortened drug plasma half-life, increased plasma-glutamyl transferase, increased urinary excretion of D-glucaric acid, increased urinary 6ß-hydroxycortisol, and increased plasma bilirubin levels. These measurements can collectively provide a reasonable indication of induction of drug metabolism in humans, although none of them can unequivocally substantiate such induction. Induction of specific liver enzymes (particularly the MFO system) may play a substantial role and have profound implications in clinical pharmacology. Inducers that modify drug metabolism, which would have the greatest effect on low-extraction drugs, would be expected to alter drug effects. A good example of this phenomenon is the impact of phenobarbitone or benzo[a]pyrene pretreatment in rats on the metabolism and duration of action of the subsequently administered muscle relaxants (e.g., zoxazolamine).

Metabolism Inhibition.   Similar to the induction of metabolism, inhibition is a well-recognized phenomenon secondary to serial drug dosing, coadministration of drugs, endogenous compounds, environmental xenobiotics, and complex multiple-ingredient drug formulations. Several mechanisms for metabolism inhibition have been noted, including the destruction of preexisting enzymes[by porphyrinogic drugs and xenobiotics containing olefinic (C=C) and acetylenic (C≡C) functions], inhibition of enzyme synthesis (by metal ions), or complexing with the hemoprotein, thereby inactivating enzymes (Table 6.11).

Compounds such as porphyrinogic drugs and xenobiotics can modify or destroy the heme component of $CytP_{450}$ to generate alkylated or substrate-heme adducts. This results in a significant and sustained drop in the level of functional $CytP_{450}$ and a concomitant

TABLE 6.11.   Mechanisms of Metabolism Inhibitors

Modify/destroy preexisting $CytP_{450}$:
  Acetylene, allobarbital, allylisopropylacetamide, aprobarbital, ethylene, norethindrone,
  secobarbital, vinyl chloride
Modulate synthesis and degradation of $CytP_{450}$ heme prosthetic group:
  Cobalt
Complexation with $CytP_{450}$:
  Amphetamine, cimetidine, diphenyhydramine, isosafrole, methadone, oleandomycin, piperonyl
  butoxide, safrole, sesamol sulfanilamide, triacetyloleandomycin

reduction in the metabolic capacity of the liver. Metabolism inhibition by these compounds depends not only on the structure of the drug itself, but also on the prevailing complement of $CytP_{450}$ isoenzymes and their substrate specificity. Many drug-drug interactions may be explained at the level of $CytP_{450}$ destruction, although interactions may also occur at other pharmacokinetic (absorption, distribution, and elimination, see Chapters 3, 4, and 5) and even pharmacodynamic levels (see Chapter 12). In contrast to the porphyrinogic drugs described above, which act primarily by modifying existing $CytP_{450}$-heme, metal ions such as cobalt exert their inhibitory effects by modulating both the synthesis and degradation of the heme prosthetic group of $CytP_{450}$ enzymes.

Formation of inactive $CytP_{450}$-inhibitor complex is another mechanism for drug metabolism inhibition. Inhibitors are usually substrates of $CytP_{450}$ and require metabolic conversion to exert their full inhibitory effects, in a manner similar to porphyrinogic drugs and xenobiotics. However, inhibitors forming complexes with hemoprotein are metabolized by $CytP_{450}$. These inhibitors can form metabolic intermediates or products that tightly bind to the hemoprotein, thereby preventing its further participation in drug metabolism.

BILIARY DRUG ELIMINATION

As an exocrine function of the liver, bile excretion is thought to be present in almost all vertebrates. The three basic physiological functions of the bile are (1) to serve as the excretory route for products of biotransformation; (2) to facilitate the intestinal absorption of ingested lipids such as fatty acids, cholesterol, lecithin, and/or monoglycerides due to the surfactant properties of bile forming mixed micelles (see Chapter 3); and (3) to serve as a major route for cholesterol elimination in order to maintain normal plasma cholesterol levels. In addition to its physiological functions, bile is also pharmacologically and toxicologically important since some heavy metals and enzymes are also excreted via the biliary system. Bile secretion is very important to chemical/drug transport and elimination under both physiological and pathological conditions. However, bile secretion has proven difficult to study, mainly due to the inaccessibility of the biliary tree for direct sampling.

The Mechanism of Bile Formation.   Bile is continuously produced by liver cells and then stored in the gall bladder, except for those species (rat, horse) lacking it. The pH level of bile ranges from 5.0 to 7.5 depending mainly on the animal species. Biliary excretion is a major route for some drugs with a molecular weight greater than 300 and a high degree of polarity. This occurs by active transport of drug and metabolites into bile; thus saturation and competition are important issues to consider. Passive diffusion of drug into bile is insignificant. Most of the compounds secreted into bile are finally excreted from the body in feces, where they may be subject to enterohepatic circulation and degradation by intestinal microflora.

Bile is formed at two sites: the ramifications of the bile duct within the portal triads and the anastomosing network of the narrow bile canaliculi in the hepatic parenchyma. The bile canaliculi are the primary secretory units of the liver. These small channels or furrows are lined by the apical membranes of the hepatocytes and thus do not have their own epithelium or basement membrane. Because hepatocytes form a canalicular lumen wherever they abut, most canaliculi communicate with each other, forming an anastomosing network. Similar to the relationship of the nephron to the kidney, the volume and composition of canalicular bile are often determined by the activity of several cords of hepatocytes.

The overall bile flow is in the opposite direction to sinusoidal blood flow, and thus solute transfer from plasma to bile involves a counterflow process (Figure 6.7). Such a blood-bile flow pattern reduces rediffusion of biliary solutes such as drugs and metabolites back into sinusoidal plasma in the portal area, which is richer in solute concentration, bathes periportal hepatocytes, and is exposed to higher canalicular concentration than any given solute (Figure 6.7). In human liver, the canalicular space accounts for 0.4% of the liver volume and has a surface area greater than 70 cm^2 per gram of tissue. Lysosomes are involved in degradation and biliary excretion of proteins. Both nutritional and metabolic changes can significantly affect this process. An intact microtubular network is essential for vesicular movement of receptor-mediated transcytosis and for biliary translocation of bile acids and other lipids. Microfilaments might serve as pump or pressure valves to control the ejection of the hepatocellular secretion into the biliary space. Three routes of fluid and drug transfer from the sinusoid to the bile canaliculus have been postulated and are shown in Figure 6.8.

Transcellular Pathway (A).   Conventionally, it was assumed that water and solutes enter (secretion) and leave (absorption) the lumen by traversing the plasma membranes of the epithelial cell (basolateral and apical regions) and the cytoplasm. Diffusive and osmotic water flow, including dissolved solutes, are recognized to enter the canalicular lumen through the lipid bilayer and/or the so-called water channels located at the protein core (polar route) of the hepatocyte plasma membrane.

Paracellular Pathway (B).   This pathway is anatomically delineated by the structures forming the tight junctions between hepatocytes and the intercellular space. Many polar nonelectrolytes (e.g., sucrose, inulin, and polyethylene glycols) can be significantly excreted in bile although they are too large to readily pass through the hepatocyte plasma membrane. Their pathway is visualized by tracing of the movement of ionic lanthanum via the paracellular shunt route without crossing the liver cell cytoplasm. In addition, the kinetics of biliary entry of liquid makers are consistent with two patterns of plasma-to-bile transfer: a long journey through the hepatocyte plasma membranes and cytoplasm (transcellular) and a relatively shorter transfer process consistent with the paracellular pathway. Therefore, the transjunctional movement of fluid between liver cells may not simply be a leak secondary to the inability of the hepatocyte tight junction to seal off the canalicular space, but instead may play an essential role in the plasma-hepatobiliary transport of fluid and drugs.

Transcytotic (Vesicular) Pathway (C).   Water and dissolved solutes are internalized within the hepatocyte cytoplasm through acidic vesicles, most of which can return to the plasma. However, others may move either into storage compartments or into the canalicular lumen. Labeled inulin studies have shown that at least 2 to 8% of the bile in the rat can originate from this mechanism, although this fraction may vary with different experimental methods. This is similar to the pinocytotic pathway in renal tubules illustrated in Figure 5.5 (see Chapter 5).

cyt- cell

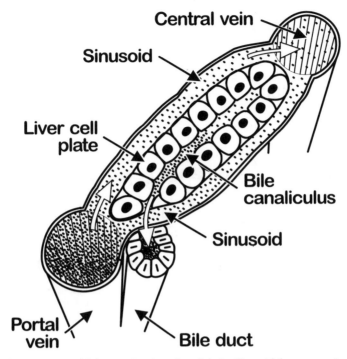

FIGURE 6.7. Gradient concept of bile secretion in a liver lobule. Sinusoidal concentration of a solute (e.g., drug, metabolite, or endogenous compound) is represented by dots that progressively decrease as blood flows from the portal to central vein. Consequently, solute concentration in the bile canaliculus increases as it courses toward the bile duct.

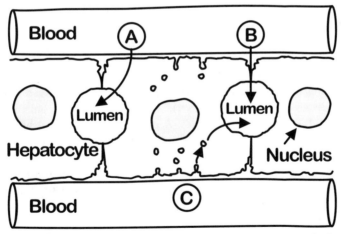

FIGURE 6.8. Three transport pathways from sinusoidal to canalicular lumen are involved in biliary excretion: A, transcellular; B, transjunctional shunt; and C, transcytotic.

Bile Acid Secretion. It has been recognized that the primary driving force for bile formation is the hepatobiliary transport of the osmotically active bile acids. Theoretically, bile acids transported across the hepatocyte allow for formation of a local osmotic gradient, which transports water by osmosis and permeable solutes by convection and/or electrochemical diffusion. This process has been traditionally referred to as *bile acid-dependent bile secretion*. Bile acid-dependent bile flow is a function of bile acid secretion

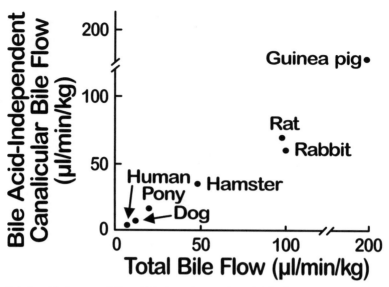

FIGURE 6.9.   Relationship between bile acid-independent and total bile flow in various species (µl/min/kg). Linearity of the relationship suggests that bile acid-independent canalicular bile flow is a constant fraction of the total bile formation over a wide range of different species.

and is regulated by both the physicochemical properties of the secreted bile acids and the factors affecting the kinetics of bile acid enterohepatic circulation. Bile acid transport mechanisms have been determined to be very efficient and specific at both the sinusoidal and canalicular poles of the hepatocyte plasma membrane. Therefore, the pool size and intestinal reabsorption efficiency are the major determinants of bile acid entry into bile. Bile acids are the most abundant anions in bile, and a direct relationship between the excretion of bile acids in bile and canalicular secretory activity has been identified in all vertebrate species studied. Alternative mechanisms have also been proposed, including an interaction of bile acids with other solute pumps, possibly a bicarbonate transport mechanism, and/or the involvement of a vesicular transport process.

Evidence for *bile acid-independent canalicular secretion* has evolved mainly from studies of bile acid-induced choleresis (bile flow), which have proved that bile flow is mathematically related to bile acid excretion rate. A positive intercept can be observed in most cases when plotting the rate of bile formation against bile acid secretion, suggesting that a fraction of bile is secreted in the absence of bile acid excretion. The importance of such bile acid-independent canalicular secretion in overall bile formation rate is animal species-dependent. More detailed signal transduction mechanisms regulating this phenomenon have been postulated at the cellular level. The bile flow stimulating effect of certain prostaglandins supports involvement of cyclic adenosine monophosphate (cAMP) in the bile acid-independent mechanism. Active secretion of bicarbonate, chloride, and/or glutathione may provide the osmotic driving force for bile secretion. Na^+-K^+-ATPase and Na^+/H^+ exchange have also been identified in hepatocytes and other preparations. Therefore, secretion of bile acid-independent canalicular bile flow is at least regulated by the cAMP cascade and also requires an intact microtubular system. Figure 6.9 illustrates the comparison of bile acid-independent and total bile flow in select species.

In summary, bile formation involves an osmotic process whereby water and dissolved solutes (drug, metabolites, xenobiotics, and physiological molecules) move from sinusoidal blood into the bile canaliculus. The only well-documented driving force for this vectorial movement of fluid is the translocation of bile acids. The reader should note the parallels with renal secretion, where sodium assumes this primary role. However, another process is also involved since significant bile secretion can occur independent of bile acid secretion. Therefore, any factor or process that affects bile acid secretion, reabsorption from the intestine, or the cAMP system can potentially alter bile formation rate and thus biliary drug excretion. If the drug being modeled in a pharmacokinetic study is excreted in the bile and can influence the rate of bile formation, this change may be reflected in the value of its pharmacokinetic parameters.

Factors Influencing Biliary Drug Elimination and Enterohepatic Recycling. Uptake and elimination kinetics of various model compounds (anions, cations, neutral steroids, and metals) in isolated perfused liver and genetically altered animal models have been used to elucidate mechanisms underlying hepatobiliary drug transport. The four major processes governing hepatic drug elimination are (1) hepatocyte uptake from blood, (2) metabolism in hepatocytes, (3) hepatobiliary excretion, and (4) intestinal reabsorption resulting in enterohepatic recirculation. Drug molecules have to be transported to hepatocytes before they can be secreted into the bile. For most drugs (except polar ones), uptake into hepatocytes across the basolateral membrane efficiently occurs via passive diffusion, with minimal reliance on carrier-mediated transport systems. In contrast, Na^+-dependent hepatic uptake of alanine and bile acids as well as Na^+-independent hepatic uptake of bilirubin and tetrabromosulfophthalein are carrier-mediated processes. The reader again should recall the similarity of this process with that described in Chapter 5 for renal tubular transport. Once inside the hepatocyte, most drugs are first metabolized and subsequently translocated back across the sinusoidal membrane into blood or delivered to the canalicular membrane for transport into the bile for fecal excretion and potential reabsorption.

Drug uptake into hepatocytes by passive diffusion is so efficient that it is rate-limited by the delivery of the drug to the liver (i.e., blood flow) rather than membrane transport per se, thereby exhibiting flow-dependent clearance. However, for highly polar molecules, passive diffusion is not an efficient mode of hepatocellular uptake, and there is an increased reliance on carrier-mediated transport systems. Drug metabolites, particularly conjugated metabolites (e.g., sulfates and glucuronides), are invariably more polar than their precursors and thus are more likely to experience hepatocyte membranes as diffusional barriers. With such a barrier, the hepatocellular export of a locally formed metabolite will depend on the presence and activity of carrier-mediated transport systems for sinusoidal efflux and biliary excretion. Transport systems of current interest (introduced in Chapter 4) include the p-glycoproteins, which are responsible for the biliary excretion of a range of organic cations, and the canalicular multispecific organic anion transporter. Intracellular trapping of metabolites formed in the liver, secondary to low membrane permeability, is clinically important as many are potentially hepatotoxic and/or capable of interfering with the hepatic transport of endogenous compounds or other drugs and metabolites. Again, this phenomenon is conceptually similar to renal tubular sequestration and has similar pharmacokinetic implications. Finally, if the metabolite is unstable, intracellular accumulation can lead to the regeneration of the precursor and so-called futile cycling within hepatocytes.

Biliary Drug Transport. Some parent drugs and numerous drug metabolites derived from hepatic metabolism are excreted in the bile into the intestinal tract. The excreted metabolites can be excreted via feces although, more commonly, they are subject to reabsorption into the blood and are eventually excreted from the body via urine. There are at least three different biliary transport pathways for organic anions, cations, and neutral compounds, although metals may also have their own transport carriers or systems. Both *organic anions* and *organic cations* can be actively transported into bile by carrier systems—again, similar to those involved in the renal tubule (see Chapter 5). Such transport systems are nonselective, and ions with similar electrical charge may compete for the same transport mechanisms. Additionally, a third carrier system, whose activity is sex-dependent, may be involved in the active transport of *steroids* and *related compounds* into bile. In contrast to renal excretion, amphipathic drugs (those having both polar and nonpolar properties) are preferentially excreted in the bile. *The drug (or metabolite) excreted into the small intestine can be reabsorbed into blood, forming the so-called drug enterohepatic cycle.* This is an important factor changing the blood:liver or liver:bile drug concentration ratios during studies of the hepatobiliary transport mechanisms and hepatic drug elimination.

The hepatobiliary excretion mechanism for bile acids has been extensively studied and expands upon concepts originally presented for renal tubular secretion. The hepatocyte is a transporting epithelial cell oriented to transfer molecules from the basolateral to the canalicular space. Basolateral localization of Na^+-K^+-ATPase creates the ion gradients essential for the other transport systems and establishes the functional polarity of the cell, much as was seen in the renal tubule cell depicted in Figure 5.4 (see Chapter 5). Bile acids such as sodium taurocholate are cotransported into hepatocytes and sinusoidal plasma membrane vesicles principally by a Na^+-dependent process. After hepatic uptake, bile acids cross the hepatocyte cytoplasm by facilitated transport systems. Conjugation of bile acids may occur and become rate-limiting.

The biliary excretion of *weak acids* is the most important mechanism in hepatic drug elimination. Bromsulfophthalein (BSP) and analogues are dyes used as diagnostic probes of liver function and model substances in studies of the hepatic uptake of organic anions. These studies suggested that hepatic anion excretion may be the main driving force for the so-called bile salt-independent bile flow (see earlier discussion in this chapter). Antibiotics such as ciprofloxacin can be actively excreted into bile in the presence of a biliary tract obstruction. Penicillin G is predominantly excreted via renal tubular secretion for organic anions (as discussed in Chapter 5) although some can be eliminated through biliary excretion and other routes. Tetracyclines, mainly excreted into urine via glomerular filtration, are also concentrated in the liver, accordingly excreted into the small intestine via the bile, and then partially reabsorbed. This reabsorbed fraction may be tetracycline type-dependent as well as affected by the concurrent ingestion or presence of other drugs, such as metal-containing formulations (aluminum, calcium, magnesium, iron, zinc), as presented in Chapter 3. This process depends on the degree of chelation of the divalent and trivalent cations with the weak acid drugs.

Glucuronides of endogenous compounds and xenobiotics, including drugs, can be actively transported from hepatocytes into bile via transport systems similar to those for organic anions. Glucuronide conjugates are very important in hepatic drug metabolism and biliary excretion. The effectiveness of biliary excretion for glucuronide conjugates can be greatly limited by enzymatic hydrolysis after the bile is mixed with the small intestine contents, thereby releasing the parent drugs to be reabsorbed and enter the enterohepatic cycle. The reabsorbed drugs and metabolites can be ultimately excreted in urine. Some drug metabolites further undergo either biotransformation in the liver or other organs or are subjected to microbiological and physicochemical degradation in the small intestine before being excreted in the feces.

Weak bases can be actively transported into bile via carrier systems similar to the renal transport processes (Chapter 5). Atropine, isoproterenol, and curare are eliminated by this mechanism, with atropine being almost equally excreted by the kidney (unchanged form) and hepatic metabolism, followed by biliary excretion. Organic cation transport is not as important as the organic anion pathway.

Neutral compounds may employ the third transport systems. Ouabain, a cardiac glycoside, is used as a model uncharged and nonmetabolized (by rat liver) compound in hepato-

TABLE 6.12. Mean Bile Flow in Selected Species

Species	Bile Flow (ml/min/kg body weight)
Cat	11
Chicken	20
Dog	4–10
Guinea pig	200
Hamster	50
Human	5–7
Monkey	10
Mouse	78
Opossum	20
Pig	9
Pony	19
Rabbit	90
Rat	50–80
Sheep	43

biliary transport studies. Organic anions and neutral steroids such as ouabain may share common mechanisms in their excretory pathways. Ouabain can be transported from blood into bile against its concentration gradient (greater than 100-fold) across both sinusoidal and canalicular membranes, suggesting active excretion processes. However, alternative nonanionic pathways may also exist, as demonstrated when the severe organic anion excretion defect in a mutant rat model was only partially expressed when ouabain was used as the probe of hepatobiliary excretion, suggesting a more complex transport process.

Inorganic metals such as lead may be transported by different mechanisms from blood into bile. Again, such processes are not as important as those for weak acid drugs, as described above. However, due to the environmental importance of lead and its adverse effects, much research has been directed to this metal toxicant.

Molecular weight is another key determinant of the extent to which drug/metabolite molecules are transported into bile. The molecular weight cutoff required for biliary excretion is much greater than that for renal tubular secretion. The threshold (in daltons) is: 325 ± 50 for rats, 400 ± 50 for guinea pigs, and 475 ± 50 for rabbits. If the molecular weight is lower (e.g., < 325 to 475 Da), the compound may be preferentially excreted in urine (see Chapter 5). Molecules with weights from 325 to 850 Da may be eliminated via both the renal and biliary routes. Excretion of molecules larger than 850 Da occurs mainly via the biliary active transport system. However, molecular weight is not the sole factor determining the route of drug excretion. Physicochemical properties of the drug (polarity/lipophilicity, structure) are also very critical to the extent of biliary excretion of a drug/metabolite, with amphipathic drugs being well secreted by the biliary route.

The specific animal species being studied is also an important factor, as can be appreciated from the differences in thresholds discussed above. Table 6.12 lists species differences in bile flow rate, which may explain some of this variation. Bile composition (acids, ions, electrolytes) also varies between species and may further explain species differences in drug biliary excretion rate and thus differences in pharmacokinetic disposition.

IN VITRO–IN VIVO CORRELATION

A good correlation between *in vivo* drug clearance and *in vitro* hepatic metabolism should occur if the drug is predominately eliminated via hepatic metabolism. The following properties of a drug are essential for an *in vivo–in vitro* correlation: (1) complete systemic absorption, (2) negligible extrahepatic metabolism, (3) first-order elimination, and (4) rapid urinary excretion of metabolite(s) without further biotransformation. Several model drugs for this have been identified in humans, including antipyrine, debrisoquine, and sparteine. Unfortunately, many other drugs do not have good *in vivo–in vitro* correlation. Therefore, *in vivo* clearance may or may not be correlated well to *in vitro* hepatic metabolism data depending upon both the drug in question and the animal species used.

PHARMACOLOGICAL AND TOXICOLOGICAL SIGNIFICANCE

Any factor affecting drug concentration at its target site can potentially alter the intensity and duration of drug action. As discussed in this chapter, drugs or xenobiotics are subject to pharmacological/toxicological activation and deactivation via the double-edged sword of biotransformation. In addition, numerous enzymes capable of metabolizing drugs have overlapping substrate specificities and can also metabolize endogenous compounds. This results in a sex-dependency in disposition of certain drugs since endogenous hormones are also metabolized by these enzyme systems. Hepatic drug metabolism also demonstrates stereoselectivity. There is a high likelihood of competition among and between drugs and endogenous substances for the same enzyme or among enzymes for the same compound. The same phenomenon was observed with renal secretion (this, and how kidney disease exacerbates these effects, will be further discussed in Chapter 15). These interactions may have profound pharmacological and toxicological consequences and are the reason many such drugs display complex pharmacokinetic profiles.

Most drugs can be deactivated by various phase I reactions, including deamination (amphetamine), side-chain hydroxylation (phenobarbitone), *N*-dealkylation (methadone), *S*-oxidation (chlorpromazine), ester hydrolysis (meperidine), and/or amide hydrolysis (procainamide). Phase II reactions generally produce pharmacologically less active metabolite(s) compared to the parent drug or to the phase I metabolite. For example, the analgesic drug paracetamol can be inactivated directly by phase II reactions such as glutathione, glucuronide, and sulfate conjugation, as illustrated in Figure 6.10.

Phase I reaction-mediated pharmacological activation, on the other hand, is the basis for pro-drug design in targeted drug delivery. For example, the pro-drug levodopa crosses the blood-brain barrier to become trapped by the neuron, where it is metabolically activated to dopamine, which exerts the pharmacological activity on the neuron as its target site. Dopamine can not be effectively delivered to its target neuronal site because it can not cross the blood-brain barrier. Obviously, there are great advantages in such pro-drug development in terms of effective drug delivery and maximal therapeutic benefits. Thus pro-drugs require metabolic activation before they can exert their pharmacological action. Another classic example identified in the 1930s is the dye Prontosil, which must be activated to liberate the pharmacologically active antibacterial agent, sulfanilamide, via the azoreduction pathway depicted in Figure 6.11. Therefore, metabolic activation can overcome difficulties encountered in drug transport from the site of administration to the target site as well as reduce the chance of site-specific biodegradation and toxicity during drug absorption and distribution.

An even more complex pairing of metabolic activation and deactivation exists with the model organophosphate pesticide, parathion. If the products of such metabolic reactions modify other disposition processes of parent parathion or its metabolites, the effect on biotransformation can be even greater. As demonstrated in our laboratory, parathion can be toxicologically activated as well as deactivated through phase I metabolism. Parathion can be activated to paraoxon (the bioactive anticholinesterase moiety) by desulfuration oxidation and deactivated to *p*-nitrophenol either directly from parathion or indirectly by hydrolysis of paraoxon by A-esterases (Figure 6.2). Phase II conjugation reactions of

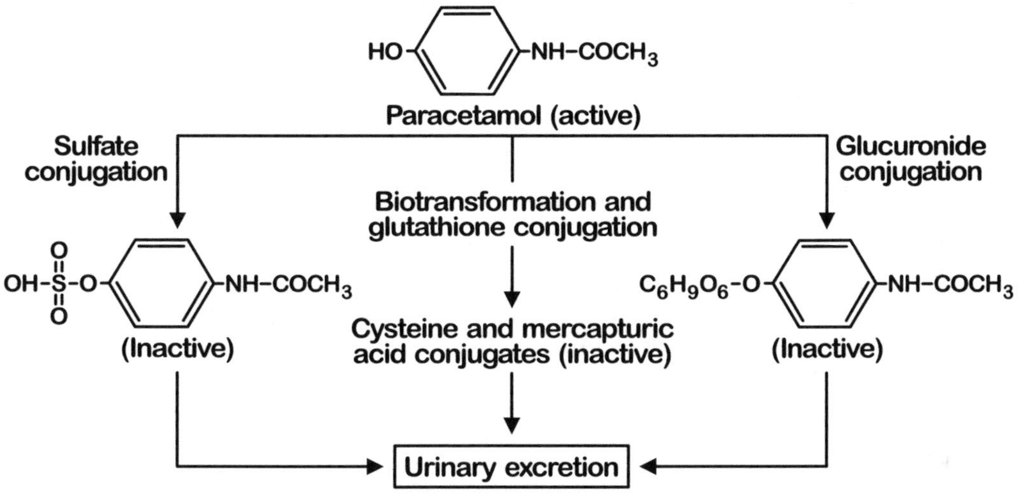

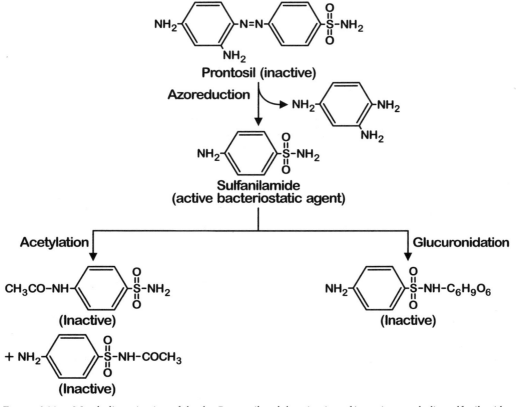

FIGURE 6.10. Direct pharmacological deactivation of paracetamol by phase II reactions.

FIGURE 6.11. Metabolic activation of the dye Prontosil and deactivation of its active metabolite sulfanilamide.

p-nitrophenol with glucuronide and sulfate can increase p-nitrophenol water solubility for a more rapid urinary excretion. *In vitro* parathion metabolism studies suggest that oxidation catalyzed by $CytP_{450}$ is the first and necessary metabolic step, with about 65% of the parathion conversion into paraoxon being contributed by the liver.

CONCLUSION

This chapter presents an overview of some essential principles regarding the classification, cellular and molecular mechanisms, and modifying factors involved in drug metabolism. Induction and inhibition of drug metabolism and mechanisms of biliary excretion are important components of interspecies extrapolations. The remaining chapters of this text will focus on the pharmacokinetic strategies needed to quantitate the processes presented in this review. Based on the heterogeneity of hepatic metabolism and biliary secretory processes, and the fact that drugs are often excreted by both renal and hepatic mechanisms, both of which may be characterized by linear and nonlinear processes, it is not surprising that drugs eliminated by these mechanisms often require the most complex pharmacokinetic models. In order to fully characterize and predict drug and xenobiotic effects, models must therefore be developed and parameters such as clearance subsequently estimated. This is the goal of conducting pharmacokinetic studies.

The concept of high- and low-extraction drugs applied to hepatic clearance is central to a complete understanding of drug disposition. The primary factors that may influence hepatic clearance are blood flow, extent of plasma protein binding, and the inherent capacity of the liver to metabolize drug, which is reflected by Cl_{int}. When metabolic capacity is low (low Cl_{int}), the drug is defined as being a low-extraction drug, and its clearance will be dependent upon the extent of protein binding. In the example of protein-binding displacement in Chapter 4, a sixfold increase in the free fraction of drug could increase hepatic metabolism by a similar amount. A low-extraction drug's clearance will be independent of hepatic blood flow. Low-extraction drugs generally have inadequate quantities of enzyme, poor biliary transport, or poor diffusion of the drug to the site of metabolism (see Figure 6.3). The disposition of these drugs is also susceptible to enzyme induction (which would increase Cl_{int}) and further enzyme inhibition.

In contrast, if Cl_{int} is high, the drug is considered to be a high-extraction compound, and its clearance is now limited to how much drug can be delivered to the organ, hence its hepatic blood flow. Changes in protein binding will not effect its clearance. For these drugs, enzyme induction will have little effect; however, enzyme inhibition may decrease Cl_{int} sufficiently to decrease the extraction ratio to the range of a moderate- to low-extraction drug. Table 6.13 lists drugs according to extraction ratios, and for comparison, also lists drugs in a similar classification that are cleared by the kidney.

The reader is encouraged to refer back to these introductory chapters to review the physiological basis of the pharmacokinetic models to be presented.

TABLE 6.13.   Classification of Drugs Based on Extraction Ratios

	Low	Intermediate	High
Liver	Diazepam	Aspirin	Isoproterenol
	Digitoxin	Codeine	Lidocaine
	Phenobarbital	Quinidine	Meperidine
	Phenylbutazone		
	Procainamide		
	Theophylline		
Kidney	Digoxin	Procainamide	Most glucuronides
	Furosemide	Penicillins	Penicillins
	Aminoglycosides	4° Ammoniums	Sulfates
	Tetracyclines		

SELECTED READINGS

Ballatori, N. 1991. Mechanisms of metal transport across liver cell plasma membranes. *Drug Metabolism Reviews.* 23:83-132.

Calabrese, E.J. 1991. *Principles of Animal Extrapolation.* Chelsea, MI: Lewis Publishers.

Caldwell, J., S.M. Winter, and A.J. Hutt. 1988. The pharmacological and toxicological significance of the stereochemistry of drug disposition. *Xenobiotica.* 18(Supplement 1):59-70.

D'Argenio, D.Z. 1995. *Advanced Methods of Pharmacokinetic and Pharmacodynamic Systems Analysis.* New York: Plenum Press.

Dutczak, W.J., T.W. Clarkson, and N. Ballatori. 1991. Biliary-hepatic recycling of a xenobiotic. *American Journal of Physiology.* 260:G873-G880.

Farrell, G.C. 1994. *Drug-Induced Liver Disease.* Edinburgh: Churchill-Livingstone.

Gibson, G.G., and P. Skett. 1994. *Introduction to Drug Metabolism,* 2ed. New York: Blackie A&P.

Halpert, J.R., F.P. Guengerich, J.R. Bend, and M.A. Correia. 1994. Contemporary issues in toxicology: Selective inhibitors of cytochrome P450. *Toxicology Applied Pharmacology.* 125:163-175.

Hawkins, D.R. 1988. *Biotransformations.* London: Royal Society of Chemistry.

Hodgson, E., and P.E. Levi. 1994. *Introduction to Biochemical Toxicology.* Norwalk, CT: Appleton and Lange.

Illing, H.P.A. 1989. *Xenobiotic Metabolism and Disposition.* Boca Raton, FL: CRC Press.

Jakoby, W.B., J.R. Bend, and J. Caldwell. 1982. *Metabolic Basis of Detoxification: Metabolism of Functional Groups.* New York: Academic Press.

Jenner, P., and B. Testa. 1981. *Concepts in Drug Metabolism.* New York: Marcel Dekker.

Kalow, W. 1992. *Pharmacogenetics of Drug Metabolism.* New York: Pergamon Press.

Klaasen, C.D. 1996. *Casarett and Doull's Toxicology: The Basic Science of Poisons,* 5ed. New York: McGraw-Hill.

Klassen, C.D., and J.B. Watkins. 1984. Mechanisms of bile formation, hepatobiliary uptake, and biliary excretion. *Pharmacology Review.* 36:1-67.

Meeks, R.G., S.D. Harrison, and R.J. Bull. 1991. *Hepatotoxicology.* Boca Raton, FL: CRC Press.

Okey, A.B. 1990. Enzyme induction in the cytochrome P450 system. *Pharmacology and Therapeutics.* 45:241-298.

Pang, K.S., and M. Rowland. 1977. Hepatic clearance of drugs. *Journal of Pharmacokinetics and Biopharmaceutics.* 5:625-653.

Qiao, G.L., and J.E. Riviere. 1995. Significant effects of application site and occlusion on the pattern of cutaneous penetration and biotransformation of parathion *in vivo* in swine. *Journal of Pharmaceutical Science.* 84:425-432.

Qiao, G.L., P.L. Williams, and J.E. Riviere. 1994. Percutaneous absorption, biotransformation and systemic disposition of parathion in vivo in swine. I. Comprehensive pharmacokinetic model. *Drug Metabolism and Disposition.* 22:459-471.

Tavoloni, N., and P.P. Berk. 1993. *Hepatic Transport and Bile Secretion: Physiology and Pathophysiology.* New York: Raven Press.

Vogelgesang, B.H., H. Echizen, E. Schmidt, and M. Eichelbaum. 1984. Stereoselective first-pass metabolism of highly cleared drugs: Studies on the bioavailability of L and D-verapamil examined with a stable isotope technique. *British Journal of Clinical Pharmacology.* 18:733-740, 1984.

Wainer, I.W., and D.E. Drayer. 1988. *Drug Stereochemistry: Analytical Methods and Pharmacology.* New York: Marcel Dekker.

Waterman, M.R., and E.F. Johnson. 1991. *Cytochrome P450. Methods in Enzymology, Volume 206.* New York: Academic Press.

Waxman, D.J., and L. Azaroff. 1992. Phenobarbital induction of cytochrome P450 gene expression. *Biochemistry Journal.* 281:577-592.

Wilkinson, G.R., and M.D. Rawlins. 1985. *Drug Metabolism and Disposition: Considerations in Clinical Pharmacology.* Boston: MTP Press.

7

Compartmental Models

The initial chapters of this text presented the underlying physiology of drug fate. The processes involved in absorption, distribution, and elimination are the primary phenomena that must be quantitated to predict the fate of a drug or toxicant in an animal. The two primary characteristics needed to adequately describe these processes are their *rate* and *extent*. In fact, this can be appreciated in the origin of the word *kinetic*, which is defined by Webster as "*of or resulting from motion.*" Many mathematical approaches to this problem have evolved over the course of the history of pharmacokinetics. In addition, hybrid as well as novel strategies are constantly being developed to quantitate these processes. However, all approaches share certain fundamental properties that are based upon estimating the rates of chemical movement. These are best illustrated using the classic models that are often considered synonymous with pharmacokinetics.

The most widely used modeling paradigm in comparative and veterinary medicine is the compartmental approach. In this analysis, the body is viewed as being composed of a number of so-called equilibrium compartments, each defined as representing nonspecific body regions where the *rates of compound disappearance* are of a similar order of magnitude. Specifically, the fraction or percent of drug eliminated per unit of time from such a defined compartment is constant. Such compartments are classified and grouped on the basis of *similar rates of drug movement* within a kinetically homogeneous but anatomically and physiologically heterogeneous group of tissues. These compartments are theoretical entities that allow formulation of mathematical models to describe a chemical's behavior over time with respect to movement within and between compartments. This concept was initially introduced in Chapter 6 with the model in Figure 6.3. Since pharmacologists and clinicians sample blood as a common and accessible biological matrix for assessing drug fate, most pharmacokinetic models are constructed with blood or plasma drug concentrations as the central reference to which other processes are related. This chapter will be restricted to the discussion of models composed of compartments defined by processes that show linear pharmacokinetic behavior, the definition of which will now be formally presented.

A PRIMER ON THE LANGUAGE OF PHARMACOKINETICS

The roots of pharmacokinetics lie in the estimation of rates. The language is that of differential calculus. It is instructive to present a brief overview of the basic principles of rate determination since the logic embedded in its syntax forms the basis of pharmacokinetic terminology.

To begin, a rate in pharmacokinetics is defined as *how fast the mass of a compound changes per unit of time*, which is expressed mathematically as the change (represented by the Greek letter delta—Δ) in mass per small unit of time (Δt). This is synonymous with the flux of drug in a system. Units of rate are thus mass/time. For the sake of convenience only, we will express this in terms of mg/min. The reader should recall that $\Delta X / \Delta t$ was the symbol used in Chapter 5 to define the rate of renal drug excretion. We will begin this discussion using mass of a compound (X), which in clinical terms would be related to the dose, rather than using concentration. As will be developed shortly, mass and concentration are easily convertible using the proportionality factor of volume of distribution.

The rate of drug excretion $\Delta X / \Delta t$ actually has two components: a constant that reflects the rate of the process and the amount of compound available for transfer:

$$\Delta X / \Delta t = KX^{n} \tag{7.1}$$

where K is the fractional rate constant (1/min), X (mg) is the mass or amount of a compound available for transfer by the process being studied, and n is the order of the process.

First-Order Rates.   For a first-order process, $n = 1$. Since $X^{1} = X$, this equation simplifies to

$$\Delta X / \Delta t = KX \tag{7.2}$$

By definition, in first-order or linear processes, K is *constant* and thus *the actual rate of the process ($\Delta X / \Delta t$) varies in direct proportion (and hence linearly) to* X. K can be viewed as the fraction of X that moves in the system being studied (absorbed, distributed, or eliminated) per unit of time. Therefore, as X increases, $\Delta X / \Delta t$ increases in direct proportion as was graphed in Figure 2.5 (see Chapter 2) for diffusion processes. This distinction is very important, for in linear models, the rate constant is fixed, but the actual rate of the process changes in direct proportion to the mass available for movement.

As can again be appreciated by examining the equation for Fick's law of diffusion (Chapter 2, equation 2.1), compounds that are absorbed, distributed, or eliminated in direct proportion to a concentration gradient are by definition first-order rate processes. The rate constants (K_{n}) modeled in pharmacokinetics are actually aggregate constants reflecting all of the membrane diffusion processes involved in the disposition parameter being studied. This includes pH partitioning phenomena in the body that exist when blood and a cellular or tissue compartment have a pH gradient that alters the fraction of X available for diffusion. Recall that it is only the unionized fraction of a weak acid or base that diffuses down its gradient across a lipid membrane. The rate constant also reflects the degree of plasma protein binding since only the free fraction of drug is available for distribution. The actual value of a K in a pharmacokinetic model thus reflects all of these variables, whose relationship defines the biological system we are attempting to quantitate. If the system is perturbed (e.g., acid-base abnormalities, altered protein binding), the K values determined in an analysis will also change. Since the majority of these transmembrane fluxes are diffusion-driven, the sum of all their individual rates can be described using linear pharmacokinetic models.

Zero-Order Rates.   For a nonlinear or zero-order process, by definition $n = 0$. Since $X^{0} = 1$, the rate equation now becomes

$$\Delta X / \Delta t = K_{0} \tag{7.3}$$

In this scenario, the *rate of excretion is fixed and thus independent of the amount of compound available, X.* K_0 now has the units of rate (mg/min) and is *not* a mass-independent fractional rate constant. Although this would appear to simplify the situation, in reality nonlinear kinetics actually complicates most models. Only when saturation occurs would nonlinear behavior become evident (recall again Figure 2.5 in Chapter 2, as well as the clearance discussions on tubular secretion in Chapter 5 or biotransformation in Chapter 6). Chapter 9 will present this subject in more detail and discuss the scenario in which the system changes from first-order to zero-order. The focus of most pharmacokinetic studies is on drugs with linear pharmacokinetics since most therapeutically active compounds are described by these models. The remainder of this chapter will be limited to linear or first-order models.

Instantaneous Rates and the Derivative. The use of $\Delta X / \Delta t$ to describe the rate of a process is experimentally and mathematically cumbersome. Calculus has been used to describe these same processes using the concept of a derivative. This tremendously increases the options available to manipulate the data and, paradoxically, to simplify applications to biological systems. Instead of describing rates in terms of some small, finite time interval (Δt), differential equations express rate in terms of the change in compound mass (dX) over an infinitesimally small time interval termed dt. Equation 7.1 could now be written as

$$dX / dt = K X \qquad (7.4)$$

The biological interpretation is identical; however, now the full power of the calculus can be used to provide tools by which these rates can be reliably estimated from biological data. Note that K and X are the same in both equations, the only change is a conceptual one in that dX / dt now describes the instantaneous rate of change in mass over time. By convention, if the amount of drug is increasing, dX / dt is positive (e.g., absorption of drug into the blood) while if it is declining (e.g., elimination or distribution from the blood), then the rate is negative or $-dX / dt$.

Graphical Representations of Rates. Recalling algebra, if a plot (Cartesian graph) is made with X on the y-axis (dependent variable; ordinate or vertical axis) and t on the x-axis (independent variable; abscissa or horizontal axis), then the rate $\Delta X / \Delta t$ is in reality the slope of a straight line, as depicted in Figure 7.1. Slopes can easily be taken from straight lines of the form $y = mx + b$, where m is the slope ($\Delta X / \Delta t$) and b is the y-intercept. Because of this simple relationship, many of the most widely employed techniques in pharmacokinetics are simply exercises in transforming the data (e.g., taking logarithms) to derive an equation in this slope-intercept form. Equations of this form will be encountered throughout this text as pharmacokinetic, pharmacodynamic, and statistical models are discussed. This approach facilitates the use of graphical techniques and is a "preprogrammed" function in most computer software packages and hand-held calculators. However, for equations that cannot be linearized, obtaining the slope is difficult since it changes with time.

Integration. The derivative is in essence the instantaneous "slope" of any function determined by taking the tangent to the curve at the time point of interest. Thus equations written as differentials allow instantaneous rates to be calculated. One may solve a differential equation through the process of integration denoted by the symbol $\int$, which transforms the equation back into terms of t rather than dt. Integration is in reality a process by which the area under the curve (AUC) defined by $\Delta X / \Delta t$, the shaded trapezoid in Figure 7.1, is taken. By repeatedly summing (Σ) these areas for the entire experi-

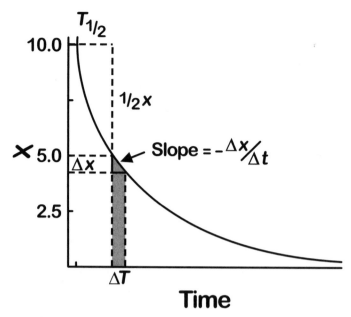

FIGURE 7.1.   Cartesian plot of the decay in drug (X) versus time. The $T^{1}/_{2}$ is defined as the time required for X to deplete to $^{1}/_{2} X$. Slope at any time is $\Delta X / \Delta T$.

mental period, the *AUC* will be obtained. We introduced this concept in Figure 3.13 (Chapter 3) when the concept of *AUC* was introduced. Analogous to the relation of a derivative to a slope, integration sums the areas under infinitesimally small regions defined by dX / dt. The *fundamental theorem of integral calculus*, developed by Sir Isaac Newton and Gottfried Leibnitz in the 17th century, linked integration to the related process of taking antiderivatives. In calculus, the rate equations may be solved using various mathematical techniques over specific time intervals, generally $t = 0$ through $t = x$ (definite integral), or through the end of an experiment estimated as $t = \infty$ (indefinite integral).

In summary, *defining rates with differentiation is analogous to taking slopes, while the inverse process of integration produces parameters that may often be expressed and numerically estimated as areas.* This basic analogy simplifies many of the concepts inherent in pharmacokinetics and, in fact, is the basis for noncompartmental modeling presented in Chapter 8.

Solving a Rate Equation.   The advantage of this approach is best illustrated by example. Let us assume that the process being studied is excretion, and thus X is declining over time. If one wants to determine the total amount of drug excretion using equation 7.1, one must sum the amount excreted during each Δt interval until the proper time is reached:

$$X = \Delta X / \Delta t_1 + \Delta X / \Delta t_2 + \Delta X / \Delta t_3 + + + = \Sigma \, \Delta X / \Delta t \qquad (7.5)$$

This requires collection of discrete timed samples and determining the *AUC*. The problem is messier if one wants to determine the rate of drug excretion. The first step required using equation 7.1 would be to measure the rates of compound decay ($-\Delta X / \Delta t$) over time. If one plotted the data as X versus time, the plot would resemble Figure 7.1. As one can see, a curve results and multiple samples would have to be collected to determine values for $\Delta X / \Delta t$ at different times that would allow determination of K. The X in equation 7.1

could be determined from equation 7.5. It is also not evident how one would easily obtain values of K, the parameter of interest.

In contrast, the situation becomes much easier if equation 7.4 is instead used and solved for K. We can use the technique of integration to solve this problem. We must integrate the equation from X at time zero (X_0) through X at time t (X_t) to obtain a formula for the mass of drug at any time.

$$\int_0^t \left(\frac{dX}{dt}\right) dt = \int_0^t (-KX)dt \tag{7.6}$$

There are numerous techniques to accomplish this integration (e.g., Laplace transformation), and the interested reader should consult a calculus textbook for further details. The result is

$$X_t = X_0 e^{-Kt} \tag{7.7}$$

where e is the base of the natural logarithm ($e = 2.713$). *It is important to realize that the process of integrating the differential equation describing rate generates the exponential term found in most linear pharmacokinetic models.* In reality, any method of pharmacokinetic analysis using exponential functions to describe physiological data implicitly assumes that a linear process is operative. Exponentials can easily be eliminated from an equation by taking their natural logarithm (ln) since the logarithm is defined as the power to which a base (in this case e) is raised. Taking the natural logarithms of equation 7.7 yields

$$\ln X_t = \ln X_0 - Kt \tag{7.8}$$

If one plots the data similar to Figure 7.1, but instead uses ln X rather than X, a straight line results (Figure 7.2). Recalling the algebraic expression for a straight line on x-y coordinates, in this case the y intercept (b) becomes X_0 and the slope of the line (m) is $-K$. The equation has been linearized providing a simple graphical method to calculate the rate constant.

The reader must realize that this equation can be linearized only because it is a first-order rate function. In theory, only two samples would have to be taken to define this line, although statistically a better estimate is obtained if more points are used. This type of plot, which is widely used throughout pharmacokinetics, is termed a semilogarithmic plot (in contrast to the Cartesian plot) since the logarithm of mass is plotted against time. Again, *when a straight line results on a semilogarithmic plot, one can assume that a linear first-order process is operative and the slope of the line is the exponent of an exponential equation.* Alternatively, a linear regression program on a computer or pocket calculator could be used to calculate K by regressing the ln X against time. Once again, the slope is $-K$ and the y-intercept is ln X_0. More sophisticated statistical techniques to solve complex linear rate equations will be presented in Chapter 13.

For those individuals more comfortable with graph that uses logarithms to the base 10 (log x) {10^x} rather than the base e (ln x){e^x}, where x is the logarithm, then the transformation of bases can be accomplished as

$$\log X = \ln X / 2.303 \tag{7.9}$$

which transforms equation 7.8 to

$$\log X_t = \log X_0 - Kt / 2.303 \tag{7.10}$$

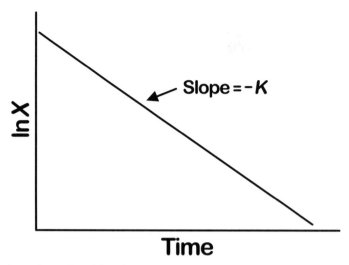

FIGURE 7.2.   Semilogarithmic plot of drug decay versus time with slope equal to $-K$.

If base 10 semilogarithmic graph paper is used to plot Figure 7.2, the slope becomes $-K / 2.303$. As this technique was in widespread use before the advent of digital computers, some workers and texts still use this approach, explaining why 2.303 appears in many pharmacokinetic equations.

This brief explanation of the derivation of exponential equations is important since all pharmacokinetic models for linear processes are expressed in these terms. These equations have certain mathematical properties (such as additivity or superposition) that greatly simplify analysis of biological data. As models become more complex, so does the process of integration, but the solutions to the equations still collapse to exponential terms that are easily analyzed using modern digital computers or graphical techniques. Thus, for the remainder of this text, the derivations and analytical solutions to the equations will not be expanded, and the reader must have faith in the author. Instead, we will focus on the proper use of the equations and the development of techniques for applying them to biological systems.

THE CONCEPT OF HALF-LIFE

The exponential equations in pharmacokinetics have another property that is central to biological applications. This is the concept of half-life $(T_{1/2})$, whose logic is central to all of this discipline. The astute biologist reading this text will have realized that equation 7.7 is the same as that used to describe population-doubling times in microbiology or ecology and to generate population growth curves, defined as the time needed for a population of organisms to double their total numbers when they are in their so-called *logarithmic* growth phase. The only difference is that since growth is described, the exponent is positive in this application. In pharmacokinetics, our perspective is a $T_{1/2}$, which is instead the time required for the amount of drug to decrease by one half, or 50%. Again we must stress that *the concept of $T_{1/2}$ is applicable only to first-order rate processes.*

Using equation 7.8, we can derive a simple equation for $T_{1/2}$. We first rearrange terms to solve for T, which yields

$$T = (\ln X_0 - \ln X_t) / K \qquad (7.11)$$

We now solve for the time at which X_t is equal to $1/2$ the initial amount X_0; that is, where $T = T_{1/2}$. Substituting these values above,

$$X_t = \frac{1}{2} X_0$$

$$
\begin{aligned}
T = T_{1/2} &= (\ln X_0 - \ln \tfrac{1}{2} X_0)/K \\
&= \ln (X_0 / \tfrac{1}{2} X_0)/K \\
&= \ln (2)/K \\
&= 0.693/K
\end{aligned}
\tag{7.12}
$$

Alternatively, we now have an equation for K, which is

$$K = 0.693 / T_{1/2} \tag{7.13}$$

It is instructive to emphasize that it is this transformation of K and $T_{1/2}$ that forces 0.693 to appear in many pharmacokinetic equations when first-order rate constants are converted to $T_{1/2}$.

What does $T_{1/2}$ really mean? This is best illustrated by returning to Figure 7.1 (remember that this is plotted on Cartesian X versus time scales). We can determine the time required for X to decrease to $1/2X$ using the original data; that is, estimating the Δt required for ΔX to be equal to $1/2X$. No matter where this is done on the concentration-time plot, the same value for Δt (e.g., $T_{1/2}$) will be obtained even though the actual rate of drug excretion ($\Delta X / \Delta t$) is decreasing at each time interval. In addition to providing a simple means of estimating $T_{1/2}$ when the data correspond to intervals of 50% decrease in X, it also clearly illustrates the meaning of $T_{1/2}$.

Assume that we start with X, decrease it by half, and repeat this process 10 times. Table 7.1 compiles these data and lists how much drug is remaining and how much has been excreted over each Δt corresponding to one $T_{1/2}$. Note that if you sum these columns, as discussed above using equation 7.5, one would have accounted for 99.9% of the original dose X. After 10 $T_{1/2}$s, 99.9% of the drug has been eliminated, or the rate process being studied has been completed. This also illustrates the logic that must be used when dealing with doses. For example, if we doubled the dose to $2X$, then after one $T_{1/2}$ we would be back to the original dose! Many "rules of thumb" used in pharmacokinetics and medicine are based on this simple fact. For therapeutic drugs, most workers assume that after 5 $T_{1/2}$s, the drug has been depleted, or the process is over since 97% of the depletion has occurred. Our experience with tissue residue depletion suggests that since the tolerance levels are so small, 10 $T_{1/2}$s of a tissue depletion may be a more appropriate estimate for some drugs. These so-called rules will be revisited in later chapters when the design of

TABLE 7.1. Relationship Between $T_{1/2}$ and Amount of Drug (A) in the Body

Number of $T_{1/2}$s	% of Drug Eliminated	% of Drug Remaining
1	50	50
2	75	25
3	87.5	12.5
4	93.75	0.625
5	96.88	0.312
6	98.44	0.156
7	99.22	0.078
8	99.61	0.039
9	99.80	0.019
10	99.90	0.0097

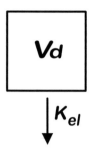

FIGURE 7.3.   One-compartment open pharmacokinetic model.

dosage regimens are considered. It now time to develop our first pharmacokinetic model using mathematical rather than physiological concepts.

ONE-COMPARTMENT OPEN MODEL

The simplest compartment model considers the body as consisting of a single homogeneous compartment; that is, the entire dose X of drug is assumed to move out of the body at a single rate. This model, depicted in Figure 7.3, is best conceptualized as instantly dissolving and homogeneously mixing the drug in a beaker from which it is eliminated by a single rate process described by the rate constant K, now termed K_{el}. Since drug leaves the system, the model is termed open. Equation 7.7 is the pharmacokinetic equation for the one-compartment open model. Although expressed in terms of the amount of drug remaining in the compartment, most experiments measure concentrations.

This requires the development of one of the so-called primary pharmacokinetic parameters, the volume of distribution (Vd) (recall equation 4.5, Chapter 4, when we discussed distribution). In terms of the one-compartment model, this would be the volume of the compartment into which the dose of drug (D) instantaneously distributes. Vd thus becomes a *proportionality factor* relating D to the observed concentration Cp by

$$Vd \, (mL) = X \, (mg) / Cp \, (mg/mL) = D/Cp \tag{7.14}$$

$$D = \text{dose of drug}, \quad Cp = \text{observed concentration}$$

Using this relation, we can now rewrite equation 7.7 in terms of concentrations, which are experimentally accessible by sampling blood, instead of the total amount of drug remaining in the body:

$$Cp = (X_0 / Vd) \, e^{-K_{el}t} = Cp_0 \, e^{-K_{el}t} \tag{7.15}$$

$$Cp = X/Vd, \quad X = X_0 \, e^{-k_{el}t}$$

A semilogarithmic plot seen after intravenous administration using this model is depicted in the top of Figure 7.4. One can easily convert between Figures 7.1 or 7.2 and 7.4 using the Vd relationship above. Vd quantitates the apparent volume into which a drug is dissolved since, recalling the discussion in Chapter 4, the true volume is determined by the physiology of the animal, the relative transmembrane diffusion coefficients, and the chemical properties of the drug being studied. A drug that is restricted to the vascular system will have a very small Vd, while one that distributes to total body water will have a very large Vd. In fact, it is this technique that was used to calculate the plasma and interstitial spaces quoted in Chapter 4.

From this simple analysis, and using the model in Figure 7.1, a number of useful pharmacokinetic parameters may be defined. Assuming that an experiment such as depicted in

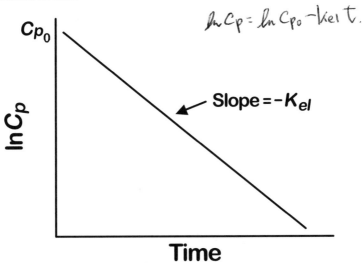

In $Cp = ln\ Cp_0 - k_{el}\ t.$

Slope $= -K_{el}$

FIGURE 7.4. Semilogarithmic concentration-time profile for a one-compartment drug with slope $-K_{el}$ and intercept Cp_0.

Figure 7.4 has been conducted using a dose of D and values for K_{el} and Vd have been determined, $T_{1/2}$ can easily be calculated from equation 7.12 above.

Clearance.   Recalling the development of clearance concepts in Chapter 5, we now can easily determine Cl_B using this information. Clearance was defined as the *volume of blood cleared of a substance by the kidney per unit of time*. If one considers the whole body, this would read as the *volume of distribution of drug in the body cleared of a substance per unit of time*. Translating this sentence to the syntax of pharmacokinetic terminology and considering whole body elimination, Vd represents the volume and K_{el} the fractional rate constant (units of 1/time). Thus, clearance is

$$Cl_B\ (\text{mL}\,/\,\text{min}) = Vd\ (\text{mL})\ K_{el}\ (1\,/\,\text{min}) \tag{7.16}$$

$Vd = $ volume, $k_{el} = $ fractional rate constant

As alluded to in the discussion on renal clearance, this equation allows one to determine glomerular filtration rate (GFR) if a glomerular filtration marker such as inulin were injected into the body and its decay plotted as in Figure 7.4. Similar logic was applied to use clearances to describe hepatic drug metabolism.

There is another method available to calculate Cl_B. In Chapter 5, clearance was also defined in equation 5.4 as the *rate of drug excretion relative to its plasma concentration.* We can also express this sentence in the syntax of pharmacokinetics and get the relation

$$Cl_B = \frac{dX\,/\,dt}{Cp} \tag{7.17}$$

$\frac{dx}{dt} = $ rate of drug excretion, $Cp = $ concentration

If we integrate both the numerator and denominator of this relation from *time* $= 0 \to \infty$, the numerator is simply the sum of the total amount of drug that has been excreted from the body; that is, the administered dose D. The denominator is the integral of the plasma concentration time profile. Since integration was analogous to taking the area under the function to be integrated over infinitesimally small time intervals (dt), the result of this operation is the *AUC*. The relation thus becomes

$\int_0^\infty \frac{dx}{dt}dt = \int_0^\infty (-kx)dt = X_0\,e^{-kt}\big|_0^\infty = X_0 = D$

$Cl_B = \frac{\int_0^\infty \frac{dx}{dt}\,dt}{\int_0^\infty Cp\,dt}$

$$Cl_B = D\,/\,AUC \tag{7.18}$$

$\int_0^\infty Cp\,dt = AUC$

$D = $ dose of drug, $AUC = $ area under the curve plasma concentration-versus-time curve

There are two approaches to calculate *AUC* that are based on determining the area under the observed concentration-time (*C-T*) profile. A common approach is to use the trapezoidal method alluded to when integration was defined. Figure 3.13 (see Chapter 3) introduced this technique, which will be presented in much greater detail in the next chapter (on noncompartmental models) since this modeling approach is based completely on calculating the *AUC*s of different functions. However, for the one-compartment open model being discussed, which generates the semilogarithmic *C-T* plot depicted in Figure 7.4, the problem is simply determining the area of the right triangle. The area of this triangle (*AUC*) is height divided by the slope of the hypotenuse, or

$$AUC = Cp_0 / K_{el} \quad (?) \tag{7.19}$$

Interpretation of Pharmacokinetic Parameters. With these equations, we now have the *three so-called primary pharmacokinetic parameters describing drug disposition in the body: $T_{1/2}$, Cl_B, and Vd.* The data required to calculate them is a knowledge of dose and an experimental derivation of either K_{el} or $T_{1/2}$.

This is a good point at which to discuss the limits of calculating parameters from such simple concentration-time profiles. Only two parameters are actually being "measured" from this analysis: the slope K_{el} and intercept Cp_0 of the semilogarithmic plot which, using equation 7.14, directly calculates Vd. The third parameter Cl is "calculated" from the two "measured" parameters. Based on the mathematical method used to calculate these, some workers suggested that K_{el} and Vd are the independent parameters in a pharmacokinetic analysis, and Cl is a derived parameter. This assertion is usually made when the statistical properties of the parameters are being defined since errors for these can be easily obtained. However, this belief is an artifact of the use of a compartmental model as a *tool* to get at values for these physiological parameters and introduces confusion when pharmacokinetic parameters are linked to physiological variables. As should be appreciated from the discussions in Chapters 4 through 6, physiologically, the truly independent parameters are the Vd and Cl, with K_{el} and thus $T_{1/2}$ becoming the dependent variables. This distinction is very important when the effects of either a species' physiology or an individual's disease state on pharmacokinetics is being estimated. From this biological perspective, the true relationship is

$$T_{1/2} = (0.693 \times Vd)/Cl \tag{7.20}$$

The observed half-life of a drug is dependent upon both the extent of a drug's distribution in the body and its rate of clearance. If the clearance of a drug is high (e.g., rapidly eliminated by the kidney), the $T_{1/2}$ will be relatively short. Logically, a slowly eliminated drug will have a prolonged $T_{1/2}$. Although not at first obvious, if a drug is extensively distributed in the body (e.g., lipid-soluble drug distributed to fat), Vd will be large *and* the $T_{1/2}$ will be relatively prolonged. In contrast, if a drug that has restricted distribution in the body (e.g., only the vascular system), the Vd will be small and thus the $T_{1/2}$ relatively short. In a disease state, $T_{1/2}$ may be prolonged by a diseased kidney; a reduced capacity for hepatic drug metabolism; or an inflammatory state, which increases capillary perfusion and permeability, thus allowing drug access to normally excluded tissue sites. *Therefore, $T_{1/2}$ is physiologically dependent on both the volume of distribution and clearance of the drug.* The basic physiological principles outlined in Chapters 4 through 6 are important to keep in mind since, as we build more complicated (but realistic) pharmacokinetic models, the calculation of Vd and Cl becomes more complex because the underlying biology dictates it.

Clearance from Intravenous Infusions. There is yet another strategy that can be used to estimate clearance in an intravenous study. This is based on the basic principle of mass balance. The strategy is to infuse a drug into the body at a constant rate R_0 (mass/time) and then measure plasma drug concentrations. By definition, when a steady-state plasma concentration is achieved, C_{ss} (mass/volume), the rate of drug input must equal the rate of clearance from the body, Cl_B:

$$R_0 \text{ (mg / min)} = C_{ss} \text{ (mg / mL)} \times Cl \text{ (mL / min)} \qquad (7.21)$$

Rearranging this equation gives a simple formula for determining Cl:

$$\begin{aligned} Cl \text{ (mL/min)} &= R_0 \text{ (mg/min)} / C_{ss} \text{ (mg/mL)} \\ &= R_0 / C_{ss} \text{ (mL/min)} \end{aligned} \qquad (7.22)$$

The Cl calculated in this manner is identical to that determined using equations 7.16 and 7.18 above, and only requires knowing the rate of infusion and assaying the achieved steady-state concentration. One may also calculate the Vd from an intravenous infusion study by the relation

$$Vd = Cl/K_{el}, \quad Cl = R_0/C_{ss}$$

$$Vd = R_0 / (C_{ss} \, K_{el}) \qquad (7.23)$$

This line of reasoning supports Cl_B as a primary parameter since it can be calculated independently of a one-compartment analysis. In fact, as discussed in Chapter 5, this is another method to estimate glomerular filtration rate using markers of renal clearance. If steady-state is assumed, then R_0 must equal the rate of excretion presented in equation 5.4 as $\Delta x / \Delta t$. Making this substitution, and using this chapter's terminology of C_{ss} in place of C_{art}, both equations are equivalent. If one knows the rate of infusion of a glomerular filtration marker such as inulin and assays the steady-state concentration, GFR can thus be estimated in a relatively robust manner since errors in time or assay will be minimized when the average C_{ss} is determined. In fact, this method holds for even more complicated pharmacokinetic models (discussed below) since as long as steady-state is achieved, the rate of infusion will always be dependent upon Cl_B.

Pharmacokinetic Analysis from Urine Data. Many of the above pharmacokinetic parameters may be obtained by analysis of urine data alone. This is often advantageous when concentrations of the compound studied are too low for assay in the blood, or when exposure in an environmental scenario results in very low absorbed doses. In these cases, the ability of the kidney to concentrate urine is taken advantage of since the kidney thereby concentrates the excreted drug. However, to use these techniques, it is important that the concepts of Cl_B and Cl_{renal} be kept distinct. In a one-compartment open model in which there is no extravascular administration or systemic metabolism, all injected drug will appear in the urine, and thus the total amount excreted over the course of an experiment (e.g., the sum of equation 7.5) is equivalent to X or D. If the drug also undergoes hepatic elimination, then $D \neq X$ since a fraction will be excreted by other routes (e.g., bile, expired, or as metabolites in urine).

These techniques all assume that some fraction of the drug is eliminated from the body by renal elimination. The compound has a C-T profile best characterized by a monoexponential decay (e.g., one-compartment open model) even though it may be eliminated by multiple organs. Recall in Chapter 5 that Cl_B is the sum of $Cl_{renal} + Cl_{hepatic} + Cl_{other}$. In an analogous fashion, since $Cl = K_{el}Vd$ and Vd is the same for drug excreted by the kidney or any organ, dividing this relationship by Vd we obtain

$$K_{el} = K_{renal} + K_{hepatic} + K_{other} = K_{renal} + K_{nonrenal} \qquad (7.24)$$

For the sake of simplicity, we will consider only renal and nonrenal routes of elimination.

In a manner analogous to analyzing the C-T profile to obtain K_{el}, we will instead analyze the rate of drug excretion in the urine. We will denote urine concentration as U_t. With the C-T profile, we are studying drug that has not yet been eliminated from the body, while in urine-based methods, we are examining the drug that has already been excreted. If bile were collected instead of urine, similar techniques could be used to model biliary drug excretion.

In many of these experiments, we are essentially measuring $\Delta X / \Delta t$ based on urine collection. It thus behooves the investigator to take great care in collecting urine specimens. For best results, one must have properly timed urine collections, and when rates are estimated, Δt should be less than one $T_{1/2}$. The assayed urine concentration is then multiplied by the collected urine volume to obtain the mass excreted in Δt, (U_t). When excretion plots are constructed as described below, the time plotted on the x-axis should be the midpoint of the Δt interval. Similarly, if a corresponding Cp is obtained, it should either be collected at the midpoint of collection or be calculated as the average of the time points defining Δt.

When data are analyzed in this manner, the rate of elimination K_{el}, and not K_{renal} alone, determines the slope of the $\ln U_t$ excretion rate profiles. Since one is measuring the rate of unchanged drug excretion into the urine, this rate will also reflect nonrenal elimination even when the drug eliminated by this route is not being excreted into the urine. This can be appreciated by examining Figure 7.3 and substituting $(K_{renal} + K_{nonrenal})$ for K_{el}. The driving concentration for elimination by both routes is the Cp in this compartment. Thus, as drug is eliminated by the kidney and other routes, its concentration will decrease at a rate proportional to the total K_{el} from this compartment. What will be dependent upon K_{renal} is the fraction of this eliminated dose, which is excreted into the urine and will effect the total urinary recovery U_∞. *Urine-based methods monitor the systemic rate of elimination.*

The technique termed the *amount remaining to be excreted (ARE)* or *sigma-minus* method is depicted in Figure 7.5. The term ARE is obtained because the y-axis is now $(U_\infty - U_t)$ or, alternatively, the amount of drug remaining to be excreted in the urine, reflecting the fact that not all of the systemically administered dose will appear in the urine. To construct this plot, for every Δt of urine collection, one plots $U_\infty - U_t$ versus the time of the midpoint of the collection interval. Note that since this is a semilogarithmic plot, the excretion profile is log-linear. The slope is then equal to $-K_{el}$. In another technique, the rate of drug excretion $(\Delta U / \Delta t)$ versus time is plotted as in Figure 7.6. The resulting slope is again $-K_{el}$.

What is different in Figures 7.5 and 7.6 compared to the plasma-based plot of Figure 7.4 is the nature of the intercept, not the rate of decay that is controlled by K_{el}. This becomes clearer from the differential rate equations for $\Delta U / \Delta t$. The formula that describes Figure 7.6 would be similar to equation 7.8:

$$\ln U_t = K_{renal} U_0 - K_{el} t \qquad (7.25)$$

U_t = urine concentration, $K_{renal} U_0$ = fraction of drug excreted in urine.

The slope of the plot is the same; however, the intercept now reflects the fraction of drug excreted in the urine. Similarly, the equation for the ARE plot would be:

$$\ln (U_\infty - U_t) = \ln U_\infty - K_{el} t \qquad (7.26)$$

Again, slopes are identical, but now the intercept reflects how much drug actually was excreted in the urine. As can be appreciated from studying these relationships, if the drug is

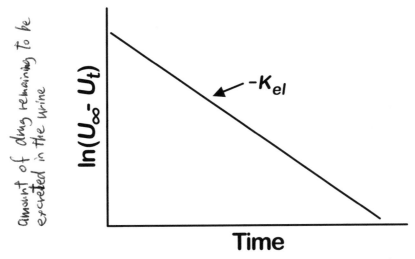

FIGURE 7.5. Pharmacokinetic analysis of urinary drug concentrations using a semilogarithmic *amount remaining to be excreted* (ARE) plot whose slope is $-K_{el}$.

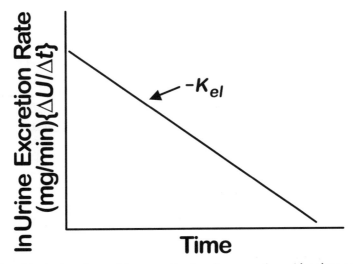

Figure 7.6. Semilogarithmic plot of rate of drug excretion in urine versus time with a slope equal to $-K_{el}$.

$$U_\infty/D = K_{renal}/K_{el}$$

totally excreted by the kidney, then $U_\infty = D$. However, if renal and nonrenal elimination routes are occurring, these data may be used to estimate the extent of nonrenal elimination since the ratio of U_∞ / D is equivalent to K_{renal} / K_{el} (also termed f in Chapter 15).

More information may be obtained if corresponding Cp versus time data is available for each $\Delta U / \Delta t$. A plot of rate of excretion on a Cartesian axis versus Cp is shown in Figure 7.7. As defined in Chapter 5 (equation 5.4), the rate of excretion relative to the blood concentration is defined as the renal clearance, and thus the slope of the line in Figure 7.7 ($\Delta U / \Delta t$ versus Cp) is Cl_{renal}. In this analysis, more information is present than with the two techniques discussed above since the rate of drug excretion in the urine is being compared to the Cp profile, which is declining with a rate constant of K_{el}. The Cp data have K_{el} information embedded within it. The clearance obtained using this technique reflects Cl_{renal} and not Cl_B. If one integrates both axes of this plot, the slope remains Cl_{renal}, but now the y-axis is the cumulative amount of drug excreted in urine and the x-axis is AUC.

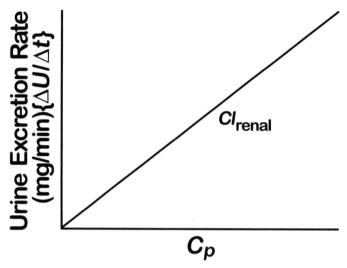

FIGURE 7.7.   Plot of rate of drug excretion in urine versus plasma concentration with slope equal to Cl_{renal}.

At any time t, the slope is cumulative U divided by AUC through time t (AUC_t), which provides a point estimate of Cl_{renal}.

The selection of which method to use is dependent upon experimental constraints and data quality. Urine excretion data are often variable and dependent upon accurate sampling. The more samples that make up an analysis, the better the estimate. Theoretically, all of the above methods will result in the same rate constant and clearance estimates. However, physiological anomalies in how the kidney handles a compound (tubular reabsorption with storage, tubular secretion with subsequent metabolism) within the tubular system may make differences in these methods evident. For example, assume drug is completely eliminated by the kidney, making any estimate of Cl_B equivalent to Cl_{renal}. However, if one of these processes occurs, Cl_B will be greater than Cl_{renal} since Cp cannot reflect what happens to the drug after filtration (see Chapter 5). Figure 7.8 illustrates this phenomenon with gentamicin. When Cl_B compared with Cl_{renal} in four separate studies, the above relation was always noted, suggesting that tubular sequestration was reducing the flux of intact drug into the urine. The same would occur if parent drug were excreted as an undetectable metabolite. However, this difference becomes a strength since these phenomena were discovered due to this discrepancy in clearances.

Additional urine techniques will only be briefly discussed in the remaining chapters since an extension of the logic presented above can be used to obtain many values formally presented only for C-T profiles. In some laboratory animal situations in which urine collection is easier than blood sampling, these approaches may prove particularly powerful as many pharmacokinetic parameters may be obtained from noninvasive urine monitoring.

ABSORPTION IN A ONE-COMPARTMENT OPEN MODEL

The above analysis assumes that the drug was injected into the body, which behaves as a single space into which the drug is uniformly dissolved. The first real-world complication occurs when the drug is administered by one of the extravascular routes discussed in Chapter 3. In this case, the drug must be absorbed from the dosing site into the blood stream. The resulting semilogarithmic concentration-time profile, depicted in Figure 7.9, now is characterized by an initial rising component that peaks and then undergoes the

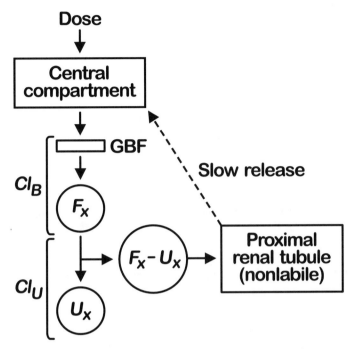

FIGURE 7.8. Difference between total body clearance calculated from plasma (Cl_B) or urine (Cl_U) due to drug that was filtered by the glomeruli (GBF) but reabsorbed and stored in the renal tubules ($F_x - U_x$) rather than being excreted in the urine. F_x is filtered drug, and U_x is drug excreted in the urine.

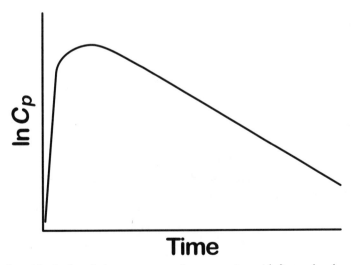

FIGURE 7.9. Semilogarithmic plot of plasma concentration versus time with first-order absorption.

same log-linear decline. The proper pharmacokinetic model for this scenario is depicted in Figure 7.10. The rate of the drug's absorption is governed by the rate constant K_a.

When the absorption process is finally complete, elimination is still described by K_{el} as depicted in Figure 7.2. The overall elimination half-life can still be calculated using K_{el} if this terminal slope is taken after the peak in the linear portion of the semilogarithmic plot (providing $K_a >> K_{el}$). However, calculation of Vd and Cl becomes more complicated since K_a is present and, unlike an intravenous injection, one is not assured that all of the

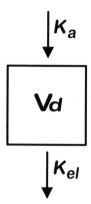

FIGURE 7.10.   One-compartment open pharmacokinetic model with first-order absorption.

drug has been absorbed into the body. In order to handle this, we must now write the differential equations to describe this process by including rate constants for absorption and elimination:

$$dX / dt = K_a D - K_{el} X \tag{7.27}$$

X = absorbed dose,   D = administered dose

where D is the administered dose driving the absorption process and X is now the amount of dose absorbed and available for excretion. The relationship between D and X is the absolute systemic availability F originally introduced in Chapter 3 (equations 3.1 and 3.2), $\{X = FD\}$. In the language of differential equations, rates are simply additive, which allows the same data sets to be described in components reflecting the different processes. As above, integrating this equation and expressing it in terms of concentrations gives the expression that describes the profile in Figure 7.9:

$D = X/F, \quad F = \dfrac{AUC_{route} / Dose_{route}}{AUC_{iv} / Dose_{iv}} \; (\%)$

$$Cp = \frac{K_a F D}{Vd (K_a - K_{el})} [e^{-K_{el}t} - e^{-K_a t}] \qquad Cp = X/Vd \tag{7.28}$$

(?)

The Concept of Curve Stripping Applied to Absorption.   This is an excellent point in the discussion to appreciate the validity of the use of multiexponential equations to describe blood C-T profiles, as the exponential terms—like the rates above from which they were derived—are simply additive. *A C-T profile is the sum of the underlying exponential terms describing the rate processes involved.* This property of superposition is the basis upon which observed C-T profiles may be "dissected" to obtain the component rates. Figure 7.11 illustrates this process, in which an observed semilogarithmic profile is plotted as a composite of its absorption phase (controlled by K_a) and the elimination phase (controlled by K_{el}). In contrast to the intravenous equation 7.15, the time zero intercept is now a more complex function, which is dependent upon the fraction of administered dose that is systemically available and thus able to be acted on by the elimination process described by the rate constant K_{el}. For this procedure to work, K_a must be greater than K_{el} so that at later time points $e^{-K_a t}$ approaches zero [exponential of a large negative number approaches zero, or expressed mathematically, as $\lim_{t \to \infty} (e^{-t}) = 0$].

This equation reduces to

$$Cp = \frac{K_a F D}{Vd (K_a - K_{el})} [e^{-K_{el}t}] \tag{7.29}$$

as $t \to$ large, $e^{-K_{el}t} \gg e^{-K_a t}$

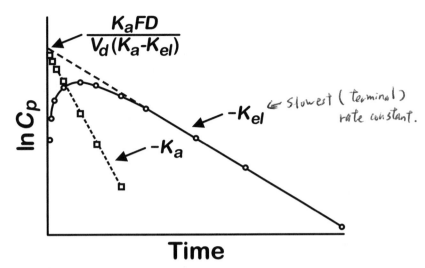

FIGURE 7.11. Semilogarithmic plot of plasma concentration versus time using a one-compartment open pharmacokinetic model with first-order absorption. The profile is decomposed into two lines with slopes $-K_a$ and $-K_{el}$.

which is the terminal phase of the C-T profile. If K_a were less than K_{el}, the same C-T profile as the one in Figure 7.9 will result; however, now the terminal slope will be K_a as it is the rate-limiting process! The intercept term would be appropriate if one just flip-flopped K_a and K_{el}. In fact, recalling the discussion in Chapter 3 on slow-release dosing formulations, we termed the resulting effect on disposition of drug in the body an example of the *flip-flop* phenomenon, the origin of which is the above relation.

In any multiexponential model, in order for multiple phases of a C-T profile to become evident, the ratio of Ks (in our example K_a and K_{el}) must be ≥ 3. The computational procedure of "stripping" the slower elimination process away from the observed composite C-T profile to generate the absorption profile (or any other faster exponential process, such as distribution) is the basis of many software algorithms presented in Chapter 13.

It is important to once again digress at this point of the discussion to stress the reason why *intravenous pharmacokinetic studies should always be conducted to define drug disposition.* If an extravascular route of administration is used, the investigator can never be certain that the C-T profile is not dependent upon a slow, and thus rate-limiting, absorptive process secondary to a formulation factor. If a depot or extended-release formulation is administered such that K_a is less than K_{el} the terminal slope will reflect the rate of absorption rather than the rate of elimination. $T_{1/2}$ may be overestimated as it will now reflect $0.693 / K_a$ rather than $0.693 / K_{el}$. Complete absorption also cannot be ensured (e.g., $F = 1$), thus one never truly knows the size of the absorbed dose. Accurate estimates of Cl and Vd, reflecting the true pharmacokinetic disposition of a drug, are required as input to determine these relations. These are best calculated after a complete intravenous injection using the equations described above.

When intravenous and extravascular dosing experiments are conducted, one can easily calculate the absolute systemic availability F for a specific formulation by determining the ratios of $AUCs$. In an intravenous study in which the total mass of drug is injected, all of the drug will have had to appear in the blood stream, and thus AUC_{iv} will reflect the maximum AUC possible. F of the extravascular dose then is the ratio of $AUC_{extravascular}$ to AUC_{iv}, the same as equation 3.1. (see Chapter 3 on absorption).

Analysis of Urine Data to Estimate Absorption Parameters.   As discussed above for intravenous administration, urine analysis may also be used to estimate absorption parameters. If the rate and pathway of metabolism is similar between both routes, F may also be simply calculated as $(U\infty)_{extravascular} / (U\infty)_{iv}$. If they are different, and the other route of elimination can be assessed (e.g., expired air, bile, feces), then absolute systemic availability becomes a ratio of the total amount excreted by both routes as depicted previously in equation 3.1 (see Chapter 3). In many cases, it is difficult to collect total urine and feces in the field, and one would like a method to assess availability (or in toxicology terms, exposure) from only one route. To accomplish this, one must know the fraction of drug that is eliminated by the route being studied. Based on our discussions of urine-based methodologies above, this is the ratio of K_{renal} / K_{el}. As shown above, this is equivalent to the ratio $(U\infty)_{iv} / D_{iv}$. Multiplication of this ratio times the $U\infty$ obtained in the intravenous study corrects it to reflect the fraction of dose absorbed that could be excreted in the urine. Bioavailability by this route is then calculated as

$$F = (U_\infty)_{extravascular} / (\text{corrected } U_\infty)_{iv} \tag{7.30}$$

The rate of absorption K_a can also be calculated from the data in Figure 7.11, but there are more efficient techniques, which will now be briefly presented. First, urine excretion data can be used to analyze for K_a in addition to F using techniques very similar to that described in equations 7.25 and 7.26 and depicted in Figures 7.5 and 7.6. The "twist" now added is that the total dose is a function of F, and the rate of absorption K_a comes into play. Thus, similar to the C-T profile in Figure 7.9, a biexponential curve in urine will result. If ARE or $\Delta U / \Delta t$ plots are used, the slopes of the line are K_a and K_{el}, with K_{el} being the terminal slope if K_a is greater than K_{el}. Again, realize that the slope of the terminal portion of a urine excretion curve reflects overall systemic elimination and not renal excretion. If a flip-flop situation is present, the terminal slope will be K_a. For a rapidly absorbed drug, it is often difficult to get good estimates of K_a from the "stripped" urine data since very short urine collection intervals are almost impossible. The intercept term is also more complex as it now reflects K_{el}, K_{renal} and K_a. However, at time infinity, the total amount excreted in urine, U_∞, reduces to $(K_{renal} F D) / K_{el}$, which is another form of the expression used to derive equation 7.30 above.

If all of these concepts are considered, and the rate of absorption may become rate-limiting, then the most widely used experimental approach for determining absolute systemic availability is based on an analysis of AUC. If different doses are applied or if the $T_{1/2}$ is different by the extravascular route being studied due to the route-effects in clearance, then F should be calculated as

$$F = \frac{(AUC_{extravascular})\,(D_{iv})\,(T_{1/2})_{iv}}{(AUC_{iv})\,(D_{extravascular})\,(T_{1/2})_{extravascular}} \tag{7.31}$$

It must be stressed that when a flip-flop absorption rate-limiting drug is studied, F must *not* be corrected for the rate limiting absorption due to flip-flop, but must be corrected for prolonged extravascular $T_{1/2}$, otherwise F will be greater than 1.0—a value that is biologically meaningless. Such "strange" values of F may also be encountered if the injected intravenous dosage form is not soluble in blood (e.g., precipitation, too lipophilic). In this case, a fraction of the intravenous dose never is truly available for systemic distribution.

Wagner-Nelson Method. The final techniques employed in bioavailability studies are designed to extract data on K_a from C-T profile analysis. The techniques above assume that K_a is a first-order process and thus may be described as an exponential process which, due to additivity, may be stripped away from a semilogarithmic C-T profile.

However, in many cases, K_a may be zero-order. The Wagner-Nelson method may be used in this situation. This technique is based on analyzing data based on percent-absorbed plots. Simply, this method assumes that the amount of drug absorbed into the systemic circulation at any time after administration (X_S) equals the sum of the amount of drug remaining in the body (X_B) plus the cumulative amount of drug that has already been eliminated (X_E) by all routes combined $\{X_S = X_B + X_E\}$. If we write a differential rate equation describing dX_S / dt, we get this rate $\{dX_S / dt = dX_B / dt + dX_E / dt\}$. We see that dX_E / dt is equivalent to equation 7.4 as X_E is the amount of drug in the body remaining to be excreted. As previously derived, this is equal to rate of drug elimination $K_{el}X$. If we express X_B in terms of Cp using the Vd relation of equation 7.14, we get

$$dX_S / dt = Vd\ C\ / dt + K_{el}\ Vd\ C \tag{7.32}$$

If one integrates this equation from time zero to t, we get

$$X_S(t) = VdC_t + K_{el}Vd\int_0^t C\ dt = VdC_t + K_{el}Vd\ AUC_t \tag{7.33}$$

where C_t is the concentration at time t and $\int C\ dt$ is the AUC from time zero through t, denoted as AUC_t. At time infinity, the total amount of drug absorbed could be calculated by integrating 7.32 from $t = 0 \to t = \infty$. In this procedure, C_t = zero for both time points. The result is

$$X_S(\infty) = K_{el}Vd\ AUC_\infty \tag{7.34}$$

Note that AUC_∞ is equivalent to the AUC calculated earlier. If we take the ratio of equations 7.33 and 7.34 and cancel common terms, we derive a relation describing the fraction of drug absorbed through time t:

$$\frac{X_S(t)}{X_S(\infty)} = \frac{C_t + K_{el}AUC_t}{K_{el}AUC_\infty} \tag{7.35}$$

This expresses the relation of the fraction of drug absorbed at any time relative to that ultimately absorbed, not the administered dose. However, from our systemic availability discussion above, $X_S(\infty) = F\ D$, a value that only can be derived using intravenous data. Wagner-Nelson plots can be now obtained as follows. Figure 7.12 shows the amount of drug absorbed as a function of time and is constructed by plotting the numerator of equation 7.35 versus time. K_{el} is obtained by the methods discussed above using a semilogarithmic C-T plot. Although many of these calculations appear at first to be cumbersome, the key is to organize collected data by time of observation such that each calculation is straightforward, a process facilitated by using a spreadsheet program in which columns are defined as

$$\text{Time} \mid \text{Observed } C_t \mid AUC_t \mid K_{el}AUC_t \mid C_t + K_{el}AUC_t$$

As seen in this plot, as time increases, the value of the function approaches $K\ AUC_\infty$. Knowing AUC_∞, a plot of the fraction absorbed calculated using equation 7.35 is depicted in Figure 7.13. It should be noted that this approach makes no assumptions about the kinetics of the absorption process since a model is never fitted to the plots. This is the power of this approach since estimates of the rate of absorption can be made for processes with zero-order (e.g., extended-release) and even more complex kinetics.

If one were to take the same data used to generate Figure 7.13 and instead plot

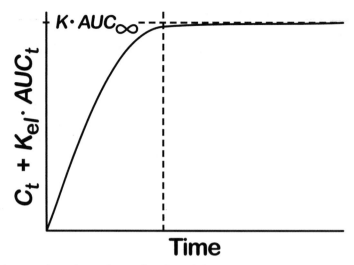

FIGURE 7.12.   Wagner-Nelson plot used to analyze drug absorption in a one-compartment model.

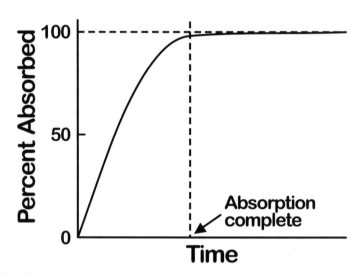

FIGURE 7.13.   Plot of percent absorbed versus time used to analyze drug absorption data.

100 (1 − % absorbed); that is, percent of drug unabsorbed, a first-order absorption process would generate a curve on ordinal plots and a straight line on a semilogarithmic plot, as in Figure 7.14 (top). In some cases in which absorption is complex and described by multiexponential equations, a curve stripping approach could be used to break this plot into its constituent rates (K_X and K_Y), as in Figure 7.14 (bottom). The Wagner-Nelson approach is generally only applicable to one-compartment data, and the Loo-Riegelman technique described below should be used in multicompartmental situations.

TWO-COMPARTMENT MODELS

Unfortunately, most drugs are not described by a simple one-compartment model since the plasma concentration-time profile is not a straight line. This reflects the biological reality that for many drugs, the body is not a single homogeneous compartment, but instead is composed of regions that are defined by having different *rates* of drug distribution. Such a

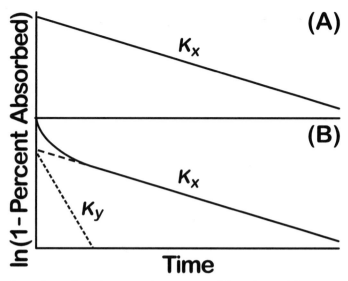

FIGURE 7.14. Semilogarithmic plots of amount of 1 − percent of drug absorbed demonstrating (A) a single absorption phase and (B) a two-component absorption phase.

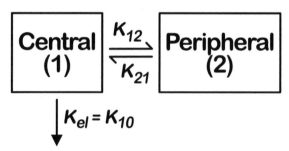

FIGURE 7.15. Generalized open two-compartment pharmacokinetic model after intravenous administration with elimination (K_{el}) from the central compartment. K_{12} and K_{21} represent intercompartmental micro-rate constants.

situation is reflected in the two-compartment model depicted in Figure 7.15. The drug initially is distributed in the central compartment and by definition is eliminated from this compartment. The difference comes because now the drug also distributes into other body regions at a rate that is different from that of the central compartment.

As presented in Chapter 4, many factors determine the rate and extent of drug distribution into a tissue (e.g., blood flow, tissue mass, blood/tissue partition coefficient). When the composite rates of these flow and diffusion processes are significantly different than K_{el}, then the C-T profile will reflect this by assuming a biexponential nature. For many drugs, the central compartment may consist of blood plasma and the extracellular fluid of highly perfused organs, such as the heart, lung, kidneys, and liver. Distribution to the remainder of the body occurs more slowly, which provides the physiological basis for a two-compartment model. Such a peripheral compartment is defined by a distribution rate constant (K_{12}) out of the central compartment and a redistribution rate constant (K_{21}) from the peripheral back into the central compartment. As discussed in Chapter 4 on distribution, depots or sinks may also occur. This is a pharmacokinetic concept whereby the distribution rate constants are significantly slower than K_{el} and thus become the rate-limiting factor defining the terminal slope of a biexponential C-T profile, a situation analogous to flip-flop in absorption studies.

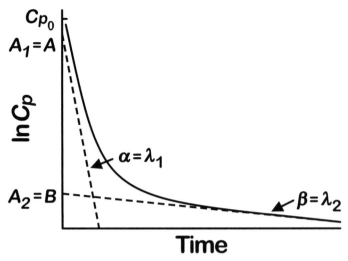

FIGURE 7.16. Semilogarithmic plasma concentration versus time profile of a drug described by a two-compartment open model. Parameters are defined in the text.

We will begin the discussion of multicompartmental models with the principles of analyzing a two-compartment model after intravenous administration (Figure 7.15). This is the most common scenario encountered in comparative medicine, and the principles translate easily to more complicated models. The fundamental principle involved is that the observed serum concentration-time profile is actually the result of two separate pharmacokinetic processes, which can be described by two separate exponential terms, commonly written as

$$C_p = Ae^{-\alpha t} + Be^{-\beta t} \qquad (7.36)$$

Note the similarity of this biexponential equation to that presented for absorption in equation 7.28. In this case we have terms with slopes (α and β) and corresponding intercepts (A and B). The C-T profile on semilogarithmic plots is depicted in Figure 7.16. By definition, $\alpha >> \beta$, and thus β is the terminal slope. If $\alpha \approx \beta$, then the slopes of the two lines would be equal and we would be back to the single line of Figure 7.2 and a one-compartment model!

Nomenclature.   When dealing with multicompartmental models, it becomes necessary to introduce new nomenclature to denote the intercept terms and slopes of the C-T profile because, as will be shown shortly, the observed slopes are no longer synonymous with the elimination and distribution rate constants as they were when we were analyzing absorption plots (Figure 7.10) for K_{el} and K_a. When these models were constructed, the defining differential rate equations could be written in terms of the mass of drug in the central compartment (X). In the two-compartment model of Figure 7.15, this equation now must describe drug movement in terms of the mass of drug in compartments one and two. As will be derived below, the solution to this differential equation is the slopes of the biexponential C-T profile giving α and β. Multicompartmental models have their own syntax: the slopes of the C-T profile are named with letters of the Greek alphabet, starting with the most rapid rate, α, for distribution, followed by β for elimination. The intercept terms are denoted using the roman alphabet, in this example A being related to α and B to β. However, this can be confusing when distribution is into a slowly equilibrating depot, where α would now reflect elimination and β distribution. This often happens when the experiment is conducted over days rather than hours, as we found in studies conducted with gentamicin.

The preferred nomenclature carries less phenomenological context and uses the Greek letter λ_n, with $n = 1, 2, 3, \ldots$, progressing from the most rapid to the slowest rate process. The corresponding intercept terms are denoted as A_n. This nomenclature describes any multicompartmental model without implying a physiological basis to the underlying mechanism responsible for the different rates observed. The biexponential equation for a two-compartment model may now be written as

$$Cp = A_1 e^{-\lambda_1 t} + A_2 e^{-\lambda_2 t} \qquad (7.37)$$

The actual rate constants describing flux between compartments are now termed micro-rate constants and denoted by k_{xy}, where compound moves from x to y. Smaller values for x and y indicate more rapid interdepartmental micro-rate constants. When the origin or destination of a compound is outside of the body, then x or y is denoted as 0, respectively. Thus, K_a becomes k_{01} and K_{el} becomes k_{10}. In order to avoid confusion, the micro-rate constants defining a multicompartmental model will be denoted as lowercase k to distinguish them from one-compartment rate constants, which are uppercase K since the latter may be obtained directly from an analysis of the C-T profile (e.g., $K_{el} = \lambda_1$). Finally, the central compartment is always denoted as 1, with higher numbers assigned to more slowly equilibrating compartments.

With a two-compartment model, three Vds may be calculated: the volume of the central compartment V_c or V_1, the peripheral compartment V_p or V_2, and the total volume of distribution in the body V_t or $V_1 + V_2$. As will be seen below, the actual Vd calculated from the data is dependent upon the method used; however, the only estimate of V_t, which can be broken into its component central and peripheral volumes, is the volume of distribution at steady-state Vd_{ss}.

When more complex models are presented in subsequent chapters, the K_{el} and K_a nomenclature may still be used to differentiate these first-order rate constants from other metabolic and pharmacodynamic effect parameters. Similarly, in some of these scenarios, α and β may still be used to denote the slopes of a biexponential model. However, most automated software packages utilize similar notation to λ_n and A_n to define the shapes of multiexponential C-T profiles and k_{xy} microconstants to define the underlying compartmental structure linked to the observed data. *When using any software package, the user should first relate the program's nomenclature to these basic parameters to ensure that the data are properly interpreted.*

Derivation of Rate Equations.   Now that we have the appropriate nomenclature, it is instructive to derive the equations for λ_n and A_n based on the microconstants that define the differential rate equation. For a two-compartment model after intravenous injection of dose D with elimination occurring from the central compartment, the following differential equation describes the rate of drug disposition:

$$dC_1 / dt = -(k_{12} + k_{10})\, C_1 + (k_{21})\, C_2 \qquad (7.38)$$

Processes that remove compound from the central compartment (k_{10} and k_{12}) are grouped together and have a negative rate since they result in a descending C-T profile. The only process that adds chemical to the central compartment (k_{21}), that is, redistribution from the peripheral compartment, is assigned a positive rate and results in an ascending C-T profile. The rate of this process is driven by the concentration of compound in the peripheral compartment. Note the similarity of this equation to the differential equation for absorption in a one-compartment model (equation 7.27). In this model, the only process that added drug to the central compartment was k_a, which therefore was assigned a positive sign, while the only process removing drug was $-K_{el}$. Similarly, as stressed throughout this text, the driving mass for this passive absorption process was the fraction of administered dose ($F\,X$) available for absorption. The power and essence of pharmacokinetic analysis is that the physiological processes driving drug disposition can be quantitated by using differential equations describing drug flux into and out of observable compartments. Most models are structured to reflect the central compartment, which is monitored via blood sampling, as the primary point of reference. Solution of the differential equation 7.38 by integration yields equations 7.36 or 7.37, which describe the biexponential C-T profile characteristic of a two-compartment open model.

The observed slopes λ_1 and λ_2 and intercepts A_1 and A_2 are related to the microconstants as

$$k_{21} = (A_1\lambda_2 + A_2\lambda_1)/(A_1 + A_2) \tag{7.39}$$

$$k_{10} = \lambda_1\lambda_2 / k_{21} \tag{7.40}$$

$$k_{12} = \lambda_1 + \lambda_2 - k_{21} - k_{10} \tag{7.41}$$

Similarly, each of the slopes now has a corresponding $T_{1/2}$ calculated as

$$T_{1/2\,\lambda_1} = 0.693 / \lambda_1 \text{ (Distribution)} \tag{7.42}$$

$$T_{1/2\,\lambda_2} = 0.693 / \lambda_2 \text{ (Elimination)} \tag{7.43}$$

The slope of the terminal phase of the C-T profile reflects the elimination $T_{1/2}$ and is the primary parameter used to calculate dosage regimens. Note that since $\lambda_1 >> \lambda_2$, $T_{1/2\,\lambda_1} << T_{1/2\,\lambda_2}$ and, at later time points (recall the five $T_{1/2}$ rule), distribution will be complete, and the biexponential equation 7.37 collapses to the monoexponential equation $Cp = A_2 e^{-\lambda_2 t}$. [Mathematically this is true because e raised to a very small negative exponent ~~t large~~ becomes zero since its limit L of (e^{-t}) as t approaches ∞ is 0]. This equation is similar in form to the one-compartment equation 7.15 except the intercept is now A_2 and not Cp_0, and the slope is $-\lambda_2$ and not K_{10}.

These differences are the basis for much confusion in pharmacokinetics when the data for a drug, truly described by a biexponential equation, are analyzed only at later post-distribution time points, and the monoexponential C-T profile observed is assumed to be described by a one-compartment model. As will be discussed below, the Vd calculated by this method erroneously uses A_2 (or B in the "$\alpha\beta$" nomenclature) as being equal to Cp_0 and thus overestimates the true Vd since A_2 or B is less than Cp_0. Dosage regimens determined using this approach will therefore administer the wrong dose since the true Vd is actually smaller.

This property of "disappearing" exponentials with large λ's at later time points provides the basis for analyzing polyexponential C-T profiles using the curve stripping approach (technically called the method of residuals) depicted in Figure 7.16 and discussed earlier in the context of absorption in Figure 7.11. To derive this residual line, one subtracts the slower process ($A_2\,e^{-\lambda_2 t}$) from the earlier time points described by the biexponential equation 7.37 ($Cp = A_1 e^{-\lambda_1 t} + A_2\,e^{-\lambda_2 t}$) to reveal the rapid component ($A_1 e^{-\lambda_2 t}$). The slopes and intercepts of these two lines can then be easily determined by the techniques described above for fitting monoexponential equations.

It is often difficult to accurately estimate distribution parameters when λ_1 is very rapid since early blood samples must be collected to determine the residual line. Recall that compartmental models assume that the drug is instantaneously distributed into the compartment being studied. Physiologically, for this to occur, drug must first circulate through the vascular system at a rate limited by the blood circulation time. In a large animal such as a horse or cow, this requires a few minutes, and thus very early samples (e.g., less than 5 minutes) will not have sufficient time for this mixing to occur. Secondly, small errors in sample timing result in a large percent error (1 minute off for a 5-minute sample; error is 20%), and thus the data obtained at very early time points are often extremely variable. In contrast, 5 minutes off for a 6-hour sample is only a 1% error, making estimates of terminal slopes much less variable.

It is important to stress that *when one is fitting an equation to a plasma concentration-time profile for pharmacokinetic purposes, this curve stripping process is assumed*. Some statisticians might elect to just split the line into two parts and determine the slopes. However, the slopes determined in this manner, which may be statistically correct, are not useful for pharmacokinetic analyses, and their insertion into all the equations presented is incorrect because the initial slope determined without stripping is in reality a composite of λ_1 and λ_2. This stripping concept arises from the principle of superposition, whereby an observed plasma concentration is the sum of all processes (absorption, distribution, elimination) involved in its disposition. These techniques will be fully discussed when their implementation in software packages is presented in Chapter 13.

C = central
P = peripheral

Volumes of Distribution.   There are three volumes of distributions to contend with: V_c or V_1, V_p or V_2, and $V_t = (V_1 + V_2)$. These are again calculated by a knowledge of intercepts and administered dose (assuming intravenous administration). The relevant intercept is Cp_0, which is now simply $A_1 + A_2$.

Vd$_{area}$, Vd (β) – estimate of Vt.

Vd = D/Cp, $V_t = V_1 + V_2 = V_{ss}$

$$V_1 = D/Cp_0 = D/(A_1 + A_2) \text{, } Cp_0 = A_1 + A_2 \tag{7.44}$$

$$Vd_{ss} = V_1 [(k_{12} + k_{21})/k_{21}] \tag{7.45}$$

$$V_2 = Vd_{ss} - V_1 \tag{7.46}$$

$$Vd(B) = D/B = D/A_2 \tag{7.47}$$

$$Vd_{area} = D/AUC \lambda_2 = D/(AUC \beta) \tag{7.48}$$

$$= Vd_\beta = (k_{10} V_1)/\lambda_2 \tag{7.49}$$

There is a great deal of debate on which volume of distribution should be used in a pharmacokinetic analysis. The answer is really dependent upon what the investigator wants to do with the data. The relationship between these estimates is

$$Vd(B) > Vd_{area} > Vd_{ss} > V_c \tag{7.50}$$

– analyzes data as one compartment

The easiest to discard is $Vd(B)$, the apparent volume of distribution by extrapolation, since it is often used when a complete analysis of the curve is avoided and only the terminal slope and its intercept A_2 is determined. As discussed above, this estimate completely ignores V_1. Similarly, V_c is defined as only the central compartment volume. It is the volume from which clearance is determined and is used in some infusion calculations.

The volume of distribution at steady state, Vd_{ss}, is the most "robust" estimate since it is mathematically and physiologically independent of any elimination process or con-

regimen - a systematic plan, esp. when designed to improve and maintain the health of a patient

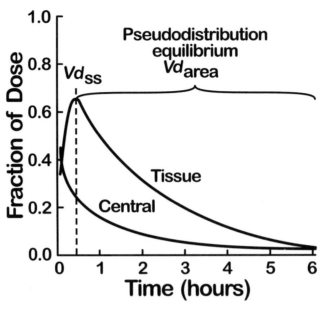

FIGURE 7.17. Relationship between Vd_{ss} and Vd_{area} for a drug described by a two-compartment model. Note that Vd_{ss} is only descriptive of the volume of distribution at the peak of the tissue compartment concentration versus time profile, while Vd_{area} describes the volume throughout the terminal elimination phase.

stant. It is the preferred Vd estimate for interspecies extrapolations and the study of the effects of altered physiology on Vd since it is independent of elimination. Theoretically, Vd_{ss} describes the Vd at only a single time point when the rate of elimination equals that of distribution. The point at which this occurs is the inflection point or bend in the C-T profile, which occurs because the more rapid tissue distribution phase has now peaked. This is best appreciated in Figure 7.17 when the concentrations in the central and tissue compartments are plotted.

Vd_{area} is often used when clinical dosage regimens are constructed (see equations 11.2, 11.6, and 11.12 in Chapter 11) because it reflects the area during the elimination phase of the curve, which predominates in any dosage regimen (see Figure 7.17). This is absolutely equivalent to Vd_β, the so-called volume of distribution at pseudodistribution equilibrium. If the rate of elimination is very prolonged (slow), as seen in severe renal disease, then the terminal slope of the concentration-time profile may approach zero (plateaus; $T_{1/2}$ becomes very long) which effectively "stretches out" the curve's inflection due to a plateau in the peripheral tissue compartment. Under this scenario, Vd_{area} becomes equal in value to Vd_{ss}

$$[\text{mathematically, } \underset{K_{el}\to 0}{L} (Vd_{area}) = Vd_{ss}].$$

$Vd_{area} \to Vd_{ss}$ as $K_{10} \to 0$

This is illustrated in Table 7.2, which shows the various Vd estimates actually determined for gentamicin in dogs with different levels of renal function using a two-compartment open model. Physiologically, Vd_{ss} actually increases in renal disease in these dogs. However, the mathematical dependence of Vd_{area} confounds this as its reduced value is secondary to the reduction in K_{el} due to reduced renal function.

Clearance. Knowing V_1, one can easily calculate the systemic clearance since Cl_B occurs from the central compartment and is essentially the same as a one-compartment model.

$$Cl = K_{10} V_1 \qquad (7.51)$$

$= K_{el} V_c$

TABLE 7.2. Pharmacokinetic Parameters for Gentamicin Administered Intravenously in Dogs with and Without Renal Disease

Parameter	Units	Normal Values	Values in Dogs with Renal Disease
Cl_B	(ml/min/kg)	3.66	1.55
k_{el}	(1/h)	1.45	1.01
$T_{1/2}$ (λ_2)	(min)	75	136
V_c	(L/kg)	0.15	0.11
Vd_{ss}	(L/kg)	0.23	0.28
Vd_{area}	(L/kg)	0.40	0.29
Vd_{area} / Vd_{ss}	–	1.74	1.03

Alternatively, Cl_B may be calculated using the intravenous infusion equation 7.22 presented earlier. The only difference is that with the more complex distribution kinetics presents in a multicompartmental model, the time to reach C_{ss} may be significantly longer.

Finally, Cl_B may also be determined using equation 7.18 based on AUC. In a two-compartment model, AUC may be calculated using slopes and intercepts by the relation

$$Cl_B = D/AUC, \qquad AUC = (A_1 / \lambda_1) + (A2 / \lambda2) \quad (?) \tag{7.52}$$

which can be generalized for a multicompartmental model to

$$AUC = \Sigma A_i / \lambda_i \tag{7.53}$$

Realize that this equation still requires fitting exponential equations to the C-T profile and, unlike other area methods discussed in Chapter 8 on noncompartmental models, first-order linear rate constants are assumed. However, this is a relatively robust technique to calculate many parameters and will be revisited where formulae for Vd_{ss} and other parameters may be determined.

Interpretation of Parameters. Using Vd_{ss} and Cl_B, equation 7.20 can again be used to calculate the overall $T_{1/2}$ of drug in the body. This $T_{1/2}$ reflects both distribution and elimination processes and is very useful as input into an interspecies allometric analysis. This is not equivalent to the terminal elimination half-life, $T_{1/2}$ (λ_2) and must be calculated from the Cl_B and Vd_{ss} parameters. Again as will be seen in Chapter 8, it is directly related to the mean residence time of drug in the body and is thus an excellent aggregate parameter for disposition.

The comparison of pharmacokinetic parameters across species brings up another concern related to parameter selection. If the elimination rate is very prolonged in a specific species (e.g., no metabolism, different type of kidneys, which restricts renal clearance), the calculated Vd_{area} between two species may be very different, while the Vd_{ss} may be the same. The disposition of a drug across species should use mathematically and physiologically independent estimates of Vd_{ss} and Cl_B. The real concern in any pharmacokinetic analysis of multicompartmental systems is that the Vd used is *appropriate* for the equation being employed to make predictions. As will be seen in Chapter 15, this is critical in the construction of dosage regimens, especially when renal disease is present.

Finally, as was presented for a one-compartment model, all of these approaches may be analyzed using urinary excretion data. The slopes in a urinary excretion plot reflect the λs determined from the C-T profile since k_{10} and not K_{renal} is rate-limiting. However, there are severe experimental restrictions on the ability to use urine data to model rapid distribution processes; it is difficult to accurately collect urine over very short time intervals since Δt should be less than the $T_{1/2}$ of the rate process being studied. When the typical $T_{1/2\ \gamma 1}$ is only a few minutes, and the distribution process starts immediately after drug administration, it is often impossible to collect accurate urine samples.

Absorption in a Two-Compartment Model. When an extravascular dose is administered as input into a two-compartment model (Figure 7.18), the differential equation defining this model is

$$V_1\, dC_1\,/\,dt = -(k_{12} + k_{10})\, C_1\, V_1 + k_{21}\, C_2\, V_2 + k_{01}\, X \qquad (7.54)$$

Note that the movement of drug in the central compartment is now driven by three different concentrations: C_1, C_2, and the fraction of the administered dose D that is available for absorption (X). There are a number of approaches to solve this model and various forms of the solution. An example of a plasma C-T profile for such a drug is depicted in Figure 7.19. The solution to this differential equation in exponential form is

$$C_p = k_{01} D\,/\,V_1[A_1{'}e^{-\lambda_1 t} + A_2{'}e^{-\lambda_2 t} - A_3{'}e^{-K_{01}t}] \qquad (7.55)$$

In this case, the intercepts $(A_n{'})$ are different from those obtained from an intravenous study (A_n) and significantly more complex since the "driving" concentrations in compartments one and two are now dependent upon the fraction absorbed in a fashion analogous to the terms of equation 7.28 seen for absorption in a one-compartment model:

$$A_1{'} = (k_{21} - \lambda_1)\,/\,[(k_{01} - \lambda_1)\,(\lambda_2 - \lambda_1)]$$
$$A_2{'} = (k_{21} - \lambda_2)\,/\,[(k_{01} - \lambda_2)\,(\lambda_1 - \lambda_2)] \qquad (7.56)$$
$$A_3{'} = (k_{21} - k_{01})\,/\,[(\lambda_1 - k_{01})\,(k_{01} - \lambda_2)]$$

Figure 7.19 depicts the C-T profile and the resulting residual lines that could be used to estimate the slopes and intercepts. However, a C-T profile such as this, which allows clear rectification of k_{01} from λ_1 is rare since even in this case, the two are of a similar order of magnitude, and independent values cannot be estimated. In fact, these residuals may only be determined from as few as two time points. Remembering that early points are often prone to large errors, even attempting this analysis may be futile. Depending on the ratio of rate constants, the C-T profile may even appear monoexponential. Workers have erroneously analyzed these profiles, neglecting to take into account the confounding of the absorption and distribution phases. The intercepts thus calculated would yield erroneous estimates of distribution volumes. The final complication is that absorption flip-flop may also occur, making selection of k_{01} and λs difficult. The only method to reliably address all of these problems is to conduct an independent intravenous bolus study using a two-compartment model and independently estimate λ_1 and λ_2 to arrive at an estimate of the absorbed dose. Even in this case, interindividual variability may make a unique model solution impossible for some drugs. This situation again supports the view that if the disposition of a drug is to be accurately modeled, the first step should be an intravenous injection so that the primary pharmacokinetic model may be unambiguously defined.

Similar to the situation with the one-compartment model above, a fractional absorption plot may be used to analyze these data. The approach used is the Loo-Riegelman method, which requires that both intravenous and extravascular dose studies be conducted in the

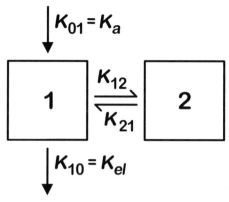

FIGURE 7.18. Generalized open two-compartment pharmacokinetic model with first-order absorption (K_{01}) into and elimination (K_{el}) from the central compartment. K_{12} and K_{21} represent intercompartmental constants reflecting distribution.

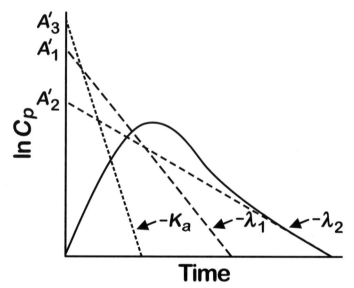

FIGURE 7.19. Semilogarithmic plasma concentration versus time profile generated using the two-compartment model in Figure 7.18.

same individual. In this case, k_{10} may be unambiguously determined from the intravenous study. The equation used to generate the fractional absorption plot is analogous to the Wagner-Nelson method (equation 7.35; Figures 7.12 and 7.13) and is as follows:

$$\frac{X_S(t)}{X_S(\infty)} = \frac{C_t + K_{10}AUC_t + (X_p)_t / V_1}{K_{10}AUC_\infty} \tag{7.57}$$

where $(X_p)_t$ is the amount of drug in the peripheral compartment at time t. Calculation of this amount requires solution of both intravenous and extravascular pharmacokinetic models using various techniques beyond the scope of this text. The advantage of this approach is that, like the Wagner-Nelson method, there is no assumption to the order of the absorption rate process, and thus complex absorption processes may be modeled.

Data Analysis and Its limitations.   Clearly, as pharmacokinetic models become more complex, the reader must question the wisdom of pursuing such analyses. In reality, there are mathematical limitations to the complexity of the model able to be fit to an experimental data set that is based on the "information density"; that is, how many data points are analyzed relative to how many parameters need to be calculated. This is similar to the statistical concept of *degrees of freedom,* which will be presented in Chapter 13 as a means of quantifying this dilemma. A primary strategy to overcome this is to simultaneously model both plasma and urine data, a process that improves estimates of all parameters. Population pharmacokinetic techniques (see Chapter 14) are also available that simultaneously can model the interindividual statistical variation.

In practice, there are better approaches to model complex absorption using noncompartmental strategies of residence times and linear system deconvolution analysis; these will be discussed in Chapter 13. The solution of differential equations into their constituent slope/intercept forms, and the definition of these in terms of the underlying micro-rate constant, are termed *analytical solution* for the model. In reality, modern software packages solve complex differential equations using techniques of *numerical integration*. The user defines the model on the basis of inputs and outputs or, in some cases, graphically defines a model such as depicted in Figures 7.3, 7.10, 7.15, and 7.18. The data are then inputted from all the sample matrices collected (e.g., plasma and urine), and the chosen model is numerically fitted to the data. Although this is easy to do, especially with modern graphical microcomputer software interfaces, one must still properly define the underlying model for the resulting analysis to make any sense.

The final consideration with two-compartmental models, and one that is even more serious for multicompartmental models, is the actual structure of the model studied. Until now, we have *assumed* that input into (absorption) and output from (elimination) the model are via the central compartment (model A) and, furthermore, that all samples are taken from this compartment and expressed as differential equations based on dC_1 / dt. Figure 7.20 illustrates other possible structures of the basic two-compartment model. Examples in which these might apply include implantation of a slow-release drug delivery device in a specific organ (model B) and when drug distributes to the organ before elimination (model C). The latter type of problem often occurs when the rate of distribution is actually slower than elimination, making the initial exponential term reflect elimination. For example, a very lipophilic chlorinated hydrocarbon may initially distribute extensively throughout the body and then slowly (periods of months) redistribute to the blood, where metabolism and elimination would then occur. The redistribution rate constant would be the rate-limiting process. All would generate C-T profiles described by the sum of exponential very similar to equation 7.55; however, realize that the equations (such as equation 7.56) that *link* these fitted parameters to the underlying micro-rate constants would be very different and, in some cases, unsolvable using analytical solutions. As will be presented in subsequent chapters, mixed-order models may be constructed in which some of the parameters are zero-order metabolic rates.

There are mathematical approaches used to quantify the uniqueness of any model relative to the data collected; that is, to determine the *structural identifiability* of the model. The reader should consult the literature to calculate the parameter (ϕ) whose value determines whether the model is uniquely identifiable, nonuniquely identifiable, or unidentifiable.

These considerations illustrate the assumptions inherent to constructing complex models that are too often forgotten when the results of such analyses are then analyzed. Models should be constructed using the principle of parsimony, whereby the fewest assumptions are made and the simplest models constructed.

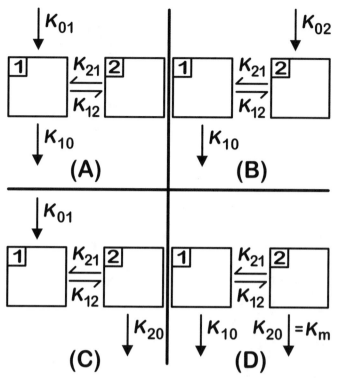

FIGURE 7.20. Four different two-compartment pharmacokinetic models. A, Absorption into and elimination from compartment 1; B, absorption into compartment 2 and elimination from compartment 1; C, absorption into compartment 1 and elimination from compartment 2; and D, intravenous administration with elimination from compartment 1 and metabolism to compartment 2.

MULTICOMPARTMENTAL MODELS

The final level of compartmental model complexity to be dealt with in this chapter is the three-compartment model depicted in Figure 7.21, which generates the C-T profile in Figure 7.22. The data are from studies conducted in the author's laboratory for the aminoglycoside antibiotic gentamicin in dogs, but the model is identical to that for similar work performed in horses and sheep. In this case, the drug distributes into two different compartments from the central compartment, one with rates faster (k_{12} / k_{21}) and the other with rates slower (k_{13} / k_{31}) than those for k_{10}. The slopes of the C-T profile for λ_1 primarily reflects the contribution of rapid distribution while λ_3, the terminal slope, primarily reflects the contribution of slower distribution into the so-called deep compartment. This model is applicable to many three-compartment drugs encountered in comparative medicine (e.g., aminoglycosides, tetracyclines, persistent chlorinated hydrocarbon pesticides). Drug elimination from the central compartment is primarily reflected in λ_2 or β and through general usage is termed the β elimination phase.

   These models are generally employed when experiments are conducted over long time frames and C-T profiles are monitored to low concentrations. If the data are truncated at earlier times, as shown in the insert in Figure 7.22, a normal two-compartment model is adequate to describe the data. However, as will be discussed in Chapter 17, the goal of a study is often to describe the tissue residue depletion profile of a drug in a food-producing animal, and thus the tissue C_3-T profile is of interest since it is the tissue used in establishing legal tolerances. As can be appreciated from Figure 7.22, each exponential phase describes the C-T profile over a specific range of concentrations and time frames. One

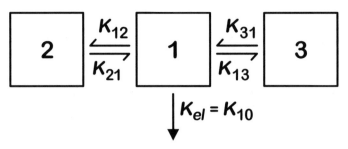

FIGURE 7.21. Three-compartment pharmacokinetic model after intravenous administration. Parameters are defined in text.

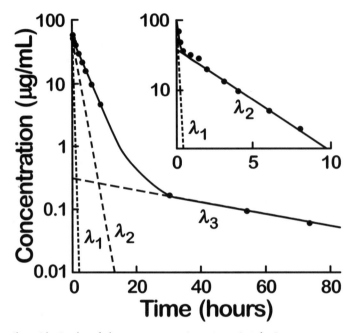

FIGURE 7.22. Semilogarithmic plot of plasma concentration versus time for intravenous gentamicin in the dog. Disposition is described by a three-compartment model when samples are collected for 80 hours and a two-compartment model when samples are collected for only 10 hours (insert).

must ensure that the appropriate parameters are used to predict the desired range of the Cp_t. If a model is misspecified and a terminal phase deleted, prediction of concentrations for a multiple dose regimen using λ_{n-1} as the rate limiting slope may underestimate the true λ_n controlling Cp since accumulation may have occurred in a deep compartment. Similarly, such misspecification will generate erroneous values for microconstants. These considerations are also important when fitting the models to the data since specific statistical weighting schemes may have to be used. An examination of Table 7.3 reveals this relation for experiments of different time frames and concentration ranges reported in the literature for gentamicin. The β phase elimination generates a $T_{1/2}$ of 0.5 to 2 hours, depending on species, which is closely correlated to renal glomerular filtration rate. Therefore, if the focus of a study is to examine effects of GFR on Cl_B, the λ_n corresponding to a β of $\approx$ 1.3 to 0.3 hours[-1] (0.693 / $T_{1/2}$) should be selected. Note here that one four-compartment model has been reported as a consequence of very early time samples detecting a very rapid distribution phase based on plasma $\rightarrow$ erythrocyte equilibration, requiring a model with two distribution components followed by elimination. In contrast,

TABLE 7.3. Correspondence of Pharmacokinetic Parameters for One-, Two-, Three-, and Four-Compartment Models for Intravenous Gentamicin

No. of Compartments	Study Duration (hours)	Slopes				Intercepts			
1	12	–	–	λ	–	–	–	A_1	–
		–	–	β	–	–	–	B	–
2	12	–	λ_1	λ_2	–	–	A_1	A_2	–
		–	α	β	–	–	A	B	–
2	$\geq \approx 50$	–	–	λ_1	λ_2	–	–	A_1	A_2
		–	–	β	γ	–	–	B	C
3	$\geq \approx 50$	–	λ_1	λ_2	λ_3	–	A_1	A_2	A_3
		–	α	β	γ	–	A	B	C
3	12	λ_1	λ_2	λ_3	–	A_1	A_2	A_3	–
		π	α	β	–	P	A	B	–
4	$\geq \approx 50$	λ_1	λ_2	λ_3	λ_4	A_1	A_2	A_3	A_4
		π	α	β	γ	P	A	B	C
4	≥ 60	λ_1	λ_2	λ_3	λ_4	A_1	A_2	A_3	A_4

the second four-compartment model is constructed with one distribution, one elimination, and two slow, deep compartment redistribution components. It is little wonder that confusion in the literature has occurred!

Models consisting of more than three compartments for unchanged parent drug have been used when the data are of sufficient quality as was the case with the four-compartment gentamicin model discussed above. In this case the drug exhibits sufficient distributional complexity that these models may be warranted. The polyexponential equation describing an *n*-compartment models is as follows:

$$Cp = \sum_{i=1}^{n} A_i e^{-\lambda_i t} \tag{7.58}$$

The differential equations needed to link these slopes and intercepts to the micro-rate constants are exceedingly complex and will not be developed here. Because of the serious concern of structural identifiability for such complex models based on plasma data alone, coupled with statistical concerns of adequate degrees of freedom based on limited plasma data, determination of micro-constants with any "real" meaning is suspect. This problem is addressed in the sample data set analysis in Chapter 13, in which even estimation of micro-constants from a two-compartment model was problematic. Complete equations for such models can be found in the Selected Readings.

The *AUC* can be calculated for an *n*-compartment model using equation 7.53, where *i* is summed from 1 to *n*. This also provides a useful method to determine how important a specific exponential phase is to overall drug disposition by dividing any component by the overall summed area ($\lambda_i / A_i \div AUC$), which becomes the fraction of the *AUC* determined by that phase. This allows one to assess just how much of an effect a terminal disposition phase may have on calculated values of Cl_B or Vd_{ss}.

In some circumstances the terminal λ may be influenced by a drug-reentry phenomenon. This is seen with drugs undergoing enterohepatic recycling (see Chapter 6) or from redistribution secondary to ion-trapping (see Chapter 4). In these cases, drug input may be intermittent, resulting in discontinuous λ slopes. Use of such confounded rate parameters would bias estimates of drug accumulation after multiple dosing (see Chapter 11), prediction of steady-state plasma concentrations, and estimation of withdrawal times.

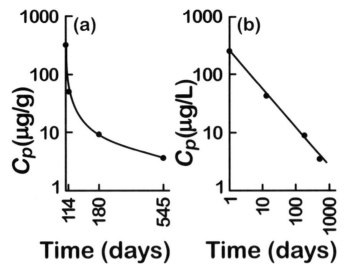

FIGURE 7.23. Semilogarithmic (left) and log-log (right) plots of gentamicin concentrations in rat kidneys, representing disposition described by exponential and power function equations, respectively.

Under these circumstances, more complex models that specifically take into account this continuous absorption should be employed.

Techniques are also available for solving these equations in terms of C_n, which becomes useful when tissue concentrations are studied. These models were once analyzed using analog computers; however, modern digital computers have made this a lost art and allow for construction of complex models using data collected from multiple matrices. This approach also increases model identifiability and increases degrees of freedom necessary for model solution.

The form of equation 7.58 can also be used to develop an alternate approach to handling models that may only be fit to an equation with a large number of exponential terms. In the gentamicin studies discussed above, we often obtained data that were best fitted by three- and four-term exponential equations. If one takes the limit of equation 7.58 as $n \to \infty$, an equation of the form results:

$$Cp = D\, At^{-a} \qquad (7.59)$$

This is a power function that forms the basis of the noncompartmental stochastic modeling approach. Figure 7.23 compares the multiexponential and power function analysis of gentamicin. The power function analysis only requires estimating two parameters and is more robust from a statistical perspective. However, its link to physiological reality is significantly different from that developed for compartmental models and is instead based on residence times (which will be introduced in Chapter 8) and the principle of "random walk." Additionally, unlike the exponential models, $T_{1/2}$ does not exist with a power exponent, and thus a different conceptual framework is needed to apply this to a clinical or field scenario.

When a tissue sample is taken, one is not measuring just concentrations in that tissue since its vascular and extracellular fluid components are actually part of the central compartment. Similar arguments can be made for other components. When one is looking at deep compartment disposition, this may be satisfactory since release from these depots is rate-limiting, making this tissue component larger than any other phase that has already reached equilibrium. Equations are available to fractionate a tissue mass into vascular, extracellular, and cellular components based again on Vd estimates. Tracers such as albumin or inulin may administered to directly derive these fractions. Protein and tissue binding may be directly assessed. Alternatively, tissue cages or microdialysis probes may be inserted into the tissue mass and extracellular kinetics directly modeled.

The dilemma facing the pharmacokineticist is determining the minimum number of exponential components to adequately describe the data. Chapter 13 will deal extensively with the statistical aspects of this curve fitting problem. However, in a compartmental framework, one is essentially asking, When are the micro-rate constants significantly different from one another such that the aggregate rates will affect the λs of the observed C-T profile? We touched upon this issue earlier when absorption was discussed in a two-compartment model. The impact on the analysis is that addition of compartments will affect the magnitude of the various volumes of distribution calculated. Recall the relation of Vd_B to Vd_{area} or Vd_{ss} in a two-compartment model when the distribution phase was ignored. The ratio of $[(k_{xy}:k_{yx}) / k_{el}]$ must generally be greater than about three for it to be distinguishable in an experiment. The construction of the actual ratio (k_{xy} / k_{yx}) or (k_{yx} / k_{xy}) determines whether the compartment could be considered rapidly versus slowly equilibrating, and thus whether it appears in the C-T profile as a λ_n greater or less than the so-called λ_β elimination slope. In some models, a biphasic elimination process could also occur if two physiologically separate mechanisms were responsible for excretion; however, the compartmental model would have to reflect this structure with two elimination rate constants k_{e1} and k_{e2} probably coming from two separate rapidly equilibrating central compartments.

There is an additional limitation inherent to the analysis of drugs with deep compartment characteristics when, over the time course of an experiment, k_{xy} / k_{yx} does not reach equilibrium. In this case, the redistribution microconstant for this compartment (k_{yx}) may be approaching zero relative to the other constants. This results in this process appearing to be the elimination from the "perspective" of the central compartment. In these cases, k_{xy} will appear as a component of k_{el} and become confounded with Cl_B. This deep compartment will not appear in Vd_{ss}. Dosage regimens that utilize these values will overestimate the Cl_B and underestimate Vd_{ss}. This was seen with drugs or xenobiotics that strongly bind to tissues (e.g., cisplatin, gentamicin). Studies over longer time frames would detect this redistribution. The sensitivity of k_{xy} to inadequate early distribution data will be addressed in Chapter 13.

Any parameter that is dependent upon the ratio of k_{el} to the distributional micro-rate constants will be sensitive to the model structure. These so-called hybrid parameters include the λ_n, A_n, V_n, and Vd_{area} or Vd_λ. In contrast, Cp_0, Vd_{ss}, and Cl_B will be independent, as will the $T_{1/2}$ calculated according to equation 7.20 using Vd_{ss} as the Vd estimate. This realization is the pharmacokinetic basis that supports the use of noncompartmental models described in the next chapter as a very powerful tool in analyzing drug disposition.

In many cases, very complex multicompartment models are solely used as a *tool* to simultaneously analyze multiple sample matrices or metabolites. Compartments are constructed specifically for metabolites (model D in Figure 7.20) since a fraction of the parent drug is eliminated from the central compartment. However, the Vd for the metabolite may be different from that of the parent drug. This was the case in the model in Figure 6.3 (see Chapter 6). Finally, as presented in subsequent chapters, when a compound is extensively bound to either plasma or tissue proteins, this binding may often be incorporated into a model since only the unbound (f) drug is distributed through these various compartments. Some workers have used compartments to model this, although Chapter 9 will develop other approaches. Partial differential equations would have to be written and numerical methods, as mentioned above, used to obtain parameter estimates. In fact, such models are often constructed solely to aid their input into packages in which multiple matrices, metabolites, and tissue binding are simultaneously modeled. Alternatively, they may be used to simulate C-T profiles to compare to the observed data so that a realistic model may then be used to analyze the drug under study.

Example of a Multi-Matrix Compartmental Analysis: Parathion in Pigs. We will conclude this chapter by illustrating a very complex model our laboratory has utilized to describe topical application of the pesticide parathion in pigs. We employed the multicompartmental scheme depicted in Figure 7.24 to analyze parathion and its metabolites paraoxon, p-nitrophenol (PNP), and PNP-glucuronide (metabolic pathway depicted in Chapter 6, Figure 6.1) in blood, urine, feces, and tissues from intravenous and topical *in vivo* studies using the CONSAAM software package. Since low concentrations of compounds were studied, metabolic rates were first-order. Additionally, we integrated these models with data from *in vitro* porcine skin models. This allowed us to probe regional absorption differences and study the effects of cutaneous metabolism on disposition and tissue residues. This modeling exercise utilized radiolabeled parathion in 20 pigs. Metabolites were separated by high-performance liquid chromatographic analysis of plasma, blood, and urine. This model is far from being mathematically unique. In order to experimentally validate this model, eight pigs were used to model intravenous and topical PNP disposition according to Figure 7.25, which was constructed to mirror the parathion model. We assumed that since PNP is the final metabolite produced in this process, that it would be most sensitive to modeling errors and structural misspecifications.

This model also illustrates many of the concepts of drug metabolism presented in Chapter 6. Metabolism in the systemic central compartments (#s 1, 11, 12, 13) was postulated on the basis of the high hepatic biotransformation capacity. It was previously demonstrated that in rat plasma, parathion was directly degraded into PNP ($k_{1,12}$ in our scheme) and was the dominant route of parathion metabolism for the first 15 to 30 minutes after intravenous administration. This is followed by activation of parathion to paraoxon and hydrolysis of parathion. The enzymes determined to be involved in blood degradation include esterases, proteases, erythrocyte cholinesterase, serum butylcholinesterase, B-esterases, and some plasma proteins. Our compartments 17 and 60 may be partially comprised of nervous tissue, such as the brain, as well as other lipophilic tissues. Previous rodent studies suggest that only parathion and paraoxon could be found in brain after intravenous administration. The pattern of cutaneous metabolism / distribution / absorption was specifically structured to reflect current understanding. Transport between compartments 2 and 1, as well as between 2 and 3, could be approximated by a one-way process since $k_{2,3} >> k_{3,2}$, and $k_{2,1} >> k_{1,2}$. Assuming this, one can calculate the relevant significance of cutaneous metabolism as compared to local skin distribution and absorption of parathion by comparing rate-constant ratios for each component. This ratio approach is a useful tool to probe the relative importance of each one-way leaving process in the overall output from a given compartment. However, if the two compartments are linked by a two-way process with similar orders of magnitude, the results may be suspect since significant back transport would affect the net flux from that compartment. This approach was also used to assess the significance of cutaneous biotransformation relative to hepatic metabolism using the ratio of the micro-rate constants as the relevant parameter.

Paraoxon produced by the liver will enter the systemic circulation and distribute to extrahepatic tissues. However, paraoxon will react with blood enzymes and stoichiometrically destroy paraoxon through phosphorylation of these nontarget sites. When paraoxon concentration is very low secondary to a very low parathion dose, hepatic protein phosphorylation constitutes the major route of paraoxon degradation. This emphasizes that factors such as parent compound dosage, relative rates of activation and degradation

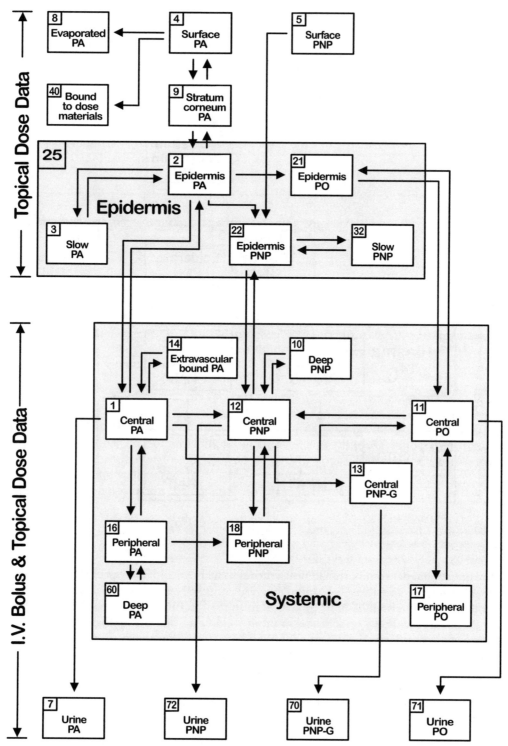

FIGURE 7.24. Multicompartmental pharmacokinetic model used to study parathion and its metabolites after topical and intravenous administration to pigs. Metabolic pathway and identity of metabolites were presented in Figure 6.2 (see Chapter 6). Topical dosing data used *in vitro–in vivo* data to model absorption. Parent and metabolite concentrations were determined in plasma, urine, and tissue at termination of the experiment. PA, parathion; PO, paraoxon; PNP, ρ-nitrophenol, PNP-G, PNP-glucuronide. (For further detail, see publications by Qiao et al in Selected Readings.)

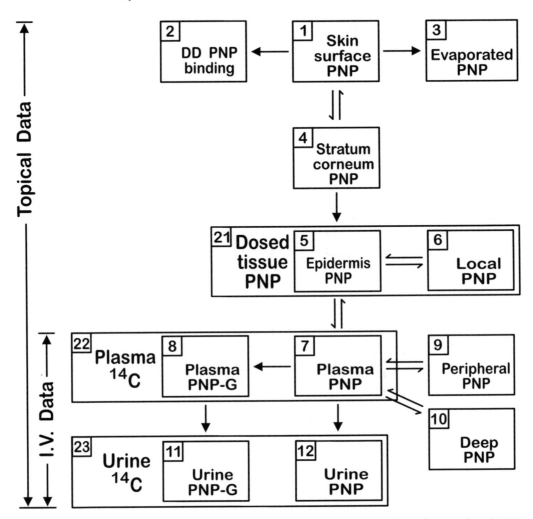

FIGURE 7.25. Multicompartmental pharmacokinetic model used to study disposition of *p*-nitrophenol (PNP) after intravenous administration in pigs. These data were used to validate PNP parameters obtained from analysis described in Figure 7.24.

of the metabolite paraoxon, transit times through the liver, and anatomical localization of the enzymes catalyzing these sequential reactions must all be taken into account when extrapolating any pharmacokinetic model to an *in vivo* setting. This is the primary reason that a model is good only under these limiting conditions, and the biological system must be "stressed" in order to validate model predictions. This was the motivation to independently study PNP disposition since it is the terminal metabolite in the parathion $\Rightarrow$ paraoxon $\Rightarrow$ PNP sequence and would be exquisitely sensitive to model misspecification. Finally, systemic availability of parathion and its metabolites in all compartments was also investigated using area methods, which will be introduced in the next chapter. The original manuscripts should be consulted for details of the modeling and data analysis.

CONCLUSION

Compartmental modeling concepts and techniques have defined the discipline of pharmacokinetics and continue to be extremely useful tools. One- and two-compartment analyses form the basis for most models used in human and comparative medicine. These two models also serve as the foundation upon which many of the other techniques now to be developed are based. Modern computers have facilitated the analysis of these data to the point that the user no longer has to derive all of the relevant differential equations. However, when compartmental schemes are assumed, the defining model is also implied, and thus the cautious investigator must be aware of the numerous caveats presented in this chapter.

SELECTED READINGS

Baggot, J.D. 1977. *Principles of Drug Disposition in Domestic Animals: The Basis of Veterinary Clinical Pharmacology.* Philadelphia: W.B. Saunders Co.

Benet, L.Z. 1972. General treatment of linear mammillary models with elimination from any compartment as used in pharmacokinetics. *Journal of Pharmaceutical Sciences.* 61:536-541.

Brown, S.A., and J.E. Riviere. 1991. Comparative pharmacokinetics of aminoglycoside antibiotics. *Journal of Veterinary Pharmacology and Therapeutics.* 14:1-35.

Brown, S.A., G.L. Coppoc, and J.E. Riviere. 1986. Effect of dose and duration of therapy on gentamicin tissue residues in sheep. *American Journal of Veterinary Research.* 47:2373-2379.

Brown, S.A., J.E. Riviere, G.L. Coppoc, and L.P. Dix. 1986. Superiority of the power function over exponential functions for prediction of renal gentamicin residues in sheep. Analysis of terminal phase gentamicin pharmacokinetic data. *Journal of Veterinary Pharmacology and Therapeutics.* 9:341-346.

Byron, P.R., and R.E. Notari. Critical analysis of "flip-flop" phenomenon in two-compartment pharmacokinetic model. *Journal of Pharmaceutical Science.* 65:1140-1144.

Chiou, W.L. 1981. The physiological significance of the apparent volume of distribution, Vd_{area} or $Vd_{ß}$, in pharmacokinetic studies. *Research Communications in Chemical Pathology and Pharmacology.* 33:499-508.

De Biasi, J. 1989. Four open mammillary and caternary compartment models for pharmacokinetic study. *Journal of Biomedical Engineering.* 11:467-470.

DiStefano, J.J., and E.M. Landaw. 1984. Multiexponential, multicompartmental, and non-compartmental modeling. I. Methodological limitations and physiological interpretations. *American Journal of Physiology.* 246:R651-R664.

Fleishaker, J.C., and R.B. Smith. 1987. Compartmental model analysis in pharmacokinetics. *Journal of Clinical Pharmacology.* 27:922-926.

Gibaldi, M., and D. Perrier. 1972. Drug elimination and apparent volume of distribution in multicompartmental systems. *Journal of Pharmaceutical Sciences.* 61:952-954.

Gibaldi, M., and D. Perrier. 1982. *Pharmacokinetics,* 2ed. New York: Marcel Dekker.

Greenblat, D.J., D.R. Abernethy, and M. Divoll. 1983. Is volume of distribution at steady state a meaningful kinetic variable? *Journal of Clinical Pharmacology.* 23:391-400.

Jacobs, J.R. 1988. Analytical solution to the three-compartment pharmacokinetic model. *IEEE Transactions on Biomedical Engineering.* 35:763-765.

Jacobs, J.R., S.L. Shafer, J.L. Larsen, and E.D. Hawkins. 1990. Two equally valid interpretations of the linear multicompartment mammillary pharmacokinetic model. *Journal of Pharmaceutical Sciences.* 79:331-333.

Jusko, W.J., and M. Gibaldi. Effects of change in elimination on various parameters of the two-compartment open model. *Journal of Pharmaceutical Sciences.* 61:1270-1273.

Labat, C., K. Mansour, M.F. Malmary, M. Terrissol, and J. Oustrin. 1987. A variable re-absorption time-delay model for pharmacokinetics of drugs. *European Journal of Drug Metabolism and Pharmacokinetics.* 12:129-133.

Loo, J.C.K., and S. Riegelman. 1968. New method for calculating the intrinsic absorption rate of drugs. *Journal Pharmaceutical Science.* 57:918-928.

Notari, R.E. 1980. *Biopharmaceutics and Clinical Pharmacokinetics,* 3ed. New York: Marcel Dekker.

O'Flaherty, E.J. 1981. *Toxicants and Drugs: Kinetics and Dynamics.* New York: John Wiley & Sons.

Pecile, A., and A. Rescigno. 1987. *Pharmacokinetics. Mathematical and Statistical Approaches to Metabolism and Distribution of Chemicals and Drugs.* New York: Plenum Press.

Qiao, G.L., and J.E. Riviere. 1995. Significant effects of application site and occlusion on the pharmacokinetics of cutaneous penetration and biotransformation of parathion in vivo in swine. *Journal of Pharmaceutical Sciences.* 84:425-432.

Qiao, G.L., P.L. Williams, and J.E. Riviere. 1994. Percutaneous absorption, biotransformation and systemic disposition of parathion in vivo in swine. I. Comprehensive pharmacokinetic model. *Drug Metabolism and Disposition.* 22:459-471.

Riegelman, J.L., and M. Rowland. 1968. Concept of a volume of distribution and possible errors in evaluation of this parameter. *Journal of Pharmaceutical Sciences.* 57:128-133.

Riegelman, J.L., and M. Rowland. 1968. Shortcomings in pharmacokinetic analysis by conceiving the body to exhibit properties of a single compartment. *Journal of Pharmaceutical Sciences.* 57:128-133.

Riviere, J.E. 1982. Paradoxical increase in aminoglycoside body clearance in renal disease when volume of distribution increases. *Journal of Pharmaceutical Sciences.* 71:720-21.

Riviere, J.E. 1982. Limitations on the physiologic interpretation of aminoglycoside body clearance derived from pharmacokinetic studies. *Research Communications in Chemical Pathology and Pharmacology.* 38:31-42.

Segre, G. 1982. Pharmacokinetics—Compartmental representation. *Pharmacology and Therapeutics.* 17:111-127.

Segre, G. 1984. Relevance, experiences, and trends in the use of compartmental models. *Drug Metabolism Reviews.* 15:7-53.

Simon, W. 1987. *Mathematical Techniques for Biology and Medicine.* New York: Dover Press.

Wagner, J.G. 1975. *Fundamentals of Clinical Pharmacokinetics.* Hamilton, IL: Drug Intelligence Publications.

Wagner, J.G. 1983. Significance of ratios of different volumes of distribution in pharmacokinetics. *Biopharmaceutics and Drug Disposition.* 4:263-270.

Wagner, J.G., and E. Nelson. 1968. Percent absorbed time plots derived from blood level and/or urinary excretion data. *Journal Pharmaceutical Sciences.* 52:610-611.

Welling, P.G., and F.L.S. Tse. 1995. *Pharmacokinetics: regulatory, Industrial, and Academic Perspectives*. New York: Marcel Dekker.

Wijnand, H.P. 1988. Pharmacokinetic model equations for the one- and two-compartment models with first-order processes in which absorption and exponential elimination or distribution rate constants are equal. *Journal of Pharmacokinetics and Biopharmaceutics*. 16:109-127.

Williams, P.L. 1990. Structural identifiability of pharmacokinetic models—Compartments and experimental design. *Journal of Veterinary Pharmacology and Therapeutics*. 13:121-131.

Williams, P.L., D. Thompson, G.L. Qiao, N.A. Monteiro-Riviere, R.L. Baynes, and J.E. Riviere. 1996. The use of mechanistically defined chemical mixtures (MDCM) to assess component effects on the percutaneous absorption and cutaneous disposition of topically-exposed chemicals. II. Development of a general dermatopharmacokinetic model for use in risk assessment. *Toxicology and Applied Pharmacology*. 141:487-496.

Zierler, K. 1981. A critique of compartmental analysis. *Annual Reviews of Biophysics and Bioengineering*. 10:531-562.

8

Noncompartmental Models

As discussed in the last chapter, compartmental models have become the primary approach to pharmacokinetics. Only in the last 15 years has there been any indication of a migration in pharmacokinetics to noncompartmental methods. Noncompartmental models were first developed and applied to radiation decay analysis and remain dominant in the physical and biological science literature for general applications. Since their first application to problems in pharmacokinetics by Yamaoka in 1979, noncompartmental methods have grown steadily in use. This relatively new approach is for the most part based on classical statistical moment theory.

Technically, the term *noncompartmental* used in reference to classical pharmacokinetics is somewhat misleading. The data that are analyzed with statistical moments are typically plasma concentration measures, which implies that at least a one- (central) compartmental model structure exists since behavior of the drug in the body is being linked to the plasma C-T profile. There is simply no way to avoid that assumption. In other words, theoretically, any "noncompartmental" analysis has a compartmental equivalent. Furthermore, when noncompartmental models are solved by fitting polyexponential equations to data, an assumption of first-order rate processes is made. In fact, some would argue that a multicompartmental structure is implied since the intercepts and slopes of the C-T profile are solutions to multicompartment differential equations. However, when the data are analyzed solely by computation of areas under curves (e.g., application of the trapezoid method), as will be presented shortly, this limitation is not present since equations are not being fitted to data. In many ways, this is the strength of this approach.

Those who prefer noncompartmental methods usually do not think of their models in terms of compartmental infrastructure, whereas those who prefer compartmental methods link their observed models to the micro-rate constants and different volumes (e.g., V_1, V_2) of constitutive compartments as discussed in Chapter 7. From a mathematical perspective, noncompartmental methods are somewhat limited in application for pharmacokinetics, but their advantage (i.e., that of obviating the necessity to deliberately commit to a specific model) is ample motivation for many investigators to use them. Additionally, as

---

Co-authored by Dr. Patrick L. Williams

discussed in the previous chapter, many multicompartmental models become too complex for the data at hand since statistically sound estimates of each slope (λ_i) and intercept (A_i) must be obtained. Solution of the micro-rate constants and volumes for individual compartments becomes ambiguous, but is not necessary if the focus of the study is an aggregate description of drug disposition, which may be obtained with estimates of Cl_B and Vd_{ss}. There are many applications in which similar endpoints are required and the assumptions inherent to defining specific compartments become unnecessary. These include, among others, the design of dosage regimens and interspecies extrapolations.

STATISTICAL MOMENT THEORY

We will begin with an overview of the basic tenets of statistical moment theory, which is a component of the more general stochastic modeling approach. Suppose one could observe a single molecule, from the time it is administered into the body $(t = 0)$ until it is eventually eliminated $(t = t_{el})$. Clearly, t_{el} is not predictable. This individual molecule could be eliminated during the first minute or could reside in the body for weeks. If, however, one looks at a large number of molecules collectively, their behavior appears much more regular. The collective, or *mean* time of residence, of all the molecules in the dose, is called the *mean residence time* (MRT; t). This is classically (and occasionally incorrectly, see below) based on plasma concentration data but has meaning for almost any mathematical function, $f(t)$. The MRT of $f(t)$ is defined as

$$MRT = \frac{\int_0^\infty t\, f(t)dt}{\int_0^\infty f(t)dt} \tag{8.1}$$

where it is assumed only that the two integrals exist. MRT can be interpreted as a mean of some variable only if $f(t)$ or

$$\frac{f(t)}{\int_0^\infty f(t)dt}$$

can be shown to be the *probability density function (pdf)* for that variable. By definition, pdf refers to a continuous random variable X [denoted $f(x)$], and must satisfy the following:

(1) $f(x) \geq 0$

(2) $\int_{-\infty}^\infty f(x)dx = 1$

(3) $\int_a^b f(x)dx = p > 0$

In pharmacokinetics applications, $f(t)$ is typically plasma concentration and in this context is commonly symbolized $C(t)$ $(= Cp_t)$. Historically, the mean residence time refers to drug in plasma. If equation 8.1 is rewritten in terms of $C(t)$,

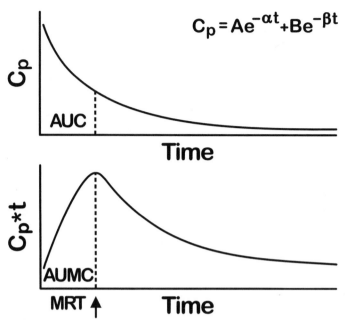

$$C_p = Ae^{-\alpha t} + Be^{-\beta t}$$

FIGURE 8.1.   Plasma concentration versus time (C-T) and its first-moment (CT-T) plots demonstrating AUC, AUMC, and MRT.

$$MRT = \frac{\int_0^\infty tC(t)dt}{\int_0^\infty C(t)dt} = \frac{AUMC}{AUC} \tag{8.2}$$

the denominator of equation 8.1 is the area under the curve (AUC), already repeatedly encountered in this text and presented in the last chapter when the plasma C-T profile was integrated to derive equation 7.18. The numerator is known as the area under the [first] moment curve (AUMC), which is the CT-T profile. AUC and AUMC are depicted in Figure 8.1.

Chanter has shown that plasma concentration may not be a mathematically legitimate function for a pdf, and thus the calculated MRT for plasma would be invalid. The problem occurs when the elimination flux (mass/time) is not proportional to C(t), or when a significant fraction of the dose either never leaves the (plasma) space or spends time in another space before being eliminated. Technically, the MRT, calculated from samples taken following an intravenous bolus injection, addresses only those molecules that are eliminated from the body at a rate proportional to C(t). Therefore, the caveat is that elimination must be at least first order, and only molecules that stay in the plasma (until elimination) and are eventually eliminated are addressed. This limitation also had applied to compartmental models for they were defined with k_{el} being a first-order elimination rate constant from the central compartment. Such assumptions also imply that sinks and temporary reservoirs are generally not mathematically permissible. As discussed in Chapter 7, this is analogous to using an n-1 compartment model when an n-compartmental model really is required. It also holds when a molecule distributes and irreversibly binds to tissue as described for drugs such as gentamicin and cisplatin. In these cases, redistribution might not be detectable from the missing deep compartment, and k_{1n} would be mistakenly interpreted as being part of the elimination process. The MRT estimate will be biased unless what is measured satisfies these requirements.

As long as the above limitations are understood (many of which apply to compartmental modeling), their application remains a powerful means of practical analysis. Furthermore, a very general (always true and applicable) definition of MRT requires only that $f(t)$ in equation 8.1 be the elimination flux (mass transfer, mass/time). Although this quantity is not typically measurable *in vivo*, it is in *ex vivo* and *in vitro* systems, which are enjoying increasing use in the forefront of research due to recent technological advances. Despite these caveats, the MRT is a very useful parameter to describe drug disposition.

The MRT could be thought of as the statistical moment analogy to the half-life ($T_{1/2}$), and it is inversely related to the first-order elimination rate of a one-compartment open model:

$$MRT_{IV} = \frac{1}{k_{el}} \qquad (8.3)$$

Rearranging demonstrates that $k_{el} = 1 / MRT_{iv}$. Recalling equation 7.12 (see Chapter 7), where $T_{1/2} = 0.693 / k_{el}$, substitution gives us

$$T_{1/2} = 0.693 \cdot MRT \qquad (8.4)$$

The MRT thus becomes an excellent parameter to describe the length of drug persistence in the body, much as the half-life is used in many linear pharmacokinetic models. The $T_{1/2}$ used in this context is the elimination $T_{1/2}$ in the body, and not that calculated from the terminal exponential phase as described in Chapter 7 for multicompartmental models.

The MRT represents the time point at which 63.2% of the drug has been eliminated from the body. If one takes the equation for a monoexponential C-T profile (see Chapter 7, equation 7.15) and solves for t = MRT, then $Cp = Cp_0 \, e^{-kel \, MRT}$. However, from equation 8.3 we know that MRT = $1/k_{el}$, thus at t = MRT, $Cp = Cp_0 \, e^{-kel \, (1 / kel)} = Cp_0 \, e^{-1} = 0.368 \, Cp_0$. Therefore, at t = MRT, 36.8% of the available dose remains in the body and 63.2% has been eliminated. Note that if all drug were excreted in the urine, one could simply estimate MRT as the time needed to recover 63.2% of the administered dose in the urine. MRT is also the time point at which the volume of distribution equals Vd_{ss}.

If the dose of drug is administered by intravenous infusion, the MRT_{iv} may be calculated as

$$MRT_{iv} = MRT_{infusion} - (\text{Infusion Time}) / 2 \qquad (8.5)$$

where $MRT_{infusion}$ is simply calculated from the observed data using equation 8.2.

MRT of zero order process is ½ of the length of the process

CALCULATION OF MOMENTS

The primary task of model-independent or noncompartmental methods is the direct estimation of the moments from data. This essentially is determining the relevant AUCs and moments from the C-T profile. *Some workers have thus referred to statistical moment analysis simply as SHAM (slopes, heights, areas, and moments) analysis to stress that these are the only data requirements for solution of these models*. However, this acronym implies that the areas are being determined using exponential-based formulae for calculating AUCs as presented in the method of Chapter 7. Other techniques ranging from trapezoidal analysis to planimetry do not require curve-fitting analysis. When the C-T profile is described by a polyexponential equation of the form $f(t) = A_i\, e^{-\lambda_i t}$, equation 7.53 (AUC $= \Sigma\, A_i\, /\, \lambda_i$)(see Chapter 7) can be generally used to determine AUC. The AUMC may then be calculated as

$$(8.6) \qquad\qquad\qquad AUMC = \Sigma\, A_i\, /\, (\lambda_i)^2$$

This technique requires fitting an exponential function to the C-T profile and, as alluded to earlier and in Chapter 7, this is equivalent to assuming a linear multicompartmental pharmacokinetic model.

Truly noncompartmental analysis uses geometrical techniques to estimate area. With planimetry, one simply plots the concentration-versus-time profile on regular graph paper, cuts out the profile and weighs the paper. A modern extension of this approach is to fit a C-T and CT-T profile (Figure 8.1) to any mathematical function (e.g., spline regression) which could determine the relevant AUC and AUMC, respectively. These techniques make no assumption about the nature of the $f(t)$ that generated the profiles; however, nuances in the statistical regression techniques used cause some problems. Finally, numerical integration techniques may be used to directly calculate these values.

The Trapezoidal Method for Estimating Areas Under Curves.   The simplest and most commonly used method for estimating area under any curve is the Trapezoidal Rule, which will be formally presented in this chapter. The application of this technique is important to master since it is the primary method used to assess bioavailability by numerous techniques as presented in Chapter 7,

$$(8.7) \qquad\qquad\qquad AUC = \sum_{n=1}^{N} \frac{C_n + C_{n+1}}{2}(t_{n+1} - t_n)$$

where the summation is over N trapezoids, formed by n + 1 data points. This algorithm is quick and, if enough data points are available, relatively accurate. It is also a simple algorithm to implement on a computer. When plasma concentration (or any observed tissue data) versus time data are plotted on a Cartesian graph, the area under each pair of connected points describes a trapezoid (except when one of the points has zero value, in which case one of the legs of the trapezoid has zero length, making a triangle) (see Chapter 3, Figure 3.13). The area under the entire curve is then the sum of the areas of the individual trapezoids, which can easily be calculated. The estimation of moments is the summed trapezoids plotted on a CT-T graph. These techniques can be effected in a simple spreadsheet application. The advantages of using computers over drawing plots by hand (few laboratories do this anymore) include speed, precision, and accuracy. A good PC application can produce areas as precise and accurate as the sampled data, whereas a hand-drawn graph often lacks precision, especially when used for planimetry.

The data in Table 8.1 and plotted in Figure 8.2 constitute a typical plasma concentration profile that might be obtained following a bolus intravenous injection of a drug with a biological half-life of 1 hour. This particular example illustrates an ideal experiment because its duration was sufficient to ensure that the concentration would fall to zero by the end of the experiment. For drugs that have long half-lives, this is often difficult or impractical, so more typically, an observed profile is open-ended. For example, Figure 8.3 illustrates such a case, outlining the trapezoids formed by the sampled points. Although there is important information in an AUC derived from a profile lacking closure, as a standard measure to be compared among several drugs, the AUC must be calculated to infinite time. Furthermore, the complete area is required for calculating plasma clearance

TABLE 8.1. Statistical Moments Calculations

Time (h)	C(t)	Actual Trap. areas	Estimated Trap. areas	Actual Cum. AUC	Estimated Cum. AUC	Actual Cum. AUMC
0.00	56.00	—	—	0.00	—	0.00
0.25	47.09	12.85	12.89	12.85	12.89	1.56
0.50	39.60	10.81	10.84	23.66	23.72	5.58
1.00	28.00	16.73	16.90	40.40	40.62	17.88
2.00	14.00	20.20	21.00	60.60	61.63	47.03
3.00	7.00	10.10	10.50	70.70	72.13	71.71
4.00	3.50	5.05	5.25	75.75	77.38	89.10
6.00	0.88	3.79	4.38	79.54	81.76	107.20
8.00	0.22	0.95	1.09	80.49	82.86	113.62
12.00	0.01	0.30	0.47	80.79	83.32	116.34

Time (h)	C(t)	Eq. 8.9 -est. Cum. AUMC	Eq. 8.11 - est. Cum. AUMC	Actual MRT (h)	Eq. 8.9 - est. MRT (h)	Eq. 8.11 - est. MRT (h)
0.00	56.00	0.00	0.00	—	—	—
0.25	47.09	1.61	1.56	0.12	0.13	0.12
0.50	39.60	5.67	5.59	0.24	0.24	0.24
1.00	28.00	18.35	18.02	0.44	0.45	0.44
2.00	14.00	49.86	48.36	0.78	0.81	0.78
3.00	7.00	76.12	74.04	1.01	1.06	1.03
4.00	3.50	94.50	92.13	1.18	1.22	1.19
6.00	0.88	116.39	113.14	1.35	1.42	1.38
8.00	0.22	124.05	120.59	1.41	1.50	1.46
12.00	0.01	128.71	124.97	1.44	1.54	1.50

Data columns from left to right: simulated blood sample times (hours); drug concentrations (mg/mL); simulated trapezoid area (mg·h/mL); estimated trapezoid area (mg·h/mL, equation 8.7); simulated cumulative AUC (mg·h/mL); estimated cumulative AUC (mg·h/mL, equation 8.7); simulated cumulative AUMC (mg·h^2/mL); estimated cumulative AUMC (mg·h^2/mL, equation 8.9); estimated cumulative AUMC (mg·h^2/mL, equation 8.11); simulated MRT (hours); estimated MRT (hours, using equation 8.9); estimated MRT (hours, using equation 8.11). Although normally only calculated at the final sample point, the MRT is calculated at each sample point here for illustration of the importance of using a complete experimental data set for statistical moments.

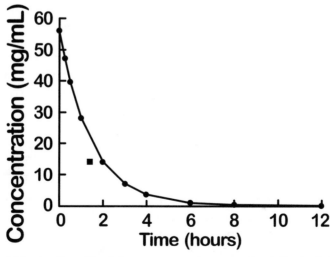

FIGURE 8.2. Typical (simulated) profile of plasma concentration versus time following bolus intravenous dose (k_{el} = 0.693 h^{-1}, C_0 = 56 mg/mL) used to generate data set in Table 8.1 and area examples in this section. The actual AUC of this C-T profile is 80.79 mg·h/mL. The single square point at (1.44,14.00) on the plot is the center of gravity (P_c) for the profile, as calculated from eq. 8.27.

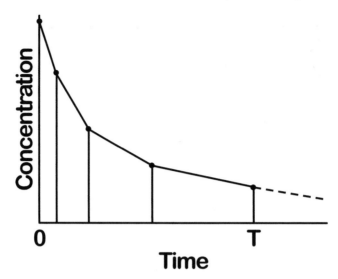

FIGURE 8.3.   Trapezoids formed from sampled concentration versus time data for calculation of areas. To estimate the total AUC, the curve must be extrapolated beyond the ultimate sample time, T, to infinity (dashed line).

and total absorption. In cases in which samples cannot be taken until the concentration drops to zero, the curve must be extrapolated to infinity.

The simplest and most common method to estimate this is by "end correction." This method involves calculating the area from the last sample measure, C_T, to infinite time and adding this value to the truncated area determined by the sum of the trapezoids. To calculate the terminal area from time, T, to infinity, this portion of the curve is treated as a separate profile. This profile is a triangle with a height of $C_0 = C_T$. The slope of the C-T profile determines the length of the base. In a monoexponential C-T situation, the elimination rate constant k_{el} is the slope, which could be calculated from these data as ln (C_n/C_{n+1}). The estimate is simply $AUC_{T\to\infty} = C_T / k_{el}$. If a polyexponential equation is used, the slope of the terminal phase λ_n should be employed, where $AUC_{T\to\infty} = C_T / \lambda_n$. This of course assumes that concentrations have been taken for sufficient time to identify and characterize k_{el} or λ_n. Various logarithmic transformations have been employed to improve the estimate of this terminal portion of the C-T profile.

Suppose the experiment exemplified in Figure 8.2 had been terminated at 2 hours. Figure 8.4 and Table 8.2 illustrates an extrapolation to t = ∞ using the truncated data. The extrapolated AUC of 81.84 mg·h/mL is a fairly good estimate of the actual value of 80.79 (Table 8.1). Unfortunately, the estimated extrapolation is subject to increasing error the further from zero the final sample is taken. Actual observed data, however, will often contain much more noise than this example used for illustration of the method, and the estimate would consequently suffer.

For exponentially descending data (such as plasma concentrations following bolus injection), the trapezoidal method will always overestimate the AUC because the linear trapezoid is greater than the convex exponential functions. Thus the estimate should be regarded as an upper limit. Other routes of administration lead to data profiles that typically begin at zero, peak later, and decline back toward zero. The trapezoidal method generally underestimates the portion of the curve that is concave down (i.e., the middle portion) and overestimates the portions that are concave up (i.e., the tails), so the biases tend to cancel, giving a potentially better overall estimate. There are several numerical integration alternatives to the linear trapezoidal method presented here, including log trapezoid, Lagrange polynomials, and spline approximations.

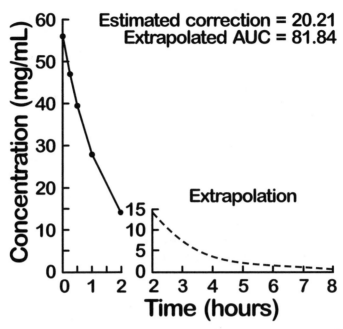

FIGURE 8.4.   Extrapolation of plasma concentration-time data from Figure 8.2 terminated at 2 hours (AUC = 61.63 hours), showing extrapolation beyond this time. AUC analysis is shown in Table 8.2.

TABLE 8.2.   Statistical Moments Calculations From a Truncated 2-Hour Data Set

Time (h)	Concentration (mg/mL)	Trapezoid areas (mg·h/mL)	Cumulative AUC
0.00	56.00	0.00	0.00
0.25	47.09	12.89	12.89
0.50	39.60	10.84	23.72
1.00	28.00	16.90	40.62
2.00	14.00	21.00	61.63
		Estimated end correction	20.21
		Extrapolated AUC	81.84

Data are the sample points for the first 2 hours, as plotted in left-hand plot of Figure 8.4. Estimated end correction simulated profile is plotted in the right-hand plot. Extrapolated AUC and total extrapolated AUC estimates were 20.21 mg·h/mL and 81.84 mg·h²/mL, respectively.

The numerical procedures for estimating AUMC are less precise than those for AUC, because the first moment is a weighted function of time, and where the trapezoids are of equal weight in the AUC determination, they are not for the AUMC. The greater time values carry correspondingly greater weight because their value is being multiplied by increasing t. Finally, the extrapolation of the terminal component of AUMC is more tenuous than that of the AUC. The area of the extrapolated curve equals $(TC_T)/\lambda + (C_T)/\lambda^2$, where λ is the terminal slope of the C-T profile and T is the time of the last measured concentration, C_T. A crude but unfortunately commonly used method for calculating AUMC is to simply multiply the area of each trapezoid by the time:

$$\text{AUMC} = \sum_{n=1}^{N} \frac{C_n + C_{n+1}}{2}(t_{n+1} - t_n)t_{n+1} \tag{8.8}$$

This algorithm can be very biased, especially for late, wide-spaced points. Using t_{n+1} overestimates the AUMC because the entire curve in the nth interval is assigned the weight t_{n+1}. Conversely, using t_n instead would underestimate the AUMC (with an even greater error). A better method is to use the linear mean time within each trapezoidal interval:

$$AUMC = \sum_{n=1}^{N} \frac{C_n + C_{n+1}}{2}(t_{n+1} - t_n)\frac{(t_n + t_{n+1})}{2} \tag{8.9}$$

This approach, which is actually based on the same considerations used in Chapter 7 to plot the midpoint of a urine excretion interval when analyzing excretion kinetics, is considerably more accurate than equation 8.8 but is still biased. Looking at the data of Table 8.1, it is evident that estimated trapezoid areas (using equation 8.7) are in greater error for the later times. This error could be mitigated with a higher sampling frequency. Since the algorithm for estimating AUMC (equation 8.9 was used for Table 8.1 estimated cumulative AUMC) is dependent on the trapezoid areas (using the same expression as equation 8.7, with the mean time factored in), the error of equation 8.7 carries over to the AUMC calculation. However, the AUMC error is not as proportionally great because the mean time term actually results in an underestimation of the AUMC of a given trapezoid, so again, there is a partial cancellation of errors.

The remaining bias in equation 8.9 is in the last term, the time (t) midpoint. It is correct to use such geometry for the AUC calculation, but not for the AUMC, because time is a weight in equation 8.8. If we substitute the equation for a straight line in the expression for AUMC (numerator of equation 8.1) for a single interval (segment), we get

$$AUMC_{t_n}^{t_{n+1}} = \int_{t_n}^{t_{n+1}} tC(t)dt = C_n \int_{t_n}^{t_{n+1}} t\,dt + \frac{C_{n+1} - C_n}{t_{n+1} - t_n} \int_{t_n}^{t_{n+1}} t(t - t_n)dt \tag{8.10}$$

then integration and some algebra admits,

$$AUMC_{t_n}^{t_{n+1}} = \frac{C_n(t_{n+1}^2 - t_n^2)}{2} + \frac{C_{n+1} - C_n}{6}(2t_{n+1}^2 - t_n t_{n+1} - t_n^2) \tag{8.11}$$

This is an exact AUMC for a trapezoid, and thus offers a much better theoretical solution than the other methods do. A similar expression can be obtained via a quadrature method. Equation 8.11 estimates of Table 8.1 are closer to the actual values for AUMC and consequently MRT. The reader is cautioned to remember, however, that the trapezoid itself is still a biased estimator of a curve's interval area, and the manifestation of that bias is a function of sampling frequency.

The attraction of statistical moment analysis to pharmacokinetics is implicit to the use of trapezoids to determine the relevant areas. No assumptions about the underlying mechanisms of drug disposition are made except for the two caveats introduced at the beginning of this chapter. One simply determines areas under the trapezoids formed from the $\Delta Ct / \Delta t$ intervals. The reader should realize that this is similar to the techniques used to analyze urine excretion data as the total amount excreted is essentially the same as determining the area of the U_t-T profile. Thus many strategies used to improve AUC or AUMC determination are directly applicable to improve urine excretion data analysis.

OTHER RESIDENCE TIMES AND PARAMETERS OF INTEREST

Three other residence times that have general application in pharmacokinetics are the mean absorption time (MAT), the mean transit time (MTT), and the variance of the residence time (VRT). MAT is technically the mean arrival time into the systemic circulation of bioavailable absorbed molecules. MAT is the statistical moment theory equivalent of estimating k_a. MAT is a computationally straightforward method to characterize the rate of drug absorption in bioavailability studies. Riegelman and Collier extended this theory using the additivity of various transit times, including the MAT, and advanced the notion that MAT is the mean time for drug molecules to remain unabsorbed.

$$MAT = MRT_{ni} - MRT_{IV} \qquad (8.12)$$

MAT is simply the difference in MRT following intravenous injection (MRT_{IV}) and another noninstantaneous administration (MRT_{ni}) by any route. Assuming absorption is described by a first-order process with an apparent rate constant of k_a,

$$K_a = 1 / MAT = 1 / (MRT_{ni} - 1/k_{el}) \qquad (8.13)$$

$, MRT_{IV} = \dfrac{1}{k_{el}}$

then the absorption half-life is, following equation 8.6,

$$T_{\frac{1}{2}[abs]} = \ln 2 \cdot MAT \qquad (8.14)$$

On the other hand, when absorption is assumed to be a zero-order process,

$$MAT = T / 2 \qquad (8.15)$$

where T is the duration of the absorption. Note the similarity to the infusion equation 8.5 above. In reality, a constant rate infusion is a zero-order absorption whose MAT is just one-half the length of the infusion. In comparisons of formulations based on intrasubject differences in MAT, the bias introduced in MRT when drug is eliminated peripherally, as noted in the caveat above, is not present in the use of MAT, but the fact remains that only those molecules that are systemically available are considered in the MAT.

The reader should recall that the determination of systemic availability expressed in equation 7.31 (see Chapter 7) is a noncompartmental analysis. AUCs should be determined by the trapezoidal methods presented in this chapter. If the point of an analysis is to determine bioequivalence between two formulations, one is actually calculating relative systemic availabilities, a concept equivalent to determining whether two formulations are therapeutically interchangeable. Bioequivalence is determined as the ratio of AUCs between the two formulations. In addition, the metric time to peak concentration and peak concentration are often compared. Comparison of MATs would also shed light on the equivalence of two formulations. The reader should consult the list of selected readings for further approaches to determining bioequivalence of human and veterinary products.

The MTT is by definition the mean time taken by drug molecules injected into the kinetic system at a given point to leave the kinetic space after first and possible subsequent entries into that space. Thus, in contrast to the MRT, which includes times spent on multiple visits of the same individual molecule to the kinetic space, MTT is the mean time spent per visit. In some stochastic modeling approaches to pharmacodynamics (Chapter 12), the MTT becomes a very useful parameter since it relates to the probability of a drug being available for causing an effect. If all molecules exit irreversibly from a kinetic space, then MTT = MRT. Note also that this is the condition mentioned above under which the MRT is a mathematically acceptable parameter for the plasma space or any other subspace of the whole body. *Statistical moment theory thus describes drug behavior based on the mean or average time an administered drug molecule spends in a kinetically homogeneous space, a concept identical to that of a compartment.* The difference again is that no specific inferences are being made about the structure of these spaces.

Another parameter that has been calculated is the variance of residence times (VRT), which is determined using the area under the second moment curve as

$$VRT = \frac{\int_0^\infty (t)^2 C dt}{\int_0^\infty C(t) dt} = \frac{\int_0^\infty (t - MRT)^2 C dt}{AUC} \tag{8.16}$$

VRT is used to calculate the coefficient of variation of residence times (CVRT) as

$$CVRT = \frac{\sqrt{VRT}}{MRT} \tag{8.17}$$

The CVRT is the dimensionless dispersion ratio and provides a measure of the dynamics and heterogeneity of drug distribution. However, as was mentioned above for determining trapezoidal areas for the AUMC, these problems are multiplied when higher moment curves are analyzed because small errors in time will be greatly magnified. This is less prone to occur with CVRT since the errors are somewhat canceled out by MRT in the denominator.

AUCs may also be used to easily estimate the fraction of a drug metabolized if the metabolite is available for a separate study. In this case, two intravenous experiments are conducted: one with the parent drug and the second with the metabolite of interest. Two C-T profiles using metabolite concentrations are then determined and the AUCs calculated. The fraction metabolized is then:

$$\text{Fraction metabolized} = AUC_{\text{drug}} \,(\textit{metabolite data}) \,/\, AUC_{\textit{metabolite}} \,(\textit{alone}) \tag{8.18}$$

Many other types of such AUC ratios may be calculated to get estimates of disposition when data from multiple routes are available. In the parathion example presented at the end of Chapter 7 (Figure 7.24), AUCs and MRTs were determined for all compartments after both intravenous and topical pesticide administration in order to probe whether metabolism occurred in the skin. To aid in this analysis, we also dosed parathion topically at two different sites using either occlusive or nonocclusive applications. Recalling discussions in Chapter 3, occlusion increases the rate and extent of absorption while the same may occur as a result of body site differences. Thus the extent (estimated by AUCs) and rates (estimated by MRTs) of parathion in the various compartments would be reflected by these differences in input to the systemic circulation. Similarly, by comparing radiolabeled parathion absorption in the central compartment estimated using AUCs and parent drug excretion in urine (bioavailability-excretion analysis), one could probe the kinetics of biotransformation with the equation:

$$\%\text{Metabolism Skin} = \frac{\sum AUC_{\text{central}} \,(\textit{Topical})}{\sum AUC_{\text{central}} \,(IV)} - \text{Parent Parathion Bioavaibilty} \tag{8.19}$$

where AUC is determined from the ^{14}C profile, and the parent parathion systemic availability is calculated in the normal manner using equation 3.2 or 7.31 (see Chapter 3). The result of this analysis yielded estimates of the ratio of cutaneous metabolism to systemic metabolism of parathion administered by these four dosing scenarios and suggested that occlusion significantly increased the amount of biotransformation occurring in the skin.

These results were similar to those determined from an analysis of micro-rate constants using classical compartmental methods.

Clearance. The determination of Cl_B is easily obtained by this approach using equation 7.18 (see Chapter 7), where $Cl_B = D / AUC$. Using the trapezoidal methods above to estimate AUC makes this a robust estimate of clearance. Cl_B can also sometimes be calculated following other routes of administration, but only if it is known that the entire dose is systemically available. For oral administration, the ratio of dose to AUC ($D_{p.o.} / AUC$) is reliably the *hepatic intrinsic clearance* only if the dose is known to be completely absorbed from the gastrointestinal tract and is eliminated exclusively by liver metabolism, an assumption difficult to make for most drugs. Clearances by other tissues and from temporal perspectives other than those assumed by D/AUC (e.g., first-pass versus repetitive-pass clearance considerations) can also be determined but are beyond the scope of the present text. If one fits the initial slope of an exponential C-T profile λ_1 and estimates V_c as described below, then a distributional clearance can be calculated as

$$Cl_D = V_c\,\lambda_1 - Cl_B \tag{8.20}$$

This allows one to define the relationship of Cl_B and Cl_D.

Volume of Distribution. The volume of the central compartment is simply equation 7.44; $V_c = D/Cp_0 = D/\Sigma\,A_i$. The volume of distribution at steady state (Vd_{ss}), according to statistical moment theory, is simply the product of MRT and Cl_B:

$$Vd_{ss} = Cl_B\,MRT \tag{8.21}$$

This, incidentally, affords an expression for half-life as a function of clearance, by solving equation 8.21 for MRT, and substitution into equation 8.6 gives

$$T_{\frac{1}{2}} = \frac{\ln 2 \cdot Vd_{ss}}{Cl_B} \qquad \begin{array}{l} T_{\frac{1}{2}} = \ln 2 \cdot MRT, \\[4pt] MRT = \dfrac{Vd_{ss}}{Cl_B}. \end{array} \tag{8.22}$$

which is the same as that derived in equation 7.20 (see Chapter 7). Continuing our investigation of distribution volume, we note that substitution of the respective expressions for MRT (equation 8.2) and Cl (equation 7.18, see Chapter 7) into equation. 8.21 yields

$$Vd_{ss} = \frac{D_{i.v.} \cdot AUMC}{AUC^2} \tag{8.23}$$

Equation 8.21 assumes a bolus intravenous dose. With a short-term constant infusion, then,

$$Vd_{ss} = \frac{R_0 T \cdot AUMC}{AUC^2} - \frac{R_0 T^2}{2 \cdot AUC} \tag{8.24}$$

where T is the length of infusion and R_0 is the zero-order infusion rate. In this case, for constant infusions, Vd_{ss} is independent of where drug is being eliminated. Another volume parameter also calculated using statistical moments used in the literature is Vd_{area}:

$$Vd_{area} = \frac{D_{i.v.}}{k_{el} \cdot AUC} \qquad , \qquad \begin{array}{l} \dot{MRT}_{iv} = \dfrac{1}{k_{el}}, \\[6pt] MRT = \dfrac{AUMC}{AUC}. \end{array} \tag{8.25}$$

TABLE 8.3. Noncompartmental Equations for Calculating Common Pharmacokinetic Parameters

$$Cl_B = Dose / AUC$$
$$Cl_D = V_c \lambda_1 - Cl_B$$
$$Vd_{ss} = (Dose \times AUMC) / AUC^2$$
$$V_c = Dose / Cp_0$$
$$MRT_{iv} = AUMC/AUC = Vd_{ss} / Cl_B$$
$$MAT = MRT_{route} - MRT_{iv}$$
$$K_a = 1 / (MRT - 1 / k_{el})$$
$$T_{1/2} = 0.693 \, MRT = 0.693 \, Vd_{ss} / Cl_B$$
$$T_{1/2} (\lambda) = 0.693 / \lambda$$
$$F = (AUC_{route}) (Dose_{iv}) / (AUC_{iv}) (Dose_{route})$$
$$= (AUC_{route}) (Dose_{iv}) (T_{1/2_{iv}}) / (AUC_{iv}) (Dose_{route}) (T_{1/2route})$$
$$AUC = \sum A_i / \lambda_i$$
$$AUMC = \sum A_i / (\lambda_i)^2$$
$$Cp_0 = \sum A_i$$

Note that AUC and AUMC could be calculated using trapezoidal analysis of areas rather than fitting curves to obtain estimates of A_i and λ_i.

and for a constant intravenous infusion,

$$Vd_{area} = \frac{R_0}{k_{el} \cdot C_{ss}} \qquad (8.26)$$

where C_{ss} is the steady-state plasma concentration as previously defined by rearrangement of equation 7.22 ($C_{ss} = R_0 / Cl_B$) (see Chapter 7). The computational advantage of Vd_{ss} over Vd_{area} is, of course, the avoidance of the need to estimate an elimination rate constant, k_{el}, but as described in Chapter 7, it is thus also independent of altered elimination. Recall that Vd_{ss} is the volume operative at the MRT.

One can appreciate that statistical moment analysis provides a powerful tool for calculating many of the common pharmacokinetic parameters that are routinely used—in the bioequivalence studies discussed above, in constructing dosage regimens (Chapter 11), in correlating disease and physiological changes to pharmacokinetic disposition (Chapters 14 and 15), and in making interspecies extrapolations (Chapter 16). As can now be even more fully appreciated, Cl_B and Vd_{ss} are truly independent parameters that quantitate distribution and excretion using computationally robust techniques based on minimal model-specific assumptions. Table 8.3 is a compilation of equations useful to calculate these parameters from an analysis of a C-T profile.

OTHER MODEL-INDEPENDENT APPROACHES

The center of gravity (or center of mass) of a curve is a single point that provides a quantitative description of a C-T profile. Veng-Pedersen defined the coordinates of this point as

$$P_c = (t_c, C_c) = \left(\frac{AUMC}{AUC}, \frac{1}{2} \cdot \frac{AUCC}{AUC} \right) \qquad (8.27)$$

where t_c is the MRT, C_c is the mean concentration, and AUCC is the area under the squared curve:

$$AUCC = \int_0^\infty [C(t)]^2 dt \qquad (8.28)$$

P_c is a simple yet powerful tool for comparing C-T profiles because it is sensitive to both the rate and extent of absorption or elimination. The square data point on the plot of Figure 8.2 at (1.44, 14.00) represents the P_c of that profile.

Another model-independent approach to analyzing pharmacokinetic data is linear systems deconvolution analysis, which actually provides a mathematical basis for the superposition principle discussed earlier. In this approach, any observed C-T profile {C(t)} can be broken down or *deconvoluted* into two mathematical functions: the *characteristic function* {F(t)}, which describes the disposition after intravenous bolus administration, and the *input* function {C'(t)}, which is an equation describing drug input as a function of time after any mode of administration. This technique is also called superposition integration and uses the observed C-T profile and the characteristic profile to determine the input profile using the relations:

$$C(t) = F(t) + C'(t) \ (convolution) \tag{8.29}$$

$$C'(t) = C(t) - F(t) \ (deconvolution) \tag{8.30}$$

There are numerous mathematical approaches to implement this. If one has intravenous data fit to a multicompartment model, then F(t) is expressed as equation 7.58. When an extravascular administration route is being studied, the C'(t) is equivalent to the shape of the absorption input profile. Thus, *this approach gives an excellent quantitative description of any absorption profile resulting from any complexity of drug delivery system*. It is a powerful tool for assessing absolute systemic availability. Although multiexponential equations are often used to describe both functions, this is not necessary, and equations of any mathematical form can be employed. The mathematical equations describing the resulting input profile may be complex, and their derivation is beyond the scope of this text.

We have used this approach to study the comparative nephrotoxicity of identical gentamicin C-T profiles in dogs with normal and impaired renal functions. We defined a target profile that is the sum of the input function and the characteristic response determined after intravenous dosing. Note that in renal disease, Cl_B and thus k_{el} are reduced compared to normal, making the achievement of identical C-T profiles in both groups impossible. However, if one uses deconvolution principles to solve for the input function required to achieve identical C-T profiles, this can be programmed into a computer-driven infusion pump to make the infusion rate-limiting. A loading dose ($C_{ss}V_c$) was first administered to rapidly achieve steady state. A steady-state infusion (mg kg^{-1}h^{-1}) was then administered for time, t, according to the equation:

$$R_{ss} = (C_{ss}V_c)\,(k_{10} + k_{12}e^{-k_{21}t}) \tag{8.31}$$

At the termination of infusion, a declining rate infusion was then administered as

$$R_{decl} = (C_{ss}V_c)\frac{(\alpha - k)(\beta - k)e^{-kt'} + (k)k_{12}e^{-k_{21}t'}}{k_{21} - k} \tag{8.32}$$

where k is the target terminal slope and t' is the length of time in the declining phase of the infusion. Figure 8.5 shows the resulting C-T profile for normal and subtotally nephrectomized dogs (see Chapter 7, Table 7.2 for pharmacokinetic parameters of the intravenous bolus dose) administered drug according to their calculated input functions. This method thus served as an excellent tool to probe the toxicokinetics of a nephrotoxic drug in diseased animals.

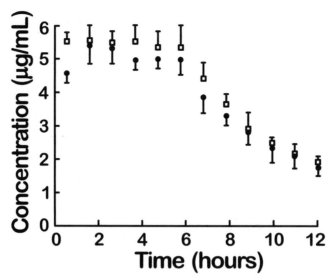

FIGURE 8.5. Plasma concentration-versus-time profiles obtained after administering computer-controlled intravenous infusions of gentamicin to normal (•) and subtotal nephrectomized (□) dogs at rates defined in equations 8.31 and 8.32.

We have also employed a similar convolution technique to model the predicted C-T profile resulting from transdermal drug delivery when the input function is experimentally determined using an isolated perfused skin preparation. In this case (depicted in Figure 8.6), the output of the skin profile could either be the experimentally observed profile or be simulated using a compartmental model to generate the terms of C′ (t). This skin model will be further developed in Chapter 10 (see text accompanying Figures 10.4 through 10.6). The characteristic response, {F(t)}, is based on a two-compartment model determined from intravenous studies (obtained after a bolus dose or modeled better with an infusion of the same duration as the transdermal input profile) conducted in the species in which the prediction is to be made. In our laboratory, we use porcine skin as the preferred human model and obtain the intravenous data from human studies. Additionally, both the input and characteristic functions may be inputted as a confidence interval to account for interindividual differences; or a "boot-strap" or "full-space" technique can be used to assess all possible combinations of input and disposition functions. This technique accurately predicts the subsequent profiles in all drugs and pesticides studied to date.

The final stochastic approach to modeling was the power function introduced in the previous chapter for gentamicin tissue disposition. Figure 8.7 depicts a power analysis of gentamicin renal cortex tissue concentrations in rats using this same general approach. This technique has been explored in much greater detail for general models and is rooted in the concept of residence times. The power function arises when a drug molecule exits the rapidly equilibrating kinetic space (e.g., normal compartments) and randomly remains nonavailable for return to this compartment because of sequestration in the so-called deep compartment. Recall that this sojourn to a peripheral compartment violated one of the basic assumptions of MRT; that is, a significant fraction of the dose never spends time in another space before being eliminated, which makes the residence time no longer proportional to the plasma Cp. This can be handled by using so-called *random walk* principles, which generate equations taking the form of a power function (equation 7.59). The concept is that drugs distribute freely into tissues until they bind to a receptor, or enter a cell, for which time they no longer can randomly reenter the exchanging kinetic

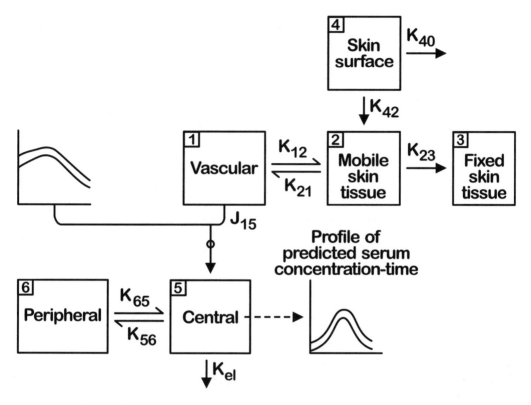

FIGURE 8.6. Pharmacokinetic strategies used to extrapolate output profiles from an *in vitro* perfused skin-flap model to predict *in vivo* concentration-time profiles. Compartments 1, 2, 3, and 4 constitute the *in vitro* model, whose output [now the input function (C′(t); upper left corner] into the *in vivo* systemic pharmacokinetic model is composed of compartments 5 and 6 [*characteristic* function, F(t)]. A derivation of a similar skin component is further developed in Figure 10.4.

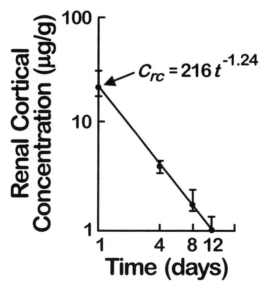

FIGURE 8.7. Power function (log C versus log T) analysis of gentamicin decay in rat renal cortex.

compartments. The distribution (pdf) of the residence times for such tissues is described by a gamma function, which implies the power dependence. Additionally, if the diffusion of the compound is described by an anatomical configuration having spherical symmetry (e.g., the liver lobule), then the equations assume the form of a power function. Significant work has been done in this area, especially applied to drug distribution in the liver (spherical diffusion) and heavy metal deposition in bone (binding). The equations for this model are beyond the scope of this introductory text since nonlinear equations are also needed to describe how the drug distributes to these sites.

AN APPLICATION OF STATISTICAL MOMENT THEORY

We will close this chapter with another application from the author's laboratory using a statistical moment approach. When absorption through skin was presented in Chapter 3, the rate-limiting factor was penetration through the stratum corneum. For many compounds in skin-absorption studies, a generally critical factor is perfusion, because the rate and extent of absorption into the general circulation (i.e., the bioavailability) of a topically applied compound is a function of (among other things, such as stratum corneum permeability and cutaneous metabolism) the extent to which the underlying skin is perfused. This is especially true with so-called active drug delivery systems (e.g., iontophoresis), which rapidly allow drug to pass the epidermal barrier. The capillary beds in the viable epidermis are normally in a dynamic state in the constant need to shunt or recruit as a function of thermoregulation. The MRT of a drug in skin following topical application may be described as

$$MRT_{skin} = \frac{PV_T}{Q_{skin}} \tag{8.33}$$

where P is the skin-to-blood partition coefficient, V_T is the volume of distribution of drug in skin, and Q_{skin} is (theoretically) the blood flow through the space where the drug is diffusing, and can be defined as

$$Q_{skin} = Q_{exchange} + Q_{shunt} \tag{8.34}$$

Thus, Q_{skin} is the sum of flow through capillaries that are exchanging with the extravascular space, and flow that has been shunted, and therefore not able to exchange (i.e., not perfused). The point is that the MRT here is dependent on two independent variables (assuming P is constant): V_T and Q_{skin}. Historically, most models in the literature assume that V_T is constant, which is not generally true since V_T is actually a direct function of $Q_{exchange}$, a dynamic variable. This leads to a dynamic MRT that is difficult to measure without knowledge of the corresponding profile of Q_{skin}.

The MTT of blood through a perfused space was estimated in a model to predict transdermal iontophoretic delivery of lidocaine. In this model, it was necessary to address the MTT (called τ_{eff} in the article, to indicate the *effective* transit time through drug-exchanging capillaries) in order to develop a mathematical expression for the flux of electrically driven drug molecules into the systemic circulation:

$$\tau_{eff} = \frac{V_{eff}}{Q_{eff}} \tag{8.35}$$

where V_{eff} and Q_{eff} are the effective vascular volume and blood flow, respectively. The subscript "eff" denotes that space through which drug diffuses in the skin, and those vessels in the proximity that have the capacity to exchange drug. This study revealed, among other things, that the state of skin vasculature is exquisitely sensitive to penetrating vasoactive compounds (i.e., tolazoline and norepinephrine as vasodilator and vasoconstrictor, respectively, in this case). Furthermore, changes in vascular state in skin have a great influence on the absorption of topically applied compounds. In the case presented, the estimated τ_{eff} for lidocaine when coadministered with tolazoline was 46 minutes, in contrast to 2 minutes when coadministered with norepinephrine (τ_{eff} for lidocaine alone was 9 minutes).

This example illustrates the power of relatively simple pharmacokinetic techniques to probe the physiological basis of drug disposition in numerous organ and experimental systems. *As stressed in the introduction of this text, pharmacokinetics is a useful tool to generate testable experimental hypotheses. There are no absolutely correct models or approaches, as many different systems may be used depending upon the availability of data and limiting assumptions.*

SELECTED READINGS

Caines, P.E. 1988. *Linear Stochastic Systems*. New York: Wiley and Sons.

Caprani, O., E. Sveindottir, and N. Lassen. 1975. SHAM, a method for biexponential curve resolution using initial slope, height, area and moment of the experimental decay type curve. *Journal of Theoretical Biology*. 52:299-315.

Chan, K.K.H., and M. Gilbaldi. 1982. Estimation of statistical moments and steady-state volume of distribution for a drug given by intravenous infusion. *Journal of Pharmacokinetics and Biopharmaceutics*. 10:551-558.

Chanter, D.O. 1985. The determination of mean residence time using statistical moments: Is it correct? *Journal of Pharmacokinetics and Biopharmaceutics*. 13:93-100.

Chiou, W.L. 1978. Critical evaluation of the potential error in pharmacokinetic studies of using the linear trapezoidal rule method for the calculation of the area under the plasma level-time curve. *Journal of Pharmacokinetics and Biopharmaceutics*. 6:539-546.

Cutler, D.J. 1978. Theory of the mean absorption time, an adjunct to conventional bioavailability studies. *Journal of Pharmacy and Pharmacology*. 30:476-478.

Cutler, D.J. 1979. A linear recirculation model for drug disposition. *Journal of Pharmacokinetics and Biopharmaceutics*. 7:101-116.

DiStefano, J. III. 1982. Noncompartmental versus compartmental analysis: Some bases for choice. *American Journal of Physiology (Regulatory Integrative Comp. Physiol. 12)* 243:R1-R6.

Dix, L.P., D.L. Frazier, M. Cooperstein, and J.E. Riviere. 1986. Exponential intravenous infusions in toxicology studies: Achieving identical serum drug concentration profiles in individuals with altered pharmacokinetic states. *Journal of Pharmaceutical Sciences*. 75:448-451.

Frazier, D.L., L.P. Dix, K.F. Bowman, C.A. Thompson, and J.E. Riviere. 1986. Increased gentamicin nephrotoxicity in normal and diseased dogs administered identical serum drug concentration profiles: Increased sensitivity in subclinical renal dysfunction. *Journal of Pharmacology and Experimental Therapeutics*. 239:946-951.

Gibaldi, M., and D. Perrier. 1982. *Pharmacokinetics*, 2ed. New York: Marcel Dekker.

Martinez, M.N. 1998. Article 1: Noncompartmental methods of drug characterization: Statistical moment theory. *Journal of the American Veterinary Medical Association* 213:974-980.

Metzler, C.M. 1989. Bioavailability / bioequivalence: Study design and statistical issues. *Journal of Clinical Pharmacology.* 29:289-292.

Nakashima, E., and L.Z. Benet. 1988. General treatment of mean residence time, clearance, and volume parameters in linear mammillary models with elimination from any compartment. *Journal of Pharmacokinetics and Biopharmaceutics.* 16:475-492.

Norwich, K.H., and S. Siu. 1982. Power functions in physiology and pharmacology. *Journal of Theoretical Biology.* 95:387-398.

Nüesch, E.A. 1984. Noncompartmental approach in pharmacokinetics using moments. *Drug Metabolism Reviews.* 15:103-131.

Pang, K.S. and M. Rowland. 1977. Hepatic clearance of drugs. I. Theoretical considerations of a "well-stirred model" and a "parallel tube" model. Influence of hepatic blood flow, plasma and blood cell binding, and the hepatocellular enzymatic activity on hepatic drug clearance. *Journal of Pharmacokinetics and Biopharmaceutics* 5:625-653.

Pecile, A., and A. Rescigno. 1987. *Pharmacokinetics. Mathematical and Statistical Approaches to Metabolism and Distribution of Chemicals and Drugs.* New York: Plenum Press.

Purves, R.D. 1994. Numerical estimation of the noncompartmental pharmacokinetic parameters variance and coefficient of variation of residence times. *Journal of Pharmaceutical Sciences.* 83:202-205.

Qiao, G.L., and J.E. Riviere. 1995. Significant effects of application site and occlusion on the pharmacokinetics of cutaneous penetration and biotransformation of parathion in vivo in swine. *Journal of Pharmaceutical Sciences.* 84:425-432.

Riegelman, S., and P. Collier. 1980. The application of statistical moment theory to the evaluation of *in vivo* dissolution time and absorption time. *Journal of Pharmacokinetics and Biopharmaceutics* 8:509-534.

Riviere, J.E., and P.L. Williams. 1992. Pharmacokinetic implications of changing blood flow in skin. *Journal of Pharmaceutical Sciences.* 81:601-602.

Riviere, J.E., P.L. Williams, R. Hillman, and L. Mishky. 1992. Quantitative prediction of transdermal iontophoretic delivery of arbutamine in humans using the in vitro isolated perfused porcine skin flap (IPPSF). *Journal of Pharmaceutical Sciences.* 81:504-507.

Riviere, J.E., N.A. Monteiro-Riviere, and P.L. Williams. 1995. Isolated perfused porcine skin flap as an in vitro model for predicting transdermal pharmacokinetics. *European Journal of Pharmacy and Biopharmaceutics.* 41:152-162.

Segre, G. 1988. The sojourn time and its prospective use in pharmacology. *Journal of Pharmacokinetics and Biopharmaceutics.* 16:657-666.

Toutain, P.L., and G.D. Koritz. 1997. Veterinary drug bioequivalence determination. *Journal of Veterinary Pharmacology and Therapeutics.* 20:79-90.

Veng-Pedersen, P. 1989. Mean time parameters in pharmacokinetics: Definition, computation and clinical implications (part I). *Clinical Pharmacokinetics.* 17:345-366.

Veng-Pedersen, P. 1989. Mean time parameters in pharmacokinetics: Definition, computation and clinical implications (part II). *Clinical Pharmacokinetics* 17:424-440.

Veng-Pedersen, P. 1991. Stochastic interpretation of linear pharmacokinetics: A linear system analysis approach. *Journal of Pharmaceutical Sciences.* 80:621-631.

Veng-Pedersen, P., and W. Gillespie. 1984. Mean residence time in peripheral tissue: A linear disposition parameter useful for evaluating a drug's tissue distribution. *Journal of Pharmacokinetics and Biopharmaceutics.* 12:535-543.

Weiss, M. 1983. Use of gamma distributed residence times in pharmacokinetics. *European Journal of Clinical Pharmacology.* 25:695-702.

Williams, P.L., and J.E. Riviere. 1993. Model describing transdermal iontophoretic delivery of lidocaine incorporating consideration of cutaneous microvascular state. *Journal of Pharmaceutical Science* 82:1080-1084.

Williams, P.L., and J.E. Riviere. 1994. A "full-space" method for predicting in vivo transdermal plasma drug profiles reflecting both cutaneous and systemic variability. *Journal of Pharmaceutical Sciences* 83:1062-1064.

Williams, P.L., and J. E. Riviere. 1994. MOMENTS, © Copyright, **1994.** Cutaneous Pharmacology and Toxicology Center, North Carolina State University, Raleigh, NC; and Polytheoretics, Inc., Wake Forest, NC. (Software for calculating statistical moments from timed data).

Yamaoka, K., T. Nakagawa, and T. Uno. 1978. Statistical moments in pharmacokinetics. *Journal of Pharmacokinetics and Biopharmaceutics.* 6:547.

Yeh, K.C., and K.C. Kwan. 1978. A comparison of numerical integrating algorithms by trapezoidal, Lagrange, and spline approximation. *Journal of Pharmacokinetics and Biopharmaceutics.* 6:79-98.

Yu, Z., and F.L.S. Tse. 1995. An evaluation of numerical integration algorithms for the estimation of area under the curve (AUC) in pharmacokinetic studies. *Biopharmaceutics and Drug Disposition.* 16:37-58.

9

Nonlinear Models

Most pharmacokinetic models incorporate the common assumption that drug elimination from the body is a first-order process, and the rate constant for elimination is assumed to be a true constant, independent of drug concentration. In such cases, the amount of drug cleared from the body per unit time is directly dose- or concentration-dependent, the percentage of body drug load that is cleared per unit time is constant, and the drug has a constant elimination half-life. Fortunately, first-order elimination (at least apparent first-order elimination) is typical in drug studies. First-order linear systems application greatly simplifies dosage design, bioavailability assessment, dose-response relationships, prediction of drug distribution and disposition, and virtually all quantitative aspects of pharmacokinetic simulation.

However, drugs most often are *not* eliminated from the body by mechanisms that are truly mathematically first-order by nature. Actual first-order elimination applies only to compounds that are eliminated exclusively by mechanisms not involving enzymatic or active transport processes (i.e., processes involving energy). As presented in Chapter 2, they are primarily driven by diffusion and obey Fick's law. The subset of drugs not requiring a transfer of energy in their elimination is restricted to those that are cleared from the body by urinary and biliary excretion and, among those, only drugs that enter the renal tubules by glomerular filtration or passive tubular diffusion. Albeit there are some minor passive excretion routes, such as saliva or sweat, these elimination routes generally account for such a small fraction of total eliminated drug that they are essentially negligible. All other important elimination processes require some form of energy-consumptive metabolic activity or transport mechanism. Thus the number of compounds that clear by truly first-order processes are very few indeed, and nonlinear elimination is therefore a potential condition for the great majority of compounds.

One might ask, then, why the elimination kinetics of so many drugs can be modeled with linear first-order processes. At clinical dosages, the majority of drugs do not reach saturation concentrations at the reaction sites, or at least not a significant fraction of the dose. One notable exception is ethanol, which is cleared from the body by oxidative metabolism at an apparent zero-order rate (indicative of a well-saturated process). There is

Co-authored by Dr. Patrick L. Williams

nothing special about ethanol *except* its low molecular weight (46 Da) relative to most drugs (> 300 Da). This means that a typical ethanol dose is actually equivalent to a relatively high molar dose that saturates metabolism. Metabolic activity operates on a molecular basis and therefore would be better expressed on the basis of the number of interacting molecules (e.g., molarity). In fact, much of the pharmacokinetic techniques already presented and their interpretation would be facilitated if molarity were employed rather than mass or concentration. However, this is rarely done.

The reason energy-involved processes are not strictly first-order is that they are generally saturable or, more specifically, *capacity limited*. That is, as the availability of finite enzyme and/or energy sources is temporarily depressed (i.e., saturated) due to acute competition among drug molecules for reaction sites, the reaction rate slows and is no longer first-order, taking on some of the properties of a zero-order process. Recalling Chapter 7 and equations 7.1 and 7.2 for first-order processes, a constant percentage of remaining drug is cleared per unit time, and the drug has a discrete, concentration-independent elimination rate constant (K) and thus half-life (or multiple half-lives for multicompartment models). For drugs eliminated by zero-order kinetics or saturated pathways (equation 7.3), however, a constant quantity of drug is eliminated per unit of time, and this quantity is drug concentration-independent, and the drug does not have a constant, characteristic elimination half-life. The potential impact of saturable elimination, leading to zero-order (versus first-order) elimination, can be profound, and its effects include altered drug concentration profiles, scope and duration of drug activity, distribution, and disposition among tissues. As discussed in Chapter 6, saturable hepatic metabolism may markedly affect drug absorption due to altered first-pass activity.

MICHAELIS-MENTEN RATE LAWS

The primary technique used to model saturable metabolic process employ the Michaelis-Menten rate laws briefly introduced in Chapter 6. Systematic studies of the effect of substrate concentration upon enzyme activity were begun in the late 19th century. The concept of the enzyme-substrate complex was introduced before any enzymes had even been purified. In fact, at the time, it was not even known that enzymes were proteins, but the idea of the enzyme-substrate complex served to launch the development of enzyme kinetics.

If one follows the appearance of product (or the disappearance of substrate in a reaction with 1:1 stoichiometry) as a function of time in an experiment, a progress curve for the reaction can be obtained (Figure 9.1). The initial rate (v_0) of the reaction is equal to the slope of the progress curve at time zero. As the reaction continues, the product continues to accumulate, but at slower rates as the supply of substrate diminishes. If a series of these experiments are effected, starting with a corresponding series of substrate concentrations, a plot of v_0 versus substrate concentration is obtained, such as shown in Figure 9.2 and explained below.

One of the most basic enzymatic reactions, first proposed by Michaelis and Menten (1913), involves a substrate S reacting with an enzyme E to form a complex SE, which in turn is converted into a product P and the enzyme. This can be represented schematically by

$$S + E \underset{k_{-1}}{\overset{k_1}{\rightleftharpoons}} SE, \quad SE \xrightarrow{k_2} P + E \tag{9.1}$$

where k_1 is a second-order reaction rate constant, and k_{-1} and k_2 are first-order reaction rate constants. Michaelis and Menten proposed that the enzymatic reaction proceeds through an enzyme-substrate complex that forms rapidly (the left reaction of equation 9.1) and is then slowly converted to product (metabolite) in the *rate-determining step* of the reaction (the right reaction in equation 9.1). The major assumption of equation 9.1

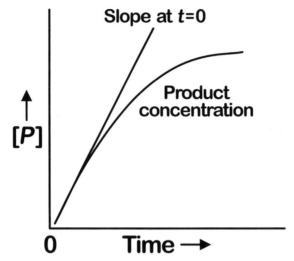

FIGURE 9.1.   Simulated enzyme-linked metabolite product formation progress curve. [P] is the concentration of product, plotted against time. The initial rate, the slope at $t = 0$ (v_0 in the text), is an important parameter for characterizing the reactions of equation 9.1 (see Figure 9.2).

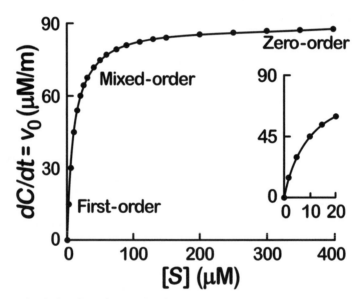

FIGURE 9.2.   A simulated plot of initial rates (dC/dt, or v_0) versus substrate concentration [S] for a reaction described by equation 9.1. With V_{max} = 90 µM/m, K_m is estimated to be 10 µM at half-maximal velocity ($V_{max}/2$ = 45 µM / m), as shown in inset.

that provides a logical basis for equation 9.2 (below) is that the enzyme and the substrate remain in thermodynamic equilibrium with the enzyme-substrate complex at all times. Michaelis-Menten kinetics are formulated for initial rates, and based on the assumption that $k_{-1} >> k_2$, which implies that, provided $[E]_t << [S]$, the concentration of enzyme-substrate complex will be small and constant. $[E]_t$ denotes the total concentration of enzyme, free and complexed, and [S] is the free substrate concentration. This is known as the *steady-state assumption*. Since only a small amount of product accumulates initially, the reverse reaction (i.e., that described by k_{-1}) can be ignored, which allows the method

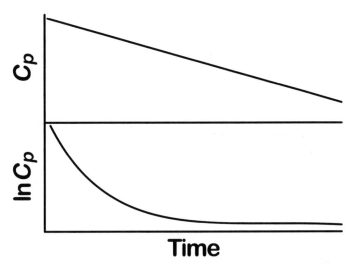

FIGURE 9.3. Plot of ln concentration (lnCp) versus time and concentration (Cp) versus time, suggesting non-linear kinetics. Recall that lnCp-T plots for linear processes result in straight terminal elimination phases as shown in the figures in Chapter 7.

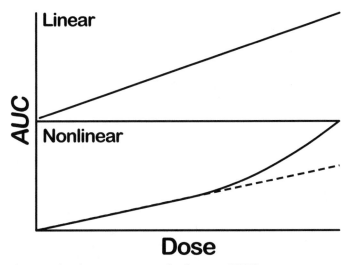

FIGURE 9.4. Linearity test using dose versus area under the curve (AUC).

used to obtain the v_0 versus [S] plot in Figure 9.2. With the above assumptions and some algebra, the Michaelis-Menten Rate Law (equation 9.2) can be derived, assuming [S] is a function of information obtained from the experimental procedures shown in Figure 9.2.

$$\frac{d[S]}{dt} = -\frac{V_{max}[S]}{K_m + [S]}$$

(9.2)

where V_{max} is the maximum velocity, or rate, of the reaction, and K_m is the Michaelis constant,

$$K_m = \frac{k_{-1} + k_2}{k_1}$$

(9.3)

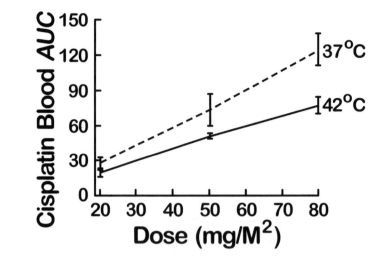

FIGURE 9.5.   Illustration of linear cisplatin disposition under normothermic (37°C) versus hyperthermic (42°C) conditions.

which represents the drug concentration at which half-maximal reaction velocity (V_{max}/2) occurs. In order to present a nomenclature consistent with the majority of the pharmacokinetics literature and the rest of this text, we will use C (referred to earlier as Cp when in plasma) in place of $[S]$ for drug or substrate concentration (i.e., $C = [S]$). Thus,

$$\frac{dC}{dt} = -\frac{V_{max}C}{K_m + C} \qquad (9.4)$$

The parameters V_{max} and K_m can be estimated from a plot like that shown in Figure 9.2, but more accuracy for *in vivo* plasma data with less experimental effort can be attained utilizing other methods. Because of the potential complexity of such models, it is prudent to use simple techniques to first test one's data for dose dependency or nonlinearity.

Testing for Nonlinearity.   Figure 9.3 depicts the simplest technique, whereby one determines if the terminal phase of the ln$C$ (or log$C$) versus time profile is a straight line using regression techniques. If this is curvilinear, then nonlinear kinetics are operative, and a plot of C versus time will often be straight. Alternatively, if multiple doses are used, one can determine the area under the curve (AUC) by a graphical technique discussed in earlier chapters and plot dose versus AUC as in Figure 9.4. If this plot is linear, then dose-independent kinetics are present, and the classical compartmental exponential or noncompartmental first-order models are appropriate. If this plot is not a straight line (in its terminal segment if a multicompartment drug), nonlinear models are required.

It is important that a true area integration technique (e.g., trapezoidal method) and not an exponential fitting equation be used to calculate AUC for this purpose, since the *use of an exponential fitting program implies linearity*. Recall that this technique was used in Table 4.1 when cisplatin tissue concentrations were normalized for systemic exposure by AUC. This was a major assumption, and the cisplatin data set was thus first tested using the approach depicted in Figure 9.5, which demonstrated that a linear dose versus AUC relation was present. Alternatively, one may determine the terminal half-life for a ln$C$ versus time profile after graduated doses. If the half-life is constant, linear kinetics are operative. If it increases with dose, then dose-dependent kinetics are present. When one's data "pass" these tests of linearity and dose-independence, then the relatively simpler

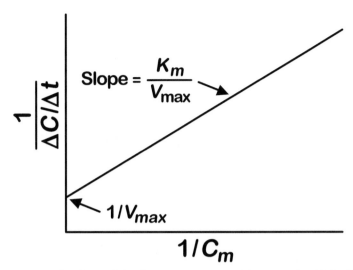

FIGURE 9.6. Lineweaver-Burke plot, as defined in equation 9.5, used for estimating Michaelis-Menten parameters K_m and V_{max}. Plotting the reciprocals of the change (decline) in drug concentrations versus the reciprocal of drug concentrations at the midpoint of the measured intervals yields a slope of K_m / V_{max} and an ordinate intercept of $1 / V_{max}$. This method is appropriate for both IV and oral administration.

techniques discussed in Chapters 7 and 8 are appropriate. If not, then more complex models (presented below) may be required.

Estimating Michaelis-Menten Parameters from Concentration-Time Data. When nonlinearity is present, one can determine the rate of change of plasma drug concentrations between successive sampling times during the postabsorptive and postdistributive phases (e.g., terminal phase) of a plasma concentration-time profile. Then the rate of change in plasma concentration, together with the drug concentration at the midpoint of each sampling period, C_m, can be incorporated into one of several appropriate expressions to solve for V_{max} and K_m. One such expression is

$$\frac{1}{\Delta C / \Delta t} = \frac{1}{V_{max}} + \frac{K_m}{V_{max} \cdot C_m} \tag{9.5}$$

This is the Lineweaver-Burke equation, which is a linear form of the Michaelis-Menten equation 9.4. In this treatment, $\Delta C / \Delta t$ and C_m represent the decline in drug concentration during a time interval and the drug concentration at the midpoint of the time interval, respectively. A plot of the left-hand side of equation 9.5 versus $1 / C_m$ yields a slope of K_m / V_{max} and an intercept of $1 / V_{max}$, as illustrated in Figure 9.6.

In another method, estimates of V_{max} and K_m are obtained directly from ln$C$ versus t data, the typical concentration-versus-time profile modeled in previous chapters. Equation 9.4 can be rearranged to

$$-dC - \frac{K_m dC}{C} = V_{max} dt \tag{9.6}$$

Integration of this result and solving for $t = 0$, where $C = C_0$, results in

$$t = \frac{C_0 - C}{V_{max}} + \frac{K_m}{V_{max}} \ln\left(\frac{C_0}{C}\right) \tag{9.7}$$

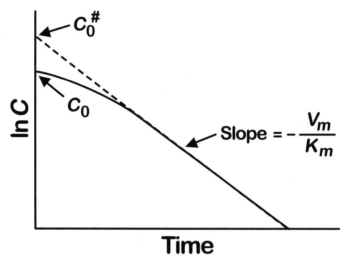

FIGURE 9.7.   Alternative method for estimating Michaelis-Menten parameters. Plotting ln concentration versus time, the terminal slope (from equation 9.9) equals $-V_{max}/(K_m)$. K_m is a function of C_0 (the initial ln drug concentration) and $C_0^\#$ (the extrapolated initial ln drug concentration). V_{max} is obtained from equation 9.13. This method is appropriate for IV administrations only.

Solving for ln C yields

$$\ln C = \frac{C_0 - C}{K_m} + \ln C_0 - \frac{V_{max}t}{K_m} \tag{9.8}$$

ln$C$ can be plotted against t for data following a bolus intravenous (IV) dose. The terminal log-linear portion of the curve (the region where apparent first-order kinetics occur) is a straight line described by

$$\ln C = \ln C_0^{\#} - \frac{V_{max}t}{K_m} \tag{9.9}$$

where $C_0^\#$ is the extrapolated intercept of C on the vertical axis, exemplified by Figure 9.7. In the log-linear region at low plasma concentrations, equation 9.9 is identical to equation 9.8 expressed as ln. These expressions can thus be equated

$$\ln C_0^{\#} - \frac{V_{max}t}{K_m} = \frac{C_0 - C}{K_m} + \ln C_0 - \frac{V_{max}t}{K_m} \tag{9.10}$$

Simplifying and rearranging yields

$$\ln \frac{C_0^{\#}}{C_0} = \frac{C_0 - C}{K_m} \tag{9.11}$$

Then, recalling that equation 9.10 specifically corresponds to the terminal phase of the drug profile (when $C << C_0$), the quantity $[C_0 - C]$ is approximately C_0. Substituting this in equation 9.11 and solving for K_m gives

$$K_m = \frac{C_0}{\ln \dfrac{C_0^{\#}}{C_0}} \tag{9.12}$$

Thus, because both C_0 and $C_0^{\#}$, the actual and extrapolated y-intercepts, respectively, can be measured, K_m can be calculated from equation 9.12, and $V_{\max}$ can be calculated as

$$V_{\max} = - [slope] \cdot K_m \tag{9.13}$$

The two methods presented above are representative of the several methods presently in use for calculating Michaelis-Menten constants from plasma data. One method uses the rates of change in plasma concentrations, which may be based on either IV or oral data; the other method is based on direct estimates from plots of ln plasma concentration-versus-time data but is restricted to IV data.

PHARMACOKINETIC IMPLICATIONS OF MICHAELIS-MENTEN KINETICS

There are two notable simplifying conditions of the Michaelis-Menten equation. If $K_m >> C$, then equation 9.4 reduces to

$$\frac{dC}{dt} = \frac{V_{\max} \cdot C}{K_m} \tag{9.14}$$

This is equivalent to first-order elimination after IV administration in a one-compartment model, where $dC / dt = - k_{el} C$. Thus, assuming elimination by a single biotransformation process, the first-order elimination rate constant k_{el} used throughout Chapter 7 is

$$k_{el} = \frac{V_{\max}}{K_m} \tag{9.15}$$

As suggested in the beginning of this chapter, since most drugs administered at normal dosages seem to obey first-order elimination kinetics, equation 9.15 supports the hypothesis that typical therapeutic dose regimens lead to drug concentrations at the active site(s) in the body that are well below the K_m of the involved associated enzymology. If $K_m << C$, then equation 9.4 collapses to

$$dC / dt = - V_{\max} = - K_0 \tag{9.16}$$

The rate in this case is independent of drug concentration (i.e., a constant), which describes a zero-order process and is exemplified by ethanol, as discussed above.

Often, drugs are found to be eliminated by both first-order and nonlinear processes in parallel. In such cases, equation 9.4 must be expanded to include the strictly first-order elimination processes:

$$\frac{dC}{dt} = -\frac{V_{\max}C}{K_m + C} - k'_{el}C \tag{9.17}$$

where k'_{el} is a rate constant representing one or several parallel first-order processes and, assuming one-compartment elimination, would be

$$k'_{el} = \sum_{j=1}^{J} k_{el,j} \tag{9.18}$$

where $k_{el,j}$ is the first-order elimination rate constant of the jth first-order elimination process from the central compartment, and the summation is over all J such defined first-order elimination processes. Similarly, we could define multiple capacity-limited processes, and the general version of equation 9.17 would be

$$\frac{dC}{dt} = -\sum_{n=1}^{N} \frac{V_{max,n}C}{K_{m,n} + C} - k'_{el}C \tag{9.19}$$

where n denotes the nth of N saturable elimination processes defined for the central compartment. Integration of equation 9.19 does not yield an explicit general solution for C, even with the benefit of the fact that first-order outputs from a single compartment (the central compartment in this case) are by their linear nature additive. Solution of equation 9.17 is less imposing, but no less refractory to a general closed solution for C. Equation 9.19 can, however, be solved for t:

$$t = \frac{1}{k'_{el}K_m + V_{max}} \left[K_m \ln \frac{C_0}{C} + \frac{V_{max}}{k'_{el}} \ln \frac{(C_0 + K_m)k'_{el} + V_{max}}{(C + K_m)k'_{el} + V_{max}} \right] \tag{9.20}$$

Assuming low concentrations (i.e., $K_m >> C$), an expression for $\ln C$ can be obtained.

$$\ln C = \ln C_0 + \frac{V_{max}}{k'_{el}K_m} \ln \frac{(C_0 + K_m)k'_{el} + V_{max}}{K_m k'_{el} + V_{max}} - (k_{el} + V_{max} / K_m)\, t \tag{9.21}$$

Various rearrangements of equation 9.21 can be effected to facilitate estimation of the first-order elimination rate constant of a drug, assuming a one-compartment model and $K_m >> C$, from a plasma concentration-versus-time plot. As can be appreciated from this illustration, the presence of mixed-order kinetics rapidly complicates a pharmacokinetic study, and the statistically valid estimation of this many parameters requires a significant number of data points based on degree-of-freedom limitations (discussed in detail in Chapter 13). Such models are rarely encountered in the clinical and comparative biomedical literature.

The organ in which metabolic saturation is most likely to occur is the liver, since most drugs are metabolized there. The reader should review the physiological basis of hepatic biotransformation in Chapter 6. Because the capacity limitation typically is important only at relatively high drug concentrations, the most likely setting for its occurrence is during absorption via the splanchnic circulation and portal vein since drug concentrations are generally much higher during this first pass into the liver than after entry into the general circulation. In those cases where metabolic activity is saturated, a greater portion of the drug gains entry into the general circulation unchanged, which leads to greater systemic availability of unchanged drug. A compound that absorbs more quickly will get a greater fraction of its dose into the general circulation (hence greater systemic availability of unchanged drug) than one that absorbs more slowly, when hepatic enzymatic processes are within the saturation range. This fact must be considered when designing timed-release formulations because the resulting lower splanchnic levels may mitigate saturation to an extent that may drastically depress systemic availability of unchanged drug.

THE IMPACT OF CAPACITY-LIMITED KINETICS AND VARIOUS PHARMACOKINETIC PARAMETERS

Elimination Half-Life.   As long as blood concentrations of the drug are in the saturable range, it will have a nonconstant half-life that will change continuously with drug concentration.

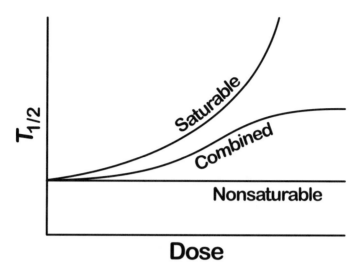

FIGURE 9.8.   Effects of drug concentration on half-life. When elimination proceeds exclusively by linear, nonsaturable elimination processes, $T_{1/2}$ is independent of dose (i.e., concentration) and is thus constant. For elimination that proceeds exclusively by saturable processes, $T_{1/2}$ rises without bound as a function of dose, whereas if both linear and nonlinear processes are operative, $T_{1/2}$ is sigmoidal.

$$T_{\frac{1}{2}} = \frac{\ln 2 (K_m + C)}{V_{\max}} \qquad (9.22)$$

The higher the concentration, the smaller the fraction cleared per unit time, and the longer the apparent half-life becomes. Thus it is in the higher concentration (dose) ranges (e.g., toxic drug overdoses) where this phenomenon is particularly important. For parallel saturable and nonsaturable processes, it can be shown that

$$T_{\frac{1}{2}} = \frac{\ln 2}{\dfrac{V_{\max}}{(K_m + C)} + k'_{el}} \qquad (9.23)$$

The extent of half-life dynamics will depend on the relative fraction of the saturable elimination pathway utilized by the drug. As drug concentrations are increased in this case, the apparent elimination half-life will tend to stabilize more or less asymptotically at a value larger than that measured at relatively low drug concentrations. The elimination half-life would ultimately become independent of concentration because the nonsaturable component becomes dominant and controls the new half-life, with negligible contribution from the saturable component. The effect of drug concentrations on the half-life of drugs that are cleared by nonsaturable, saturable, and combined parallel saturable and nonsaturable pathways is illustrated in Figure 9.8. One potentially profound consequence of the increase in apparent half-life with increasing drug concentrations is increased and prolonged drug accumulation with repeated dosing, and an increase in time to reach steady state.

Area Under the Curve.   For a one-compartment model drug obeying linear first-order kinetics, we have seen in Chapters 7 and 8 that *AUC* is directly proportional to dose (Figure 9.4):

$$AUC = \frac{D}{V_d k_{el}} = \frac{D}{Cl} \qquad (9.24)$$

where D is the available dose and V_d is the volume of distribution. Unfortunately, non-linear elimination processes generally destroy this proportionality between dose and AUC. In this situation, the AUC following an IV bolus injection of a drug that is eliminated by a single capacity-limited pathway is given by

$$AUC = \frac{C_0}{V_{max}}\left(K_m + \frac{C_0}{2}\right) \tag{9.25}$$

When the initial drug concentration, C_0, is much less than K_m (i.e., $C_0 << K_m$), this reduces to

$$AUC = \frac{C_0 K_m}{V_{max}} = \frac{D}{V_d k_{el}} \tag{9.26}$$

which is again identical to the nonsaturable situation of equation 9.24. On the other hand, if $C_0 >> K_m$, then equation 9.25 collapses to

$$AUC = \frac{C_0{}^2}{2V_{max}} = \frac{D^2}{2V_d{}^2 V_{max}} \tag{9.27}$$

since in equation 7.14 (see Chapter 7) for a one-compartment system, C_0 is simply the IV dose (amount, D) divided by the apparent volume of distribution (V_d). Here, the AUC is proportional to the square of the dose and inversely proportional to the square of the distribution volume. V_d should remain constant and should not influence drug levels from different doses. Therefore, drug concentrations within the saturable range lead to disproportionately increasing AUC with increasing dose, as seen in the bottom of Figure 9.4.

Systemic Availability.   Systemic availability is generally determined by comparing the AUC resulting from the administration of some test dosage form to the AUC from the administration of a standard. Thus, such a nonlinear change in AUC with dose becomes important and invalidates using the simple test for comparison of AUC presented in Chapter 3 (equation 3.2) for estimating availability. A commonly used method for estimation of bioavailability of drugs eliminated by saturable processes starts with integration of $-dC/dt$:

$$\int_0^\infty -\frac{dC}{dt}\,dt = \int_0^\infty -dC = C_0 = \frac{D}{V_d} \tag{9.28}$$

where C_0 is the plasma concentration at $t = 0$ following IV administration. A plot of the left side of equation 9.28 versus C_0 or D/V_d will be linear and pass through the origin regardless of the linearity of the model. C_0 or D/V_d can be estimated by numerical differentiation of IV plasma concentration-versus time data, and calculation of the AUC resulting from a plot of $-dC/dt$ versus time. Following oral administration, for example, the rate of drug elimination from the body is given by

$$\frac{1}{V_d}\frac{dD_E}{dt} = k'_{el} + \frac{V_{max}C}{K_m + C} \tag{9.29}$$

where D_E denotes the part of the dose eliminated up to time T. If all absorbed drug is ultimately eliminated (i.e., if $(D_E)_\infty = FD$, where F is the fraction of dose ultimately absorbed), then

$$\frac{1}{V_d}\int_0^\infty \frac{dD_E}{dt}dt = \int_0^\infty \left(k'_{el} + \frac{V_{max}C}{K_m + C}\right)dt = \frac{FD}{V_d} \tag{9.30}$$

since the integral on the left is simply $(D_E)_\infty$. Dividing equation 9.30 by equation 9.28 admits

$$\frac{FD/V_d}{D/V_d} = \frac{[V_d^{-1}\int_0^\infty (dD_E/dt)dt]_{oral}}{[-\int_0^\infty (dC/dt)dt]_{IV}} \tag{9.31}$$

If the *oral* and *IV* doses are equal, assuming V_d remains constant, then

$$F = \frac{[V_d^{-1}\int_0^\infty (dD_E/dt)dt]_{oral}}{[-\int_0^\infty (dC/dt)dt]_{IV}} \tag{9.32}$$

Thus in practice, the absolute systemic availability of an *oral* dose can be estimated by calculating the AUC of a $-dC/dt$-versus-time plot using *IV* data (the denominator of equation 9.32) and using equation 9.29 to generate points of $(dD_E/dt)/V_d$ versus time from oral data. The AUC of the latter is then calculated as the numerator of equation 9.32.

Clearance. For nonlinear elimination processes, such as Michaelis-Menten kinetics, clearance is a nonconstant function of drug concentration. In the case of a one-compartment model with elimination by Michaelis-Menten processes and first-order processes in parallel,

$$Cl = \frac{V_{max}V_d}{K_m + C} + k'_{el}V_d \tag{9.33}$$

clearance decreases as the concentration increases, until at very high drug concentrations, Cl asymptotically reaches a lower limit of $k'_{el}V_d$. Figure 9.9 illustrates this behavior of clearance as a function of drug concentration under the influence of parallel capacity-limited and noncapacity-limited elimination processes by simulating equation 9.33.

This was previously discussed in Chapter 6. When hepatic capacity is exceeded, and the drug has a *low extraction ratio*, total body clearance becomes independent of hepatic blood flow but sensitive to the extent of plasma protein binding. In contrast, when biotransformation is not saturated, the drug has a *high extraction ratio*, and clearance is independent of protein binding (as all drug can be extracted and metabolized) but is dependent upon hepatic blood flow. The discussion in Chapter 6 on intrinsic hepatic clearance (Cl_{int}) (equations 6.4 through 6.7) should now be revisited since the pharmacokinetics of nonlinear elimination have been presented.

Other Nonlinear Elimination Processes
Renal Excretion. Other nonlinear elimination processes can be important for some drugs. As presented in Chapter 5, urinary excretion can be dose-dependent when a drug

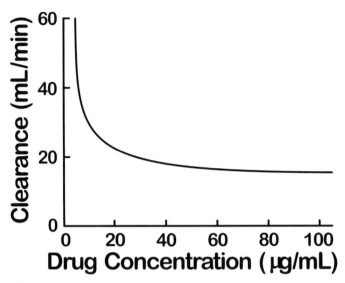

FIGURE 9.9.   Bimodal clearance as a function of drug concentration. As concentration increases, clearance decreases due to the nonlinear processes until, at very high concentrations, it asymptotically approaches a lower limit of $k'_{el}V_d$, the linear elimination processes. The simulation assigned the following values in equation 9.33: k'_{el} = 0.2 min^{-1}; V_d = 60 mL; K_m = 1.5 µg/mL; V_{max} = 2 µg/mL/min.

TABLE **9.1.**   Percutaneous Absorption of Topical Parathion on Pig Skin Demonstrating Nonlinear Absorption As Evidenced by Decreased Percent Dose Absorbed at Higher Applied Surface Concentrations

Dose	4 µg/cm²	40 µg/cm²	400 µg/cm²
Mass (µg/cm²/8 h)	0.32 ± 0.02	0.77 ± 0.11	1.86 ± 0.14
Percent dose/8 h	7.91 ± 0.38	1.91 ± 0.28	0.46 ± 0.04

Data are mean ± standard deviation.

is partly reabsorbed from renal tubules by a saturable process. Thus the elimination (urinary excretion) of large doses can be proportionally faster than smaller doses, and clearance may become a function of dose.

Absorption.   As presented in Chapter 4, there are many processes involved with extravascular drug administration in which nonlinearities may be involved, invalidating the use of linear pharmacokinetic models for data analysis. This can easily be tested by plotting percent dose absorbed after multiple dose administration. If absorption is linear, the percentage absorbed will be constant, while if saturation is present, a lower percent dose will be absorbed at higher doses, as is seen in the saturable topical absorption of parathion in pigs (Table 9.1). In such a case, pharmacokinetic models such as those described above must be employed.

Our laboratory has spent significant effort in studying topical drug and pesticide absorption, and we have constructed complex pharmacokinetic models to describe these phenomena. Presentation of such models is well beyond the scope of this text; however, the interested reader should consult the Selected Readings on parathion absorption and metabolism for application of many of these principles in both *in vitro* and *in vivo* systems.

Enzyme Induction.   Some drugs influence their own clearance (and that of other substrates, in some cases) by directly or indirectly activating (inducing) the gene(s) that codes for the enzyme that metabolizes them. This type of kinetic negative feedback, called enzyme induction and discussed in Chapter 6, is especially interesting because, in contrast to most pharmacokinetic parameters that are concentration-dependent or dose-dependent, this phenomenon is now time-dependent, and results from real time dynamic biochemical or physiological changes in the body (i.e., unscheduled protein synthesis in this case). An early model developed in 1965 by Berlin and Schimke described time-dependent enzyme concentration, $E(t)$, following induction using the following expression:

$$E(t) = \frac{S}{k} - \left(\frac{S}{k} - \frac{S_0}{k_0}\right)e^{-kt} \tag{9.34}$$

where S_0 = initial (steady-state, before induction) zero-order rate of enzyme synthesis; S = new (steady-state, after induction) zero-order rate of enzyme synthesis; k_0 = initial (steady-state, before induction) first-order rate constant for enzyme degradation; and k = new (steady-state, after induction) first-order rate constant for enzyme degradation.

Note that, prior to induction ($t = 0$),

$$E(0) = \frac{S_0}{k_0} \tag{9.35}$$

and, at the new steady-state following induction ($t = \infty$),

$$E(\infty) = \frac{S}{k} \tag{9.36}$$

The pharmacokinetic implications of enzyme induction are important. It can be shown that the change in V_{max} during induction can be described by

$$V_{max}(t) = V'_{max} - [V'_{max} - V_{max}(0)]e^{-kt} \tag{9.37}$$

where V'_{max} = the new (steady-state following induction) value at $t = \infty$ and $V_{max}(0)$ = the preinduction steady-state value at $t = 0$. Similarly, the change in systemic clearance, $Cl(t)$, of a drug following self-induction can be described by

$$Cl(t) = Cl' - [Cl' - Cl_0]e^{-kt} \tag{9.38}$$

where Cl' = the new (steady-state following induction) value at $t = \infty$ and
Cl_0 = the preinduction steady-state value at $t = 0$.

The plasma drug concentration profile under the influence of self-induction can be described for a one-compartment model where the drug is infused at constant rate R_0 and eliminated otherwise by first-order processes.

$$C(t) = \frac{R_0}{Cl_0}\left[1 - e^{-\frac{Cl_0 t}{V_d}}\right] \tag{9.39}$$

Note that when induction begins, Cl_0 in equation 9.39 will be replaced by $Cl(t)$ (equation 9.38). Figure 9.10 illustrates this by simulating equations. 9.38 and 9.39.

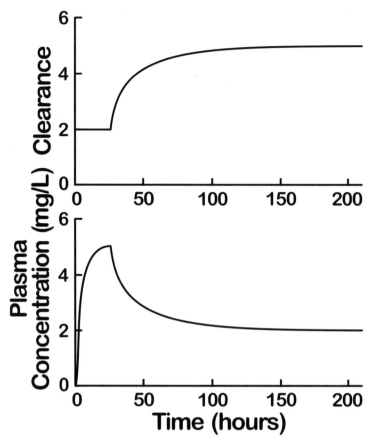

FIGURE 9.10. Illustration of the influence of enzyme induction on clearance (upper plot, equation 9.38) and plasma concentration (lower plot, equation 9.39) profiles during an IV infusion. Induction occurs at $t = 20$ h. Clearance rises and plasma concentration falls sharply at induction, before asymptotically approaching new steady-state values. Values assigned were preinduction clearance = $Cl_0 = 2$ L/h; drug infusion rate = $R_0 = 10$ mg/min; $V_d = 7$ L; postinduction steady-state clearance = $Cl' = 5$ L/h; postinduction first-order enzyme degradation rate constant = $k = .03$ h^{-1}.

Enzyme induction becomes an important factor with chronic drug administration and with many examples of environmental and occupational exposure to toxicants (see Chapter 6, Tables 6.6, 6.9, and 6.10). If experiments are conducted such that multiple pharmacokinetic trials can be done at similar doses over a prolonged period, the extent of induction can be quantitated.

Other examples of time-dependent pharmacokinetic events include circadian rhythms and disease onset or chemical-induced toxicity in an organ of elimination. These events are often difficult to detect unless full metabolic studies are conducted or independent markers of toxicity are examined. Our laboratory has encountered two such cases. The first was nonlinearity in the clearance of aminoglycoside antibiotics induced by direct drug toxicity to the kidney. In this case, high doses of gentamicin resulted in decreased clearance shown by drug accumulation and nonlinear dose versus *AUC* plots. Similarly, in percutaneous absorption studies of the chemical vesicant sulfur mustard (*bis* 2-chloroethyl sulfide), severe vascular damage occurred as the compound was absorbed, necessitating constructing a toxicokinetic model that specifically altered vascular volume in proportion to absorbed chemical.

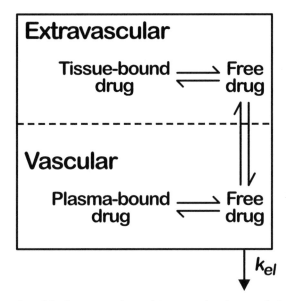

FIGURE 9.11. Schematic of model of extravascular and intravascular tissue and plasma protein binding, respectively. The model assumes elimination (k_{el}) of free drug from the plasma space exclusively, and only free drug is able to traverse vascular epithelia.

PROTEIN AND TISSUE BINDING

It is typically assumed that drug binding to plasma proteins and extravascular tissues is constant and independent of concentration at the binding site. However, as presented in Chapter 4, protein binding is also saturable, and thus nonlinear pharmacokinetics may become operative. We will now discuss the implications of both plasma and tissue binding to pharmacokinetic models.

Figure 9.11 depicts two major types of tissue as binding sites, vascular (e.g., plasma binding to albumin) and nonvascular tissue spaces, and assumes as in most compartmental models that elimination exclusively occurs from the vascular space. In the vascular space, protein binds drug, forming a drug-protein complex as previously described by equation 4.1 (see Chapter 4), and now reformulated in equation 9.40:

$$[f]+[p] \underset{k_{-1}}{\overset{k_1}{\rightleftharpoons}} [b]$$ (9.40)

where f = free drug in the vascular space ($[T]_F$ in Chapter 4); b = bound drug in vascular space ($[T]_B$ in Chapter 4); p = free protein binding sites; and k_1, k_{-1} are rate constants.

The brackets [] indicate molar concentration. Then

$$\frac{d[f]}{dt} = k_{-1}[b] - k_1[f][p]$$ (9.41)

The steady-state assumption (i.e., $d[f]/dt = 0$) implies

$$\frac{k_{-1}}{k_1} = k_d = \frac{[f][p]}{[b]}$$ (9.42)

where k_d is the dissociation constant (in units of concentration) for the protein-drug complex. If n = the number of binding sites per protein molecule, and $[P_r]$ is the molarity of protein, then the total concentration of vascular protein binding sites is

$$n[P_r] = [f] + [b] \tag{9.43}$$

Equation 9.43 can be solved for $[f]$ and its result substituted into equation 9.42, giving

$$k_d = \frac{[f](n[P_r] - [b])}{[b]} \tag{9.44}$$

and solving for [b] yields

$$[b] = \frac{[f]n[P_r]}{k_d + [f]} \tag{9.45}$$

By definition,

$$C_{vasc} = [f] + [b] \tag{9.46}$$

where C_{vasc} is the total concentration of drug in the vascular space, which is simply the sum of the concentrations of free and bound drug. Substitution of equation 9.45 into 9.46 then gives

$$C_{vasc} = [f] + \frac{[f]n[P_r]}{k_d + [f]} \tag{9.47}$$

A corresponding expression for total extravascular (tissue) drug concentration can be derived analogously, resulting in equation 9.48:

$$C_{tiss} = [f] + \frac{[f]q[P_T]}{k_d^T + [f]} \tag{9.48}$$

where q and $[P_T]$ are analogously the number of binding sites per tissue-binding molecule and the molarity, respectively, and the superscript T on k_d denotes the dissociation constant for tissue-drug complexes.

If we define a new variable for the fraction free in the vascular space (referred to by some authors as $[fu]_b$),

$$\varphi_V = \frac{[f]}{C_{vasc}} \tag{9.49}$$

and the corresponding one for the extravascular space (often referred to as $[fu]_T$),

$$\varphi_T = \frac{[f]}{C_{Tiss}} \tag{9.50}$$

then the following expressions, which take into account both plasma and tissue protein binding, can be derived for volume of distribution,

$$V_d = V_v + \frac{\varphi_V}{\varphi_T} V_T \tag{9.51}$$

and clearance,

$$Cl = Q \frac{\varphi_V Cl_I}{Q + \varphi_V Cl_I} \tag{9.52}$$

where Cl_I is the intrinsic clearance of free drug from the blood, Q is blood flow to the eliminating organ(s), V_v is the intravascular (blood) volume, and V_T is the extravascular (tissue) volume. For drugs with low intrinsic clearance (i.e., $Q >> \varphi_V Cl_I$) and with intravascular nonlinear binding, the decrease in free fraction as intravascular drug concentration decreases will cause a corresponding decrease in clearance and volume of distribution. These techniques are often used in constructing physiologically based pharmacokinetic models (presented in Chapter 10), where using the *in vitro* binding techniques presented in Chapter 4 and constructing models on an organ-by-organ basis, accurate descriptions of a drug's disposition may be obtained.

Recalling equations 7.20 and 8.22 (see Chapters 7 and 8),

$$T_{\frac{1}{2}} = \frac{0.693 \, V_d}{Cl} \tag{9.53}$$

it is easy to see that, given the effect nonlinear binding has on distribution and clearance, half-life should suffer corresponding dynamic influences, and the resulting plasma concentration-versus-time profile will reflect this. This makes the analysis of drugs with extensive binding characteristics a difficult task, unfortunately a problem often encountered in the modeling of tissue residues.

The problem, as the astute reader probably has gathered, is the extensive experimental data required for adequate solution of these models. Therefore, assumptions are often made, and simpler linear approaches are used. However, when such approaches generate inconsistent and confounding data, the above principles may be operative, thereby invalidating these simplifying assumptions. The simple tests for nonlinearity would save much "modeler anxiety."

It is instructive to see what the effects of plasma and tissue binding have on disposition. Here, numerical simulation techniques are useful. Equations 9.47 through 9.52 are plotted against arbitrary ranges of independent variables in Figure 9.12. The reader should be reminded that these simulations, though instructive, are "snapshots" of the sensitivity of the various parameters when all but one variable on the x-axis are held constant. Unfortunately, in the intact animal this simple scenario may not always be the case.

NONLINEAR PHARMACOKINETICS: A CAVEAT

The theory developed in this chapter is based on the assumption of a one-compartment model, but it enjoys general application regardless of model structure. One caveat, however, should be raised here. In certain cases where single compartment kinetics are erroneously assumed, the estimation of K_m and V_{max} can be flawed. Since the elimination rate constant $k_{el} = V_{max} / K_m$, the estimate of V_{max} would be low because the estimated k_{el} would be lower than the actual value.

Sometimes it is difficult to distinguish between nonlinear processes and linear ones as they are manifested in the plasma concentration-versus-time profiles. An actual nonlinear

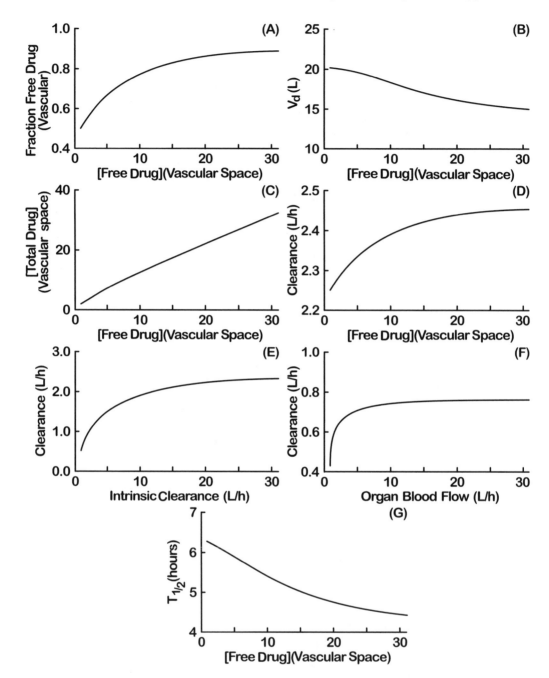

FIGURE 9.12.   Nonlinear binding illustrations of equations developed in the text. Initial assigned default values: $n = 2$; $P_r = 2$ mM; $k_d = 3$ mM; $V_v = 10$ L; $V_T = 2$ L; $q = 8$; $P_T = 8$ mM; $k_d^T = 6$ mM; $Q = 2.5$ mL/m; $Cl_I = 45$ mL/m.; $[f] = (1–30$ mM). Note on nomenclature: the unit mM denotes molar concentration (molarity), i.e., mM = mmol/L. (A): Fraction free drug, φ_v, in vascular space as a function of free vascular drug concentration, $[f]$ (mM), from equation 9.49. (B): V_d profile simulated as a function of intravascular space, from equation 9.51. (C): Total drug concentration in the vascular space (C_{vasc}, mM) as a function of $[f]$, from equation 9.49. (D): Clearance (L/h) as a function of $[f]$, from equation 9.52. (E): Clearance as a function of intrinsic clearance, Cl_I ($1–40$ L/h), from equation 9.52. (F): Clearance as a function of organ blood flow, Q ($1–30$ L/h), from equation 9.52. (G): Half-life, $T_{1/2}$, as a function of $[f]$, from equation 9.53 using appropriate substitutions from earlier relations.

mechanism (especially nonlinear binding) can be misinterpreted as a multiexponential or compartmental structure (e.g., an additional exponential term or compartment, respectively), or a nonlinear plasma protein binding influence could mistakenly be subsumed under in a Michaelis-Menten construct. Conversely, the distribution characteristics of a drug could be misinterpreted as one or more nonlinear phenomena. Often it is prudent to invest in additional experimentation to separate and rule out certain model structures. Normally, linear processes can be separated from nonlinear ones by analyzing various dosages with both bolus and infusion profiles, as discussed above. As will be repeatedly stressed in Chapter 13 on experimental design, it is often cost-effective to conduct pilot studies to help select the proper model. *As is too often the case, the use of pharmacokinetics is judged erroneous when inconsistent results are obtained, when in reality the problem is often use of an inappropriate modeling strategy.* A simple one- or two-compartmental or noncompartmental analysis of single-dose plasma data is often not sufficient to define models for drugs that undergo extensive biotransformation or tissue binding. Thus extrapolations using these approaches will neither be robust nor predict subsequent *in vivo* behavior. Similarly, when dealing with interspecies extrapolations, peculiarities in metabolism or binding may only occur in a single species, and without knowledge of these differences, erroneous extrapolations may be made. Simple multidose IV pilot studies may prevent these pitfalls.

SELECTED READINGS

(*The Selected Readings listed in Chapter 6 should also be consulted for pharmacokinetic modeling of drugs undergoing nonlinear hepatic metabolism.*)

Berlin, C.M., and R.T. Schimke. 1965. Influence of turnover rates on the responses of enzymes to cortisone. *Molecular Pharmacology*. 1:149.

Chang, S.K., W.C. Dauterman, and J.E. Riviere. 1994. Percutaneous absorption of parathion and its metabolites paraoxon and *p*-nitrophenol administered alone or in combination: In vitro flow through diffusion cell system. *Pesticide Biochemistry and Physiology*. 48:56-62.

Cheng, H. 1991. A method for calculating the mean residence times of caternary metabolites. *Biopharmaceutics and Drug Disposition*. 12:335-342.

Cheng, H., and W.J. Jusko. 1988. Mean residence time concepts for pharmacokinetic systems with nonlinear drug elimination described by the Michaelis-Menten equation. *Pharmaceutical Research*. 5:156-164.

Cheng, H., and W.J. Jusko. 1989. Mean residence time of drugs showing simultaneous first-order and Michaelis-Menten kinetics. *Pharmaceutical Research*. 6:258-261.

Cheng, H., and W.J. Jusko. 1990. Mean residence times of multicompartmental drugs undergoing reversible metabolism. *Pharmaceutical Research*. 7:103-107.

Gibaldi, M., and D. Perrier. 1982. *Pharmacokinetics*, 2ed. New York:Marcel Dekker.

Jusko, W.J., J.R. Koup, and G. Alvan. 1976. Nonlinear assessment of phenytoin bioavailability. *Journal of Pharmacokinetics and Biopharmaceutics*. 4:327.

Michaelis, L. and M.I. Menten. 1913. Die Kinetik der Intertinwirkung. *Biochemikal Z*. 49:333-369.

Qiao, G.L., and J.E. Riviere. 1995. Significant effects of application site and occlusion on the pharmacokinetics of cutaneous penetration and biotransformation of parathion *in vivo* in swine. *Journal of Pharmaceutical Sciences*. 84:425-432.

Qiao, G.L., P.L. Williams, and J.E. Riviere. 1994. Percutaneous absorption, biotransformation and systemic disposition of parathion *in vivo* in swine. I. Comprehensive pharmacokinetic model. *Drug Metabolism and Disposition*. 22:459-471.

Qiao, G.L., J.D. Brooks, R.E. Baynes, N.A. Monteiro-Riviere, P.L. Williams, and J.E. Riviere. 1996. The use of mechanistically defined chemical mixtures (MDCM) to assess mixture component effects on the percutaneous absorption and cutaneous disposition of topically exposed chemicals. I. Studies with parathion mixtures in isolated perfused porcine skin. *Toxicology and Applied Pharmacology*. 141:473-486.

Riviere, J.E., J.D. Brooks, P.L. Williams, and N.A. Monteiro-Riviere. 1995. Toxicokinetics of topical sulfur-mustard penetration, disposition and vascular toxicity in isolated perfused porcine skin. *Toxicology and Applied Pharmacology*. 135:25-34.

Sedman, A.J., and J.G. Wagner. 1974. Quantitative pooling of Michaelis-Menten equations in models with parallel metabolite formation paths. *Journal of Pharmacokinetics and Biopharmaceutics*. 2:149.

St-Pierre, M.V., D. van den Berg, and K.S. Pang. 1990. Physiological modeling of drug and metabolite:Disposition of oxazapam and oxazepam glucuronides in the recirculating perfused mouse liver preparation. *Journal of Pharmacokinetics and Biopharmaceutics*.18:423-448.

Williams, P.L., and J.E. Riviere, J.E. 1995. A biophysically based dermatopharmacokinetic compartment model for quantifying percutaneous penetration and absorption of topically applied agents. I. Theory. *Journal of Pharmaceutical Sciences*. 84:599-608.

Williams, P.L., D. Thompson, G.L. Qiao, N.A. Monteiro-Riviere, R.E. Baynes, and J.E. Riviere. 1996. The use of mechanistically defined chemical mixtures (MDCM) to assess mixture component effects on the percutaneous absorption and cutaneous disposition of topically exposed chemicals. II. Development of a general dermatopharmacokinetic model for use in risk assessment. *Toxicology and Applied Pharmacology*. 141:487-496.

10

Physiological Models

All of the pharmacokinetic modeling strategies presented up to this point have assumed that the defining criteria for a *compartment* or *kinetic space* was an anatomically heterogeneous group of tissues that could be described by single-rate equations since the disposition of drug within these areas had homogeneous rates. In compartmental terms, drug in these spaces could be characterized by a specific volume of distribution (Vd) and pairs of intercompartmental micro-rate constants (k_{xy} / k_{yx}). Noncompartmental models made no assumptions about underlying anatomy nor physiology. The infrastructure of the compartments were based on rates and were not unique (recall Figure 7.20 in Chapter 7 for the possible configurations of a two-compartment model).

INTRODUCTION

Physiologically based pharmacokinetic (PBPK) modeling builds models based on compartments that mirror the anatomical and physiological structure of the body. A PBPK model is constructed as a series of organ systems interconnected by the circulatory system as depicted in Figure 10.1. Specific organs are included in parallel in the model based upon their relative importance in determining drug disposition for the compound being studied. Compartments are connected to one another by arterial and venous blood supplies. If the lung is included in a model, it is placed in series with the plasma compartment since it receives the total of cardiac output via the right heart, while the rest of the tissues receive the output from the left heart. Thus, all drug will circulate through the pulmonary circulation before it enters the systemic circulation.

The route of administration is also included as input into the relevant compartment. In the scheme depicted, the compound distributes to red blood cells, the kidney, and the liver and, furthermore, is eliminated by the latter two organs. The model is structured to handle either oral or topical administration. Inhalational administration would include a lung compartment placed in series with the blood. All other sites of compound distribution are pooled into a general tissue compartment. Each tissue is modeled as being composed of plasma and interstitial and intracellular components.

It is important to reflect upon the nature of these models for they are essentially an attempt to create a mathematical structure that quantitates the processes described in Figure 2.1 (see Chapter 2). All of the physiological factors that impact on drug distribution

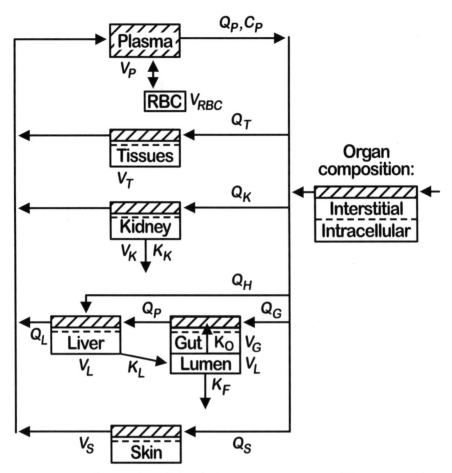

FIGURE 10.1.   Structure of a physiologically based pharmacokinetic (PBPK) model incorporating disposition in plasma, liver, kidney, skin, and gastrointestinal tract. Elimination from the body occurs from the kidney (K_K), liver (K_L) and gut lumen in feces (K_F). Oral absorption (K_O) is allowed. V refers to organ volumes of distribution and Q to organ blood flows.

and elimination, discussed in Chapters 4 through 6, may be incorporated into the model. If a drug primarily distributes to the muscle, then it would be included as a tissue compartment. If the model were constructed to predict drug concentrations in a specific organ, that organ would be included. In most models, the liver and kidney are incorporated since their high blood flow:tissue mass ratio coupled with their function as eliminating organs dictate that they are determining factors in predicting the overall disposition of the drug in the body.

The other major advantage of this approach is that many factors that can be experimentally assessed in a specific organ may be incorporated easily into that organ's disposition. PBPK models easily allow the incorporation of such data from *in vitro* systems. These include factors such as tissue binding, active enzyme transport systems, local metabolism, and even pharmacodynamic effects on blood flow. For example, if plasma and tissue binding were included, a component such as depicted in Figure 9.11 (see Chapter 9) could be incorporated. The strategy is to describe these models on an individual organ basis and then link them, using blood flow through the organs, to develop an overall model for disposition in the body.

MODEL CONSTRUCTION

The model is constructed by defining the rate of plasma flow (Q) and Vd of drug in each organ and then writing a mass balance equation describing the rate of drug input and output for each organ. The major assumption is that distribution between organs in the model are limited by blood flow to each organ. The basic form of these equations is based on the same principle as that of Fick's law of diffusion (described in Chapter 5) for determining the renal clearance of a drug based on blood flow and extraction ratio (E) outlined in equation 5.2 (see Chapter 5). In this case, E is expressed in terms of an equilibrium ratio or partition coefficient (R) as

$$R_{tissue} = R_t = C_{tissue} / C_{blood} \qquad (10.1)$$

where C_{tissue} (C_t) is the concentration of drug in the tissue at equilibrium, which is equal to the C_{ven}, and C_{blood} (Cp in previous chapters in which plasma concentrations were analyzed) is the concentration of drug in blood entering the organ or C_{art} of equation 5.2. Simple algebra yields $R = 1 - E$. The differential equation describing the rate of change in drug concentration for any organ is simply the rate in minus the rate out. For any noneliminating organ, this becomes

$$dC_t / dt = (\text{Rate in}) - (\text{Rate out}) \; \{Noneliminating\ Organ\}$$
$$= [Q_t(Cp) - Q_t(C_t / R_t)] / V_t \qquad , \quad C_{blood} = C_t / R_t \qquad (10.2)$$
$$= Q_t[Cp - C_t / R_t] / V_t$$

where V_t is the drug Vd in the tissue that converts mass to concentration.

If the organ is an eliminating organ, then some fraction of drug will be removed through this process, thus reducing the venous output. This will be related to the clearance of the drug in that organ (Cl_{organ}) and C_t. This can be expressed as

$$dC_t / dt = \frac{\{Q_t[(Cp - C_t / R_t)]\}}{V_t} - C_t Cl_{organ} \; \{Eliminating\ Organ\} \qquad (10.3)$$

These equations describe the disposition of the drug in each organ component of the model. All that is now needed is to write an equation describing the rate of change of drug concentration in the blood, which is the sum of the contributions of all organs:

$$dCp / dt = \frac{Dose + \Sigma Q_t(C_t / R_t) - (\Sigma Q_t)Cp}{V_{vascular}} \qquad (10.4)$$

As discussed in the distribution chapter, only free drug is distributed out of the vascular space into tissue, and thus Cp should be expressed as the free concentration f. Equations 9.46 to 9.52 presented in Chapter 9 on plasma and tissue protein binding may be directly incorporated into these PBPK models if the drug's characteristics warrant it.

Similarly, if a drug is metabolized in an organ, the Michaelis-Menton concepts introduced in Chapter 6 and presented in Chapter 9 may be utilized in place of the Cl_{organ} term of equation 10.3. For the liver, this would be

$$dC_1 / dt = \frac{\{Q_1[(Cp - C_1 / R_1)]\} - V_m f_1 / (Km_f + f_1)}{V_t} \qquad (10.5)$$

where f_1 is the free blood concentration in the liver and Km_f is the Michaelis constant expressed in terms of free drug. Depending on the compound, the metabolite may be entered back into a parallel PBPK model that describes the metabolite's disposition in the body (needed because the metabolite will have independent elimination and distribution characteristics from the parent drug as originally presented in Chapter 6, Figure 6.3) or is excreted in the bile back to the gastrointestinal tract. The complexity of this compartment is dependent upon how much data are available to handle biliary excretion, enterohepatic recycling, and first-pass metabolism. Some workers have modeled drug transit through the gut as a function of gastrointestinal content flow and absorption from each region of the digestive tract. This results in a more complex model, providing input into the portal vein. The physiological basis for some of these models were presented in Chapter 6, in which the hybrid PBPK model was introduced in Figure 6.3.

In a PBPK model, the overall volume of distribution Vd_{ss} is easily expressed as the sum of the Vd for plasma and all tissues, or

$$Vd_{ss} = V_p + \Sigma V_t R_t \tag{10.6}$$

Finally, if absorption occurs in an organ, a term relating the administered dose to the amount and rate of absorption must also be included. When this occurs after oral absorption, the equation for the liver is often written in terms of absorption from the portal vein as a positive term adding drug input to the liver ($k_a FD$). $X = FD$

For topical delivery, a simple absorption rate may be added to the skin compartment, or the skin may be modeled in terms of stratum corneum penetration and dermal distribution. Our laboratory has used the output flux from the isolated perfused skin-flap model to serve as the skin compartment of a PBPK model (recall Figure 8.6 in Chapter 8), with the complexity of the skin component reflecting the design of the specific experiment. In fact, this is a strength of this modeling approach, for *in vitro* organ studies may often be directly used in a whole-body model. Isolated perfused livers are often used to define the Michaelis-Menten kinetics of a drug. Some modeling systems administer volatile drug via inhalation, obtain data on the rate of chemical uptake from the inspired air, and then collect tissue samples after equilibrium has occurred. To solve these models, air-to-tissue partition coefficients are determined.

For most tissues, equilibration among the plasma, interstitial fluid, and cellular spaces is assumed to be rapid, and thus the V_t and R_t become a composite estimate for that organ. This could also be assessed *in situ* by use of microdialysis probes to directly assess interstitial fluid concentrations. If diffusional barriers exist (organ is membrane-limited rather than flow-limited as assumed above), or if extensive tissue binding occurs (e.g., consider Chapter 9, Figure 9.11 again), then such organs can be modeled with appropriate equations. The description of tissue concentration as being composed of vascular, extravascular, and tissue components is well handled by PBPK models for, as stressed in Chapter 7 on compartmental models, tissue concentrations may not correlate directly to a peripheral compartment prediction since they are actually composed of multiple compartments. In a PBPK model, this integration is implicit to the model. As an example of non–flow-limited behavior, if diffusion from plasma to a tissue compartment is rate-limiting, a first-order diffusion rate constant may be added to that organ's equation {$k(Cp - C_t)$} to reflect the fraction of drug that will diffuse into the space as a function of the driving concentration.

In most cases, only specific organs are of interest and sampled in any study; the remainder are grouped as a general tissue compartment. If tissues composing this group have heterogeneous kinetic behavior for the compound being studied, two compartments may be added, reflecting this kinetic difference (e.g., slowly and rapidly equilibrating). In many cases, a specific tissue may be added because it is the target tissue for the drug of concern even if it has a minor influence on the total disposition of the drug in the body.

ANALYSIS

A complete PBPK model is then constructed using the differential equations for the plasma compartment and each tissue component modeled. The complete model thus consists of a series of differential equations, written in terms of Cp, that must be simultaneously solved. This allows all compartments to be linked to one another. The data required to solve these are the Cp versus time data, as well as estimates of organ blood flows, organ distribution volumes, and partition coefficients for the drug in each organ. Recall that these equations assume that equilibrium has occurred within each organ, such that C_{ven} reflects C_t. One does not "curve-fit" plasma and tissue data in a PBPK model experiment; rather, one conducts experiments to estimate these components and then simulates the entire model to assess how well the predicted concentration profiles in plasma, urine, and tissues match observed data. *This is conceptually very different from all of the previous modeling approaches discussed.* The models are simulated using various software packages, including Advanced Continuous Simulation Language (ACSL), SimuSolv, routines in Windows NONLIN, and many other FORTRAN-based simulation programs. All of these modeling approaches use numerical integration algorithms embedded in the software to calculate time estimates of each component equation and reiterate until an optimal model solution is achieved. PBPK models had their roots in chemical engineering, and thus many approaches use software developed from this discipline.

The techniques used to obtain these parameter values are varied and determine the experimental design. Organ blood flows and volumes are usually taken from historical sources such as those tabulated in Table 10.1. The sum of all organ blood flows (excluding the lung which, recall, is in series with the systemic circulation and thus has a total pulmonary blood flow equal to the cardiac output) must equal the overall cardiac output of the animal. In other cases, blood flows may be directly determined using microsphere, laser Doppler velocimetry (LDV), or tracer dilution techniques. In contrast, the sum of all tissue volumes may be less than total body weight since some tissues are not perfused (e.g., fur, teeth, bone matrix). Again, the lung is not included in these calculations. The benefit of using data collected from the same animals as in the experimental study is to reduce variability, as individual differences in any of these major parameters will confound the result. Organs with large blood flows or distribution volumes will have more influence on the overall fit to the model predictions than those with smaller flows or volumes making the overall goodness of fit of the model heavily dependent upon these organs (e.g., liver, kidney).

The major data needed for a PBPK model are estimates of R_t, for which there are a number of approaches. The most robust method is to use an intravenous infusion to achieve steady-state blood concentrations. The animals are then sacrificed, and R_t is simply as defined in equation 10.1 above. Alternatively, if a volatile compound is being studied, tissue:air and blood:air partition coefficients may be experimentally determined, with their quotient being used as the estimate of R_t (C_t:C_a ÷ Cp:C_a). Intravenous dose bolus studies may also be used if simultaneous blood and tissue samples are collected for analysis after distribution pseudoequilibrium has occurred. Blood and tissue concentrations are then plotted on a Cartesian plot, and a constrained linear regression through the origin is used to fit the data. The slope of this line is used as the estimate of R_t for that tissue (Figure 10.2). Severe deviations from linearity would be indicative of tissue binding or complex diffusion, which would require accounting for these phenomena in the differential equations for that organ. Finally, if no independent estimate of R_t is available, then the PBPK model itself may be used to vary R_t to determine the best fit to the data.

TABLE 10.1. Physiological Parameters for Four Species

Parameter	Mouse	Rat	Dog	Human
Body Weight (g)	22	500	12,000	70,000
Volume (mL)				
Plasma	1.0	19.6	500	3,000
Muscle	10.0	245	5530	35,000
Kidney	0.34	3.6	60	280
Liver	1.3	19.6	480	1,350
Gut	1.5	11.2	480	2,100
Heart	0.10	1.2	120	300
Spleen	0.10	1.3	36	160
Blood flow (mL/min)				
Plasma	4.4	84.6	512	3,670
Muscle	0.5	22.4	138	420
Kidney	0.8	12.8	90	700
Liver	1.1	4.7	60	800
Gut	0.9	14.6	82	700
Heart	0.3	1.6	60	150
Spleen	0.1	1.0	14	240

Adapted from *Gerlowski and Jain. 1983. Journal of Pharmaceutical Sciences. 72:1103-1126.*

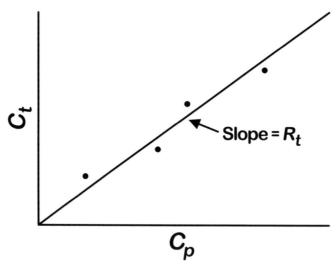

FIGURE 10.2. Estimation of effective tissue:blood partition coefficients (R_t) at steady-state using a C_t versus Cp plot.

Many investigators use multiple doses of drugs to determine R_t to ensure that non-linear behavior is not evident or, if it is present, to write equations that account for it. Whatever the method used to calculate ratios, R_t for an eliminating organ that has high intrinsic Cl_{organ} relative to Q_{organ} may be misleading. However, if clearance is low compared to organ blood flow, the steady-state estimates are good approximations. Finally, R_ts calculated for one species may not always be applicable to another because of species differences in tissue composition. This question may be assessed using some of the allometric principles covered in Chapter 16. The prudent investigator will determine these

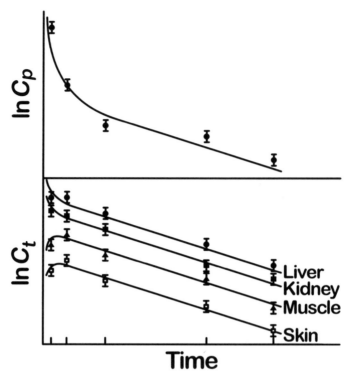

FIGURE 10.3.   Observed versus model predicted (mean ± SEM) concentration versus time profiles of drug in all organs modeled using a PBPK model structured according to Figure 10.1.

parameters for the species of interest to reduce extrapolation error, although PBPK modeling is probably the best approach to interspecies pharmacokinetics available at this point.

Tissue and plasma protein binding may be experimentally determined by the methods outlined in Chapter 4 and 9. As mentioned earlier, estimates of V_{max} and K_m may be efficiently determined using many *in vitro* tissue preparations. The nature of the elimination of the drug by the kidney could be assessed using many of the principles presented in Chapter 5.

The final result of a PBPK exercise is a properly parameterized model that adequately fits all of the observed data. The output of such a model is a list of R_ts and simulated versus observed C-T and tissue versus time profiles, as simulated for a hypothetical drug in Figure 10.3. Note that the drug concentrations vary in magnitude as a function of the tissue, with liver and kidney typically showing the highest values. In this example, there is a peak in the muscle and skin profiles, indicating the time required to reach distribution equilibrium, a slower process for skin in this example. If the model does not reasonably predict concentrations for a specific organ, the structure of the equations for that compartment must be investigated. If a lack of fit occurred in a primary organ such as the liver or kidney, the entire model would be unsatisfactory since they have such a large influence on overall disposition.

Most often the problem resides in an inappropriate or nonlinear R_t, tissue binding or diffusion-limited distribution. Various hybrid models could be constructed to address this problem by using empirical functions for R_t obtained by fitting equation to the C_t versus C_B data plots. The nature of these functions could then help define the type of processes needed to be incorporated into the PBPK model.

ADVANTAGES

The most obvious advantage to the PBPK approach is that the model is based upon both anatomical and physiological reality. It is very powerful technique since concentration-time profiles can be simulated in different tissues of interest. It is also evident that inter-species differences in drug disposition can be easily tested by changing the organ-related parameters listed in Table 10.1, running a simulation and comparing the predictions against limited experimental data points. If the fit is reasonable, then one may be assured that no major species-specific factors are involved in the disposition process. Alternatively, one can easily incorporate *in vitro* data into the model to improve fit. These models also allow one to use experimentally simpler *in vitro* systems to assess impact on *in vivo* disposition by inserting the *in vitro* system directly into a model.

The other major advantage to PBPK models is that the effects of altered physiology are easily simulated by just changing the organ parameters in a model. This type of modeling has been extensively used in cancer chemotherapy to target drugs specifically to tumor sites. It is also a useful tool to extrapolate rodent data to humans for toxicology risk assessment. The limitations to its widespread adoption are based on the extensive data required to adequately create a model and on difficulties with assessing statistical properties of fit and interindividual differences. Finally, these models may be linked to pharmacodynamic (PD) effect models (see Chapter 12) to derive PB-PK-PD models. The advantage to this approach is that the tissue in which the receptors for activity are located may be specifically modeled as the *biophase* or *effect compartment*, making pharmacodynamic linkages easier to construct and physiologically more realistic.

AN APPLICATION APPLIED TO A HYBRID MODEL

Now that the primary types of pharmacokinetic models have been presented, it is instructive to see how these various approaches can be combined using the basic construct of a PBPK model. We will close this chapter with an example of dermal absorption used by our laboratory. In the case of topical drug delivery, diffusion is the primary rate-limiting process governing drug movement across the stratum corneum and through the avascular regions of the epidermis and basement membrane zone. However, once the drug is in the dermal domain, flow-dependent vascular uptake predominates. The approach presented was necessary for certain transdermal drugs because both diffusion-limited and perfusion-limited scenarios may occur. PBPK models are better suited to describe flow-dependent processes, while compartmental schemes are often ideal to handle diffusion-limited disposition.

To follow up on the development of skin models previously presented in this book, we will describe a "hybrid" model, in which a compartmental scheme is used to describe the disposition in the epidermis, and a flow-limited physiologically based model is used to link this to the systemic circulation. We have used such a strategy (see Figure 10.4) to describe drug disposition within isolated perfused skin flaps after arterial drug administration. A version of this model was previously presented as the "skin output" component in Figure 8.6 (see Chapter 8). As one can see, this scheme also can be easily substituted for the skin component of Figure 10.1 as it is constructed with arterial inputs and venous output fluxes. This model was constructed to study cisplatin disposition, which demonstrated a membrane-limited disposition within skin and extensive nonreversible covalent tissue binding, modeled here as a slowly equilibrating compartment. The volumes of the vascular compartments were independently determined using dual radiolabeled inulin/albumin infusion studies and analyzing these data using noncompartmental methods presented in Chapter 8. Similar studies were done to model drug-induced changes in capillary permeability (albumin/inulin volumes) when drugs induced vascular changes.

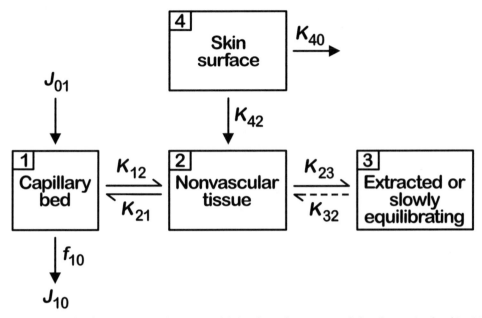

FIGURE 10.4. Hybrid compartmental/PBPK model for drug absorption and distribution in the skin. Note similarity to that presented in Figure 8.6 (see Chapter 8) if arterial fluxes into the skin are assumed negligible ($J_{01} \cong 0$).

The absorption component may also be included to cover transdermal delivery. In this case, the output from this model assumes no arterial recirculation and thus is represented as a drug flux into the systemic model as depicted in Figure 8.6 (see Chapter 8). Note the difference in the model structure for skin in Figure 10.4, which is based on vascular flux into and out of the dermis, versus Figure 8.6, which only allows unidirectional flux out of skin. However, if extensive redistribution occurs back to the skin, the elevated arterial drug concentrations may affect these processes, a scenario very difficult to account for in other modeling schemes. This is especially critical when drug has an affinity for the skin.

The true absorption profile of a compound is also dependent upon the solvent in which it is dosed. By again using a compartmental scheme to develop this model, compound flux into and through skin may be specifically linked to relevant biophysical properties of the skin and penetrating compound, links that require some of the nonlinear models presented in Chapter 9. Such a model is structured as shown in Figure 10.5.

The compartments on the left represent the solvent; and the rest represent the primary compound of interest. This flux is then modeled using a variant of Fick's law of diffusion (equation 2.1, Chapter 2) rewritten to reflect a variable diffusion "constant" and the experimental data available in our studies. Intercompartmental transfer rates are constants, except for those designated as functions of t by $k_{ij}(t)$. $J_{92}(t)$ is a mass transfer function (flux), and is defined as

$$J_{92}(t) = \frac{AD(t)[K_{sv}C_v(t) - K_{sw}C_T(t)]}{L} \tag{10.7}$$

where A = area dosed; $D(t)$ = effective time-dependent diffusion coefficient that is a function of the inverses of the amounts of solvent (vehicle) (compartment 23) and solute (compartment 9) in stratum corneum (SC); K_{sv} = SC/vehicle partition coefficient; K_{sw} = SC/water partition coefficient; $C_v(t)$ = $M_4(t)$ / $V_4(t)$ = surface drug concentration

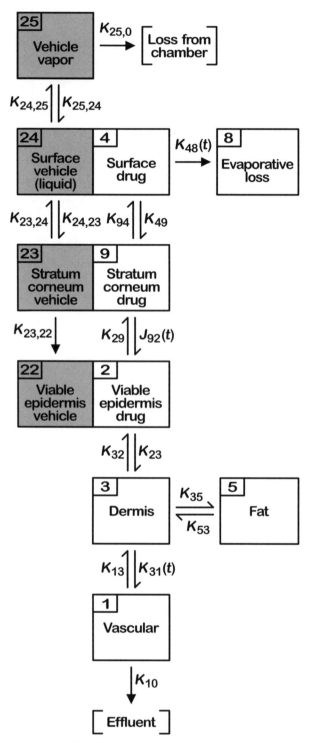

FIGURE 10.5.   Hybrid compartmental/PBPK model for drug and vehicle absorption and distribution in the skin. The compartments on the left (shaded) represent solvent/vehicle; those on the right represent the solute or compound of interest. The k_{ij} or k_{ji} denote intercompartmental transfer rate constants between compartment i and compartment j, while the $k_{ij}(t)$ denote nonlinear mass transfer rate functions. The two nonlinear rates defined are $k_{48}(t)$ and $k_{31}(t)$ for processes of evaporation of solute and dermal absorption of solute, respectively. $J_{92}(t)$ describes flux (mass/time) of solute from compartment 9 (stratum corneum) to compartment 2 (viable epidermis). This is a dynamic function of relative concentrations in compartments 4 (surface) and 2, and a function of the dynamic effective diffusion coefficient, which is in turn a function of amounts of solvent and solute in stratum corneum (compartments 23 and 9, respectively).

(compartment 4); $C_T(t) = M_2(t) / V_2(t)$ = drug concentration in viable epidermis (compartment 2); and L = length of path followed by diffusing molecules.

As presented in Chapter 3, the stratum corneum is generally the rate-limiting diffusional medium in percutaneous penetration and is kinetically very complex. A simple first-order rate constant reflecting a constant D lacks the generality to address all but very specific experimental designs. In response to this complexity, instead of a rate constant describing transfer of drug from compartment 9 (SC) to compartment 2 (viable epidermis), this model assigns a nonlinear flux. As discussed in Chapter 3, vehicles may alter intercellular lipid fluidity, which would change the drug's permeability constant. Vehicle to stratum corneum partition coefficients were determined by experimentally measuring vehicle-to-water and water-to-stratum corneum partitioning and then applying a ratio approach similar to that earlier described for estimating the R_t from partition coefficients of volatile chemicals. Nonlinear rate functions of time were also assigned to two other intercompartmental rates in this model:

$$k_{48}(t) = se^{-qt} \qquad (10.8)$$

where $k_{48}(t)$ is the time-dependent rate from compartment 4 (surface) to compartment 8 (surface loss, or evaporation) and s and q are constants, and

$$k_{31}(t) = \alpha p(t) \qquad (10.9)$$

where $k_{31}(t)$ is the time-dependent rate from compartment 3 (dermis) to compartment 1 (vascular space or capillary beds), α is a constant, and $p(t)$ is the involved capillary surface area (i.e., the effective surface area of exchanging capillaries introduced in Chapter 8). The surface evaporation rates were independently estimated in separate skin experiments. Figure 10.6 illustrates a simulation of this model with phenol in ethanol, showing calculated versus observed isolated perfused porcine skin-flap (IPPSF) venous flux profiles, simulated profiles for compartments 1 and 2, and the calculated time-dependent diffusion coefficient, $D(t)$, profile.

The use of such a hybrid model allows one to probe the effects of solvent on the penetrating kinetics of a topically applied drug as well as to directly incorporate vascular changes detected as the experiment progresses. This model is fit to the data by iterations much as was described above for PBPK models, with the goodness of fit judged by how well the model predicts drug concentrations in all compartments sampled. The use of an *in vitro* experimental tool such as the IPPSF allows cutaneous efflux profiles to be simultaneously modeled with stratum corneum concentrations, skin depth of penetration data, and complete mass balance data collected in a single experiment. The predictions of this model may then be tested in a systemic pharmacokinetic experiment based on how well the input flux matches the observed C-T profile. These models are used as tools to investigate the underlying biology of chemical disposition in skin, and to study the effects of chemical enhancers on the absorption kinetics of transdermal drugs.

As is clearly seen in this example, no one approach (compartmental, noncompartmental, PBPK) is optimal for all biological situations. However, if one understands the basic assumptions, the approaches can easily be combined to facilitate the description of the underlying biology, the true goal of any pharmacokinetic study.

SELECTED READINGS

Andersen, M.E. 1989. Tissue dosimetry, physiologically based pharmacokinetic modeling, and cancer risk assessment. *Cell Biology and Toxicology.* 5:405-416.

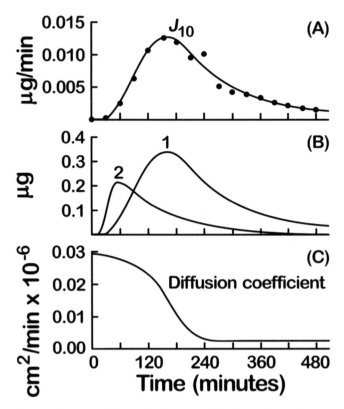

FIGURE 10.6.   Results of application of the model of Figure 10.5 to data obtained from a study of percutaneous penetration and absorption of phenol following topical application of phenol in ethanol to the isolated perfused porcine skin flap. A, Predicted (line) and measured (solid circles) venous flux (μg/min) of phenol from the IPPSF; B, predicted mass (μg) profiles in compartments 1 (capillary space under dosed area) and 2 (viable epidermis); C, simulated effective diffusion coefficient (cm²/min) profile.

SELECTED READINGS

Andersen, M.E. 1991. Physiological modelling of organic compounds. *Annals of Occupational Hygiene.* 35:309-321.

Bernareggi, A. and M. Rowland. 1991. Physiologic modeling of cyclosporin kinetics in rat and man. *Journal of Pharmacokinetics and Biopharmaceutics.* 19:21-50.

Bischoff, K.B. 1980. Current applications of physiological pharmacokinetics. *Federation Proceedings.* 39:2456-2459.

Bischoff, K.B. 1986. Physiological pharmacokinetics. *Bulletin of Mathematical Biology.* 48:309-322.

Clewell, H.J. III, and M.E. Andersen. 1994. Physiologically based pharmacokinetic modeling and bioactivation of xenobiotics. *Journal of Toxicology and Industrial Health.* 10:1-24.

Colburn, W.A. 1988. Physiologic pharmacokinetic modeling. *Journal of Clinical Pharmacology.* 28:673-677.

Gargas, M.L., M.E. Andersen, and H.J. Clewell III. 1986. A physiologically based simulation approach for determining metabolic constants from gas uptake data. *Toxicology and Applied Pharmacology.* 86:341-352.

Gargas, M.L., R.J. Burgess, D.E. Voisard, G.H. Cason, and M.E. Andersen. 1989. Partition coefficients of low-molecular-weight volatile chemicals in various liquids and tissues. *Toxicology and Applied Pharmacology.* 98:87-99.

Gearhart, J.M., D.A. Mahle, R.J. Greene, C.S. Seckel, C.D. Flemming, J.W. Fisher, and H.J. Clewell III. 1993. Variability of physiologically based pharmacokinetic (PBPK) model parameters and their effects on PBPK model predictions in a risk assessment for perchloroethylene (PCE). *Toxicology Letters* 68:131-144.

Gelman, A., F. Bois, and J. Jiang. 1996. Physiological pharmacokinetic analysis using population modeling and informative prior distributions. *Journal of the American Statistical Association.* 91:1400-1412.

Gerlowski, L.E., and R.K. Jain. 1983. Physiologically based pharmacokinetic modeling: Principles and applications. *Journal of Pharmaceutical Sciences.* 72:1103-1126.

Leung, H.W. 1991. Development and utilization of physiologically based pharmacokinetic models for toxicological applications. *Journal of Toxicology and Environmental Health.* 32:247-267.

Luecke, R.H., W.D. Wosilait, B.A. Pearce, and J.F. Young. 1994. A physiologically based pharmacokinetic computer model for human pregnancy. *Teratology* 49:90-103.

Marzulli, F.N., and H.I. Maibach. 1996. *Dermatotoxicology,* 5ed. Washington, D.C.: Taylor & Francis.

Ritschel, W.A., and P.S. Banerjee. 1986. Physiological pharmacokinetic models: Principles, applications, limitations and outlook. *Methods and Findings in Experimental and Clinical Pharmacology.* 8:603-614.

Rowland, M. 1984. Physiologic pharmacokinetic models: Relevance, experience, and future trends. *Drug Metabolism Reviews.* 15:55-74.

Spear, R.C., and F.Y. Bois. 1994. Parameter variability and the interpretation of physiologically based pharmacokinetic modeling results. *Environmental Health Perspectives.* 102(Supplement 11):61-66.

Verotta, D., L.B. Sheiner, W.F. Ebling, and D.R. Stanski. 1989. A semiparametric approach to physiological flow models. *Journal of Pharmacokinetics and Biopharmaceutics.* 17:463-491.

Vinegar, A., R.J. Williams, J.W. Fisher, and J.N. McDougal. 1994. Dose-dependent metabolism of 2,2-dichloro-1,1,1-trifluoroethane: A physiologically based pharmacokinetic model in the male Fisher 344 rat. *Toxicology and Applied Pharmacology.* 129:103-113.

Williams, P.L., J.D. Brooks, A.L. Inman, N.A. Monteiro-Riviere, and J.E. Riviere. 1994. Determination of physiochemical properties of phenol, paranitrophenol, acetone and ethanol relevant to quantitating their percutaneous absorption in porcine skin. *Research Communications in Chemical Pathology and Pharmacology.* 83:61-75.

Williams, P.L., Carver, M.P., and J.E. Riviere. 1990. A physiologically relevant pharmacokinetic model of xenobiotic percutaneous absorption utilizing the isolated perfused porcine skin flap. *Journal of Pharmaceutical Sciences.* 79:305-311.

Williams, P.L., and J.E. Riviere, J.E. 1995. A biophysically based dermatopharmacokinetic compartment model for quantifying percutaneous penetration and absorption of topically applied agents. I. Theory. *Journal of Pharmaceutical Sciences.* 84:599-608.

11

Dosage Regimens

The primary use of pharmacokinetics in a clinical setting is to calculate safe and effective drug dosage regimens for patients. These are generally based on target plasma drug concentrations that are believed to be therapeutically effective. The dose required to achieve and then maintain these target concentrations must be calculated using a knowledge of the drug's pharmacokinetic parameters in the individual animals.

DOSAGE REGIMEN DESCRIPTORS

This concept is best addressed by visualizing the drug's concentration-time (C-T) profile after multiple dose administration, as depicted in Figure 11.1. There are two descriptors of the *dosage regimen* that are important to describe a multiple-dose regimen. These are the dose and dosage interval (τ). The dose is further classified as the initial or *loading dose* (D_L) required to rapidly achieve an effective plasma concentration and the *maintenance dose* (D_M) needed to sustain these concentrations. The resulting profile is characterized by *peak* (Cp^{max}) and *trough* (Cp^{min}) plasma concentrations, which result after the animal has achieved a steady-state condition.

The shape of such a multiple dosage regimen is dependent upon the relationship between the $T_{1/2}$ of the drug and the length of the dosage interval, τ. Assuming that a single dose of drug is administered to an animal, the resulting C-T profile after extravascular administration will resemble that depicted in Chapter 7, Figure 7.9 (plotted on a semilog C-T axis), which (plotted on a Cartesian C-T axis) is the first shaded profile in the left of Figures 11.1 and 11.2. The *AUC* of this C-T segment describes the quantity of drug cleared from the body (recall Chapter 7, equation 7.18). If a second dose of drug was given after the first dose was completely eliminated (e.g., approximately 5 $T_{1/2}$s), then this profile would be repeated, as depicted in Figure 11.2. This dosage regimen, where τ is $>>$ 5 $T_{1/2}$s, does not result in any drug accumulation in the body.

The peak and trough plasma concentrations of this multiple-dose regimen is the same as seen after a single dose, and equations 7.15 and 7.28 (see Chapter 7) for an intravenous and extravascular dose, respectively, may be used to describe the profile. The dose required to achieve a specific peak concentration, or Cp^{max}, after administering a very rapidly absorbed preparation is essentially obtained by rearranging the equation for volume of distribution (equation 7.14), which becomes

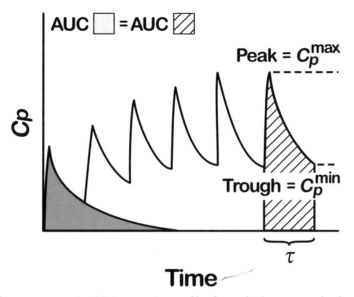

FIGURE 11.1. Plasma concentration (Cp) versus time profile after multiple extravascular drug administrations demonstrating accumulation. Peak and trough concentrations represent those after achievement of steady-state, at which the area under the curve (AUC) under a dosing interval τ (hatched area) is equal to that after a single dose (shaded area).

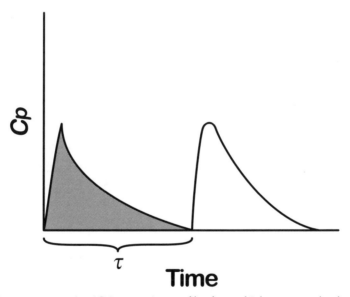

FIGURE 11.2. Plasma concentration (Cp) versus time profile after multiple extravascular drug administration, with no accumulation resulting in independent pharmacokinetics described by two single-dose profiles.

$$\text{Dose} = (Cp^{\text{max}})\, Vd \tag{11.1}$$

If the drug is not completely bioavailable (e.g., $F < 1$), then this equation is divided by the systemic availability F. Administering this dose at every τ will result in the same C-T profile characterized by Cp^{max} and a Cp^{min} of essentially zero.

However, the more likely scenario is that depicted in Figure 11.1, in which a second dose is administered before the first dose is completely eliminated from the body. In this

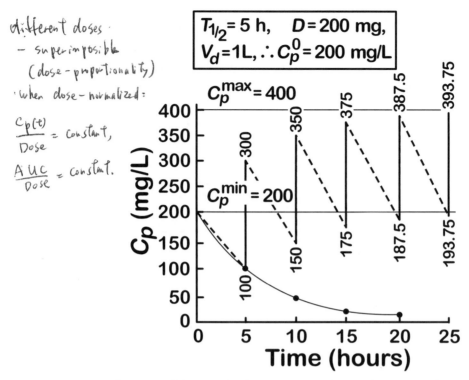

different doses ·
— superimposible
(dose – proportionality)
· when dose – normalized :

$$\frac{C_p(t)}{Dose} = Constant,$$

$$\frac{AUC}{Dose} = Constant.$$

Box in figure:
$T_{1/2} = 5$ h, $D = 200$ mg,
$V_d = 1$ L, $\therefore C_p^0 = 200$ mg/L

$C_p^{max} = 400$

$C_p^{min} = 200$

FIGURE 11.3.   Illustration of the principle of superposition and accumulation to steady-state. (See text for full description).

case, the drug concentrations will accumulate with continued dosing. This accumulation will stop or reach a steady-state when the amount of drug administered at the start of each dosing interval is equal to the amount eliminated during that interval. This can be appreciated since at steady-state the *AUC* under one dosing interval is equal to that after a single dose administration. In fact, steady-state could be defined as the dosing interval in which the *AUC* for that interval is equal to the single-dose *AUC*. Administering repeated doses at a τ defined in this manner will continuously produce a C-T profile with the same peak and trough plasma concentrations.

PRINCIPLE OF SUPERPOSITION *(dose proportionality)*

This principle can be simply illustrated using a straightforward graphic approach, as first presented to the author by Dr. Gary Koritz of the University of Illinois. Figure 11.3 illustrates this procedure. To simplify the presentation, assume that we have a drug with a *Vd* of 1 L given at a dose of 200 mg. This would result in a Cp^0 of 200 mg/L. If the $T_{1/2}$ is 5 hours and τ also is 5 hours, then 50% of the drug would be eliminated in one dosing interval, resulting in a trough concentration at 5 hours equal to 100 mg/L. If a second dose is then administered, *Cp* now becomes 300 mg/L (100 + 200) and the trough after two doses becomes 150 mg/L (300 / 2). If this process continues, the peak and trough will approach their true steady-state values of a Cp^{max} equal to 400 and a Cp^{min} equal to 200 since at these concentrations, 200 mg would be eliminated during each dosing level, requiring 200 to be administered to replace this amount. Note that after 5 dosing intervals (25 hours in Figure 11.3), the peak and trough concentrations are at 98% of their steady-state levels.

This simple graphical approach, often referred to as the principle of superposition, may be used to plot the resulting C-T profile seen after any multiple dose administration. However, I believe its main strength lies in its use to visualize what actually happens after multiple drug administration. For example, if one wanted to rapidly achieve the steady-state concentrations, one could administer a loading dose (D_L) that would start this process at a Cp of 400 mg/L. This dose would be calculated using equation 11.1 as

$$D_L = (400 \text{ mg} / \text{L}) (1 \text{ L}) = 400 \text{ mg}$$

After one dosing interval, the trough concentration would now be 400 / 2 = 200 mg/L, and the maintenance dose (D_M) of 200 mg could be administered to immediately achieve the steady-state profile! The average concentration of this profile at steady-state (Cp^{avg}) would be 300 mg/L {(400 + 200) / 2}.

The final dosage regimen would be characterized as follows:

$$D_L = 400 \text{ mg}$$
$$D_M = 200 \text{ mg}$$
$$\tau = 5 \text{ hours}$$
$$Cp^{\text{max}} = 400 \text{ mg} / \text{L}$$
$$Cp^{\text{min}} = 200 \text{ mg} / \text{L}$$

Recall from Chapter 7 that since log-linear decay (e.g., first-order kinetics) is governing this C-T profile, the average concentration obtained must be determined logarithmically; therefore,

$$Cp^{\text{avg}} = e^{(\ln 400 + \ln 200)/2} \cong 283 \text{ mg} / \text{L}$$

DOSAGE REGIMEN FORMULAE

This essentially is the strategy needed to calculate any multiple dose regimen; unfortunately, in most cases the numbers are not so easily obtained from a graphical analysis, and τ is not always equal to $T_{1/2}$. There are a series of simple formulae derived from the principles outlined in Chapter 7 that can be used to precisely derive these profiles.

The first is to determine Cp^{avg}, which is a function of Vd and the ratio $T_{1/2}/\tau$, where

$$Cp^{\text{avg}} = \frac{(1.44) \, (F) \, (D)}{Vd_{\text{area}}} \times \frac{T_{\frac{1}{2}}}{\tau} = \frac{Cp^{\text{max}} - Cp^{\text{min}}}{\ln \, (Cp^{\text{max}} / Cp^{\text{min}})} \qquad (11.2)$$

Recalling the relationship between $T_{1/2}$, Cl, and Vd presented in Chapter 7, and rearranging equation 7.20 $(1/Cl = 1.44 \, T_{1/2} / Vd_{\text{area}})$, the first part of equation 11.2 is now

$$Cp^{\text{avg}} = \frac{F}{Cl} \times \frac{D}{\tau} \qquad (11.3)$$

The derivation of the second part of equation 11.2 is evident in the discussion that follows (or by substituting equations 11.9 and 11.12 solved for 1.44 $T_{1/2}/\tau$ and FD/Vd_{area}, respectively, in the first part of equation 11.2). Another relationship becomes evident. We learned in Chapter 7 that Cl is D / AUC (equation 7.18), which allows equation 11.3 to be algebraically expressed as $Cp^{\text{avg}} = (F) \, (AUC) / \tau$. This relation quantitates the observation presented earlier that the AUC under any dosing interval τ will always be the same when steady-state conditions are achieved.

Accumulation. Two factors that are important in designing dosage regimens also emerge from equations 11.2 and 11.3. The ratio D/τ can be defined as the *dosage rate* and is the *major determinant under the control of the clinician, which determines the amount of drug that will accumulate in the body.* The ratio $T_{1/2}/\tau$ is a proportion relating the relative length of the dosing interval to the half-life of the drug. If the inverse of this ratio is taken, the *relative dosage interval ε* may be defined as $\varepsilon = \tau/T_{1/2}$. As will be discussed later, these two ratios provide useful parameters to gauge the shape and height of the C-T profile produced by a tailored dosage regimen.

The primary factor governing the extent of drug accumulation in a multiple-dose regimen is the fraction of a dose eliminated in one dosing interval termed f_{el}. This can be easily calculated by first determining the amount of drug remaining at the end of a dosing interval, f_r. We showed earlier that the amount of drug in the body at any time t is given by the exponential (Chapter 7, equation 7.7) relation $X_t = X_0 e^{-kt}$. If one substitutes τ for t at the end of a dosing interval, then f_r is defined as

$$f_r = 1 - f_{el} = X_\tau / X_0 = e^{-k\tau} = e^{-\lambda\tau} \tag{11.4}$$

where k is the fractional elimination constant or the relevant slope of the terminal phase (λ) of the C-T profile governing the disposition of the drug (Chapter 7, Table 7.3). Therefore,

$$f_{el} = 1 - f_r = 1 - e^{-\lambda\tau} = 1 - e^{-0.693(\tau/T_{1/2})} = 1 - e^{-0.693\varepsilon} \tag{11.5}$$

(It is instructive when studying these relations to recall that 0.693 is the ln 2, and 1.44 is $1/\ln 2$.} Using f_{el}, the peak and trough concentrations may be calculated as

$$Cp^{\max} = \frac{(F)\,(D)}{(Vd_{area})\,(f_{el})} \tag{11.6}$$

$$Cp^{\min} = (Cp^{\max})\,(1 - f_{el}) \tag{11.7}$$

If these formulae are used to characterize the C-T profile in Figure 11.3 ($D = 200$ mg, $Vd = 1$L, $\tau = 5$ hours, $T_{1/2} = 5$ hours, $F = 1$), the following parameters could be calculated:

$$\lambda = .693/5 = 0.1386 \text{ hours}$$
$$f_{el} = 1 - e^{-(0.1386)(5)} = 1 - e^{-0.693} = 1 - 0.5 = 0.5$$
$$Cp^{avg} = [(1.44)(200)(5)/(1)(5)] = 288 \text{ mg}/L$$
$$Cp^{\max} = 200/(1)(0.5) = 400 \text{ mg}/L$$
$$Cp^{\min} = (400)(1 - 0.5) = 200 \text{ mg}/L$$

The ratio of the fluctuation in $Cp^{\max}$ and $Cp^{\min}$ can be determined using an approach similar to the one used to derive equation 11.4 from equation 7.7 (see Chapter 7) but instead calculate the ratio X_0/X_t, which removes the negative sign from the exponential term ($X_0/X_t = e^{\lambda\tau}$); therefore,

$$Cp^{\max}/Cp^{\min} = e^{0.693(\tau/T_{1/2})}$$

and thus

$$\ln (Cp^{max} / Cp^{min}) = 0.693 \; (\tau) / (T_{1/2}) = 0.693 \; \varepsilon \tag{11.8}$$

The dosing interval (τ) required to keep Cp within a desired maximum and minimum window is obtained by solving for τ as

$$\tau = 1.44 \; T_{1/2} \ln (Cp^{max} / Cp^{min}) \tag{11.9}$$

These extremely powerful relationships demonstrate that the magnitude of fluctuations in a C-T profile is directly related to the *relative* dosage interval ε. As either τ increases or $T_{1/2}$ decreases, this ratio will get larger and result in a greater fluctuation in drug concentrations. Again, using the law of exponentials $(e^x = 1/e^{-x})$, equation 11.8 is equivalent to

$$Cp^{max} / Cp^{min} = 1 / e^{-0.693 \; \tau / T_{1/2}} \tag{11.10}$$

However, we have seen from rearrangement of equations 11.4 and 11.5 that $e^{-0.693 \; \tau / T_{1/2}}$ is also equivalent to $1 - f_{el}$. Thus this ratio can be written in a form preferred by some authors as

$$Cp^{max} / Cp^{min} = 1 / (1 - f_{el}) = 1 / f_r \tag{11.11}$$

This ratio reflects the amount of accumulation that occurs in a multiple-dose regimen. In our example above, when the drug was dosed at an interval equal to the half-life, the accumulation at steady-state was twofold.

Calculation of Dosage Regimens. Using these relationships, and rearranging equation 11.6 to solve for dose, one can now derive the dosage formulae required to achieve a C-T profile with specified target peak and trough concentrations.

$$\begin{aligned} D_M &= (f_{el}) \; (Vd_{area}) \; (Cp^{max}) / F \\ &= Vd_{area} \; (Cp^{max} - Cp^{min}) / F \end{aligned} \tag{11.12}$$

$$\begin{aligned} D_L &= (D_M)/(f_{el}) \\ &= \frac{(Vd_{area}) \; (Cp^{max})}{F} \end{aligned} \tag{11.13}$$

Equation 11.9 above is used to determine the appropriate τ. Thus, to construct a dosage regimen, the only parameters that are required are the Vd_{area} and $T_{1/2}$ (and hence λ or k_{el}) of the drug, which are needed to calculate f_{el} . If one is targeting only the average plasma concentration, then equation 11.2 can be solved for dose as

$$\begin{aligned} D_M &= \frac{(Cp^{avg}) \; (Vd_{area})}{(1.44) \; (F)} \times \frac{\tau}{T_{1/2}} \\ &= \frac{(0.693) \; (Cp^{avg}) \; (Vd_{area})}{F} \times \frac{\tau}{T_{1/2}} \\ &= \frac{(Cp^{avg}) \; (Cl) \; (\tau)}{F} \end{aligned} \tag{11.14}$$

As discussed earlier, the magnitude of f_{el} is a good estimate of the degree of fluctuation that occurs between the peak and trough concentration at steady-state. As the ratio of $\tau / T_{1/2}$ or ε approaches zero in equation 11.5, f_{el} approaches zero, and the amount of fluctuation in a dosage interval is minimal. (This can also be seen by examining equations 11.8 through 11.11.) In contrast, when this ratio is large, f_{el} approaches 1, and the peak and trough concentrations have a large degree of fluctuation.

When f_{el} is very small, Cp^{max} approaches Cp^{min} since f_{el} approaches zero when τ approaches zero (see equation 11.5 and recall that the limit of e^{-x} as $x \to 0 = 1$). The resulting C-T profile becomes characterized by Cp^{avg}. This occurs when the drug is given as an intravenous infusion. The rate of an intravenous infusion (R mg/min) is essentially an *instantaneous* dose rate and is equivalent to D/τ. When R is inserted in equation 11.3 for D/τ and F is set equal to 1 (since an intravenous dose is by definition 100% systemically available),

$$Cp^{avg} = R / Cl \qquad (11.15)$$

$$R \ (mg / min) = (Cp^{avg}) \ (Cl) \qquad (11.16)$$

which is identical to equation 7.21 (see Chapter 7) for the steady-state plasma concentration (C^{ss}) obtained after administering an intravenous infusion. If one desires that concentration be achieved immediately, then a loading dose may be calculated as

$$D_L = (Cp^{avg}) \ (Vd) \qquad (11.17)$$

Comparing equations 11.2 and 11.15 is instructive since it demonstrates the dependence of the average steady-state concentration on the rate of drug input (R or D / τ) in mass/time and the rate of drug elimination exemplified by the clearance. When constructing and comparing dosage regimens, the Cp^{avg} of any two regimens will always be the same as long as D / τ is constant. This factor becomes very important in Chapter 15, in which dosage regimens are constructed for patients with impaired clearance due to renal disease. The larger the f_{el} or ε is in a single dosage interval τ, the greater the fluctuation in plasma concentrations. To minimize fluctuation but maintain a constant Cp^{avg}, smaller maintenance doses (D_M) must be administered at shorter dosage intervals.

It is also important to stress at this point that the length of time required to achieve steady-state for any dosage regimen is solely based on the rate-controlling λ or $T_{1/2}$ of the drug in the clinical situation. Thus, with drugs having a prolonged half-life, a loading dose may often have to be administered to rapidly achieve therapeutically effective plasma concentrations. The more complex the distribution kinetics are, the more difficult it will be to rapidly achieve the target plasma concentration since the tissue compartment must first be loaded before the plasma compartment can reach an equilibrium (revisit Chapter 7, Figure 7.17). The only way to precisely counteract this is through the administration of an intravenous infusion protocol based on both distribution and elimination pharmacokinetics, as in the text discussion of Figure 8.5 and equations 8.31 and 8.32.

The principles presented in this chapter may be widely applied for a number of therapeutic situations. They will be revisited in Chapter 15, which discusses dosage regimens for individuals with impaired renal function. Similarly, equations developed in this chapter will form the basis for calculating the withdrawal time needed to ensure that drug is completely eliminated from a food-producing animal before its edible tissues are consumed. In this case the problem is conceptualized as constructing a dosage regimen whereby tissue depletion data are used, the final trough or Cp^{min} is set as the legal tolerance of drug for that tissue, and the final dosage interval τ is actually the withdrawal time.

Other Considerations. The astute reader should realize that the equations developed above are strictly applicable only to a drug having a disposition described by a one-compartment pharmacokinetic model. These relations will hold if the proper set of pharmacokinetic parameters for the time and concentration range of the targeted C-T profile are employed (see Chapter 7, Table 7.3). For most drugs employed in a therapeutic setting, the relevant $T_{1/2}$ will be that governing the elimination (or so-called β phase) of the drug's C-T profile. Similarly, the slope of the C-T profile λ will often be β. This assumption is valid as long as the distribution rate constants (λ_1 or α) are much greater (more rapid, shorter $T_{1/2}$) than the elimination rate constants (λ_2 or β). This works since, as discussed extensively in Chapter 7, the initial exponential term will disappear as time increases. However, when such parameters are employed, the proper volume of distribution term must be used (Vd_{area}) since the multicompartment characteristics of a drug will influence this parameter (recall relations presented in Chapter 7, equation 7.50). If a *deep compartment* (e.g., λ_3 or γ phase) exists and is not accounted for, the actual measured Cp^{min} will be greater than that predicted using λ_2 or β. Finally, for drugs that undergo biotransformation, Chapter 9 should be consulted for equations relevant for these scenarios. The problem with drugs exhibiting nonlinear pharmacokinetic properties is that as drug accumulates, saturation may occur and the clearance operative at low Cps may be reduced at the higher concentrations seen at steady-state. Similarly, if the drug induces its own metabolism, the disposition and thus required dosage regimen may be different after chronic use.

Other considerations are operative when administering extravascular drugs with relatively slow rates of absorption. In many cases, the governing rate process may be the absorption phase (k_a), and a *flip-flop* situation will occur. In this case, it will take five *absorption $T_{1/2}$s* to reach steady-state, but Cp^{avg} will still be predicted from equations 11.2 and 11.3. The best approach to handle this is to use the actual equations governing the shape of the C-T profile (e.g., equation 7.55, see Chapter 7, if a model is available) and solve for dose. These approaches are implemented in all major clinical pharmacokinetic software packages available today. It must be stressed that the principles involved are identical to those presented above except for the added computation burden introduced by the multiexponential equations employed.

These approaches to constructing dosage regimens are ideally suited when pharmacokinetic parameters are obtained from the noncompartmental models presented in Chapter 8. In these cases, the same equations may be used. Similarly, the approaches presented above will be extensively revisited in Chapter 14 on population pharmacokinetics.

SOME COMMENTS ON EFFICACY AND SAFETY

The final point to consider is the relationship between the target Cp^{max} and Cp^{min} concentrations and therapeutic or toxic effect. This relation is best presented in Figure 11.4, which depicts a hypothetical C-T profile versus various target Cps for efficacy and toxicity. The precise relationship between a pharmacokinetic profile and pharmacodynamic or toxicodynamic effects will be presented in greater detail in Chapter 12. However, it is instructive to realize that the form of a C-T profile is by itself only dependent upon the dosage regimen parameters (D / τ) and the pharmacokinetics of the drug in the patient. The resulting efficacy or toxicity of the profile is dependent upon the underlying pharmacology and toxicology of the drug. These biological effects are often, though not always, correlated to plasma concentrations. Thus, for a specific drug, one might have data indicating that efficacy would occur when Cp is maintained above the *effective low* concentration in Figure 11.4, and toxicity would be expected to occur only if concentration exceeded the *toxic high* level plotted. In this case, the dosage regimen that produced this

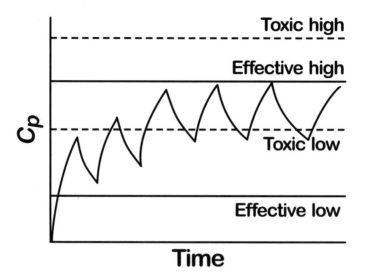

FIGURE 11.4.   Relationship between a multiple-dose plasma concentration versus time profile and thresholds for efficacy and toxicity that define the therapeutic benefit-risk ratio for the drug.

C-T profile would be considered optimal since at steady-state it is well within the *therapeutic window* defined by these two thresholds. However, if the efficacy of the drug was defined by the *effective high* threshold plotted, the regimen would not be therapeutically effective. Similarly, if the relevant toxicological threshold were the *toxic low* line in this figure, one would predict that this regimen would be unsafe to administer.

It is important to realize that the mechanism of action for the pharmacological and toxicological endpoints represented by these thresholds may be different, and thus some drugs may actually have toxic thresholds that are less than their effective levels. Such an example would be administering a nephrotoxic aminoglycoside antimicrobial drug to treat a pathogen that is moderately resistant to this class of drugs as indicated by a high minimum inhibitory concentration (MIC).

A more likely scenario often encountered in infectious disease therapy is administering a specific antibiotic regimen *according to label conditions* in patients infected with pathogens having different MICs. Figure 11.5 illustrates this scenario with an antimicrobial used against pathogens with an MIC of 1 µg/mL versus one with 5 µg/mL. The steady-state C-T profiles plotted represent dosages of this drug administered (A) 6.6 mg/kg every 12 hours, (B) 11 mg/kg every 6 hours, (C) 15 mg/kg every 8 hours, and (D) 22 mg/kg every 12 hours. It is obvious that all four dosage regimens would be effective against a pathogen with a lower MIC; however, regimen (A) may not be effective against the pathogen with the higher MIC. If the drug required maintenance of effective plasma concentrations throughout a dosage interval, then one would opt for regimen (B) and possibly (C). However, if efficacy was clearly associated with high peak plasma concentrations (e.g., an aminoglycoside), then regimen (C) or (D) might be preferred. It is instructive to realize that the total daily dose for the latter three regimens are all approximately 44 to 45 mg per day. A great deal of work is in progress on defining what are the relative endpoints for antimicrobial therapy. For concentration-dependent antimicrobials such as the aminoglycosides, the peak concentration best correlates to efficacy. For other drugs, such as some bacteriostatic and beta-lactam antimicrobials, the time that plasma concentrations remain above the MIC seems important. For others, efficacy has been correlated to the ratio of *AUC/MIC*.

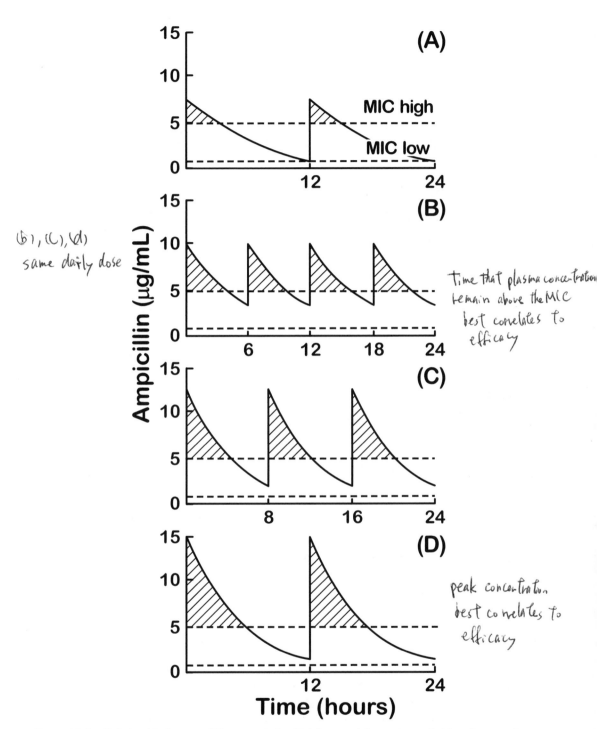

(b), (c), (d)
same daily dose

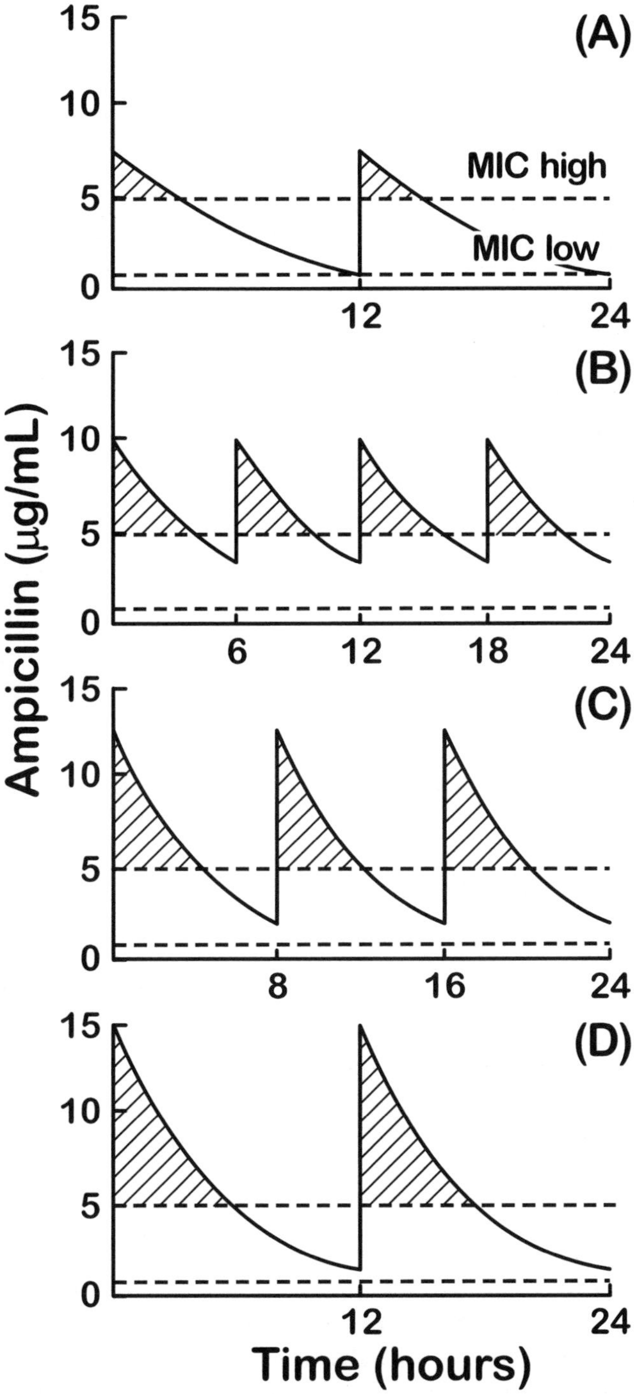

Time that plasma concentration remain above the MIC best correlates to efficacy

peak concentration best correlates to efficacy

FIGURE 11.5. Relationship between different antimicrobial doses and dosage intervals (τ) against a pathogen with a high or low minimum inhibitory concentration (MIC). Dosage conditions are (A) 6.6 mg/kg every 12 hours, (B) 11 mg/kg every 6 hours, (C) 15 mg/kg every 8 hours, and (D) 22 mg/kg every 12 hours. Hatched areas of the profiles are time greater than MIC.

The toxicity of such a regimen (e.g., an aminoglycoside) might also come into play when selecting the optimal strategy. The consensus among investigators is that aminoglycoside nephrotoxicity is best correlated to the trough (Cp^{min}) plasma concentration achieved at the end of a dosing interval, and not the peak concentration achieved or total exposure to the substance (assessed by AUC). In this light, regimens (A) and (D) would be selected based on toxicological criteria. Fortunately for this class of drugs, high peak concentrations correlate with efficacy and low trough concentrations with lack of toxicity, suggesting that regimen (D) may actually be the optimal approach. However, this decision is *drug-specific*, and for those antimicrobials for which time above MIC is required for efficacy (e.g., penicillin) and peak concentrations correlate to toxicity, regimen (B) would be optimal. This could also be a function of the site of the infection (fibrous plaque in the heart versus a renal medulla infection) and the distribution characteristics of the drug (see Chapter 4). Similar considerations occur for other classes of drugs in which efficacy and toxicity may be dependent upon different characteristics of the C-T profile. A complete discussion of the specific approaches required for different drugs and clinical syndromes is well beyond the scope of this pharmacokinetics text. A text on clinical pharmacology should be consulted.

A number of descriptive parameters are used to describe such C-T profiles for discussions related to efficacy and toxicity. The most obvious are those already mentioned, including peak (Cp^{max}), trough (Cp^{min}), time to peak and AUC. Additionally, some drugs are correlated to the time the C-T profile is greater than some pharmacologic or toxicologic endpoint. This is indicated in Figure 11.5 by the shaded areas of the C-T profile, where concentrations exceed the MIC. This could be expressed as % AUC > MIC or the time of the dosage intervals where AUC > MIC. As these descriptive pharmacokinetic parameters are determined in the process of conducting clinical trials, such correlations will become more commonplace, allowing dosage regimens to be constructed with these parameters as targets.

Similar considerations are applied when the bioavailability of two pharmaceutical products are compared for therapeutic equivalence. In this case, a new product's bioavailability is statistically compared to the innovator's product. If these products have statistically comparable bioavailabilities, they are considered *bioequivalent*. The parameters usually compared are Cp^{max}, time to Cp^{max}, and AUC after single-dose administration. Some workers also evaluate the terminal λ of the C-T profile, and others suggest that multiple-dose regimens should be compared if that is the predicted clinical use. Our laboratory conducted a simulation study of comparative bioavailabilities of drugs with complex absorptive properties that illustrate many of these concepts.

CONCLUSION

This chapter presented the fundamental concepts used to apply basic pharmacokinetic models to the selection and construction of dosage regimens. Other texts and references are available that provide equations for the more complex pharmacokinetic scenarios that may be encountered. However, it is the author's firm conviction that most workers in this field will use various commercially available software packages or "home-grown" spreadsheets to calculate dosage regimens. Whatever the complexity of the resulting dosage regimens obtained using these tools, the principles outlined above relating to dosage rate, accumulation, time to steady-state, and C-T fluctuations will be operative and must be taken into consideration before administering them to a clinical patient. If the desired effects or untoward adverse effects occur, then the first diagnostic technique performed should be to evaluate one's assumptions concerning the underlying pharmacokinetics before other actions are taken.

SELECTED READINGS

The basic pharmacokinetic texts in Selected Readings, Chapter 7, should be consulted for discussions on pharmacokinetics of multiple-dose administration and the design of clinical dosage regimens.

Baggot, J.D. 1992. Clinical pharmacokinetics in veterinary medicine. *Clinical Pharmacokinetics*. 22:254-273.

Benet, L.Z., N. Massoud, and J.G. Gambertoglio. 1984. *Pharmacokinetic Basis for Drug Treatment*. New York: Raven Press.

Burton, M.E., M.R. Vasko, and D.C. Brater. Comparison of drug dosing methods. *Clinical Pharmacokinetics*. 10:1-37.

Colburn, W.A., D. Shen, and M. Gibaldi. 1976. Pharmacokinetic analysis of drug concentration data obtained during repetitive drug administration. *Journal of Pharmacokinetics and Biopharmaceutics*. 4:469-486.

DeVane, C.L., and W.J. Jusko. 1982. Dosage regimen design. *Pharmacology and Therapeutics*. 17:143-163.

Frazier, D.L., and J.E. Riviere. 1987. Gentamicin dosing strategies for dogs with subclinical renal dysfunction. *Antimicrobial Agents Chemotherapy*. 31:1929-1934.

Gibaldi, M. 1991. *Biopharmaceutics and Clinical Pharmacokinetics*. Philadelphia: Lea and Febiger.

Gumbleton, M. and W. Sneader. 1994. Pharmacokinetics considerations in rational drug design. *Clinical Pharmacokinetics*. 26:161-168.

Martinez, M.N., and J.E. Riviere. 1994. Review of the 1993 veterinary drug bioequivalence workshop. *Journal of Veterinary Pharmacology and Therapeutics*. 17:85-119.

Martinez, M.N. , J.E. Riviere, and G. Koritz. 1995. Review of the first interactive workshop on professional flexible labeling. *Journal of the American Veterinary Medical Association*. 207:865-914.

Mungall, D.R. 1983. *Applied Clinical Pharmacokinetics*. New York: Raven Press.

Riviere, J.E. 1994. Influence of compounding on bioavailability. *Journal of the American Veterinary Medical Association*. 205:226-231.

Riviere, J.E., M.P. Carver, G.L. Coppoc, W.W. Carlton, G.C. Lantz, and J.S. Shy-Modjeska. 1984. Pharmacokinetics and comparative nephrotoxicity of fixed-dose versus fixed-interval reduction of gentamicin dosage in subtotal nephrectomized dogs. *Toxicology and Applied Pharmacology*. 75:496-509.

Riviere, J.E., D.L. Frazier, and W.L. Tippitt. 1988. Pharmacokinetic estimation of therapeutic dosage regimens (PETDR): A software program designed to determine drug dosage regimens for veterinary applications. *Journal of Veterinary Pharmacology and Therapeutics*. 11:390-396.

Rowland, M., and T.N. Tozer. 1995. *Clinical Pharmacokinetics: Concepts and Applications,* 3ed. Baltimore: Williams & Wilkins.

Ruckebusch, Y., P.L. Toutain, and G.D. Koritz. 1983. *Veterinary Pharmacology and Toxicology*. Westport, CT.: Avi Publishing Co.

Traver, D.S., and J.E. Riviere. 1981. Penicillin and ampicillin therapy in horses. *Journal of the American Veterinary Medical Association.* 178:1186-1189.

Vogelman, B., S. Gundmundsson, J. Legget, J. Turnidge, S. Ebert, and W.A. Craig. 1988. Correlation of antimicrobial pharmacokinetic parameters with therapeutic efficacy in an animal model. *Journal of Infectious Diseases.* 158:831-847.

Winter, M.E. 1988. *Basic Clinical Pharmacokinetics,* 2ed. Spokane, WA: Applied Therapeutics, Inc.

12

Simultaneous Pharmacokinetic–Pharmacodynamic Modeling

The initial chapters of this text covered the pharmaceutical and pharmacokinetic (PK) phases of drug disposition encompassed in quantitating absorption, distribution, metabolism and elimination (ADME). The final phase of modeling involves the coupling of the concentration of drug at the active site to its biological effect. This phase is defined as pharmacodynamics (PD). The present chapter will discuss quantitative approaches to link these processes into complete models of drug disposition and action, an approach referred to as PK-PD modeling.

For the parent drug molecule and its active metabolites to elicit a pharmacodynamic effect, they must reach the site of action, referred to as the *biophase*, which is represented in PK-PD modeling as an effector-compartment (E-Comp). The active molecules are then able to interact with a specific receptor to trigger an effect cascade (signal transduction) resulting in an observable pharmacodynamic effect. This is often the endpoint of *in vitro* bioassays. Pharmaceutical, pharmacokinetic, and pharmacodynamic processes are interactively linked during drug therapy (Figure 12.1), although for convenience they are often studied separately. To predict and adjust maintenance doses in a clinical setting by applying feedback (e.g., drug therapeutic outcome) from previous drug administration, one may utilize experience-based methodologies and/or theoretical PK-PD modeling. The conventional experience-based approaches, introduced in Chapter 11, utilize a researcher's or physician's experience to adjust dosages. The PK-PD modeling approach, however, is systematic and theoretically based, and often results in better quantitative predictions.

The final goal of drug administration is to achieve therapeutic effect. Unfortunately, pharmacokinetics is too often viewed as the end rather than a means to an end. Findings of increased $T_{1/2}$, altered Vd, modified K_a, and changed AUC are not always accompanied by the obvious question "*What is the clinical relevance of these findings*"? There is thus a need to somehow bridge the gap between a pharmacokinetic study and its clinical application. A mechanistically integrated PK-PD model can provide such a tool. With progress in drug effect quantitation arising from developments in enzymology and cellular and molecular biology, it has become much easier to continuously measure drug effect while meeting certain criteria that satisfy pharmacodynamic modeling requirements.

Co-authored by Dr. Gui Lin Qiao

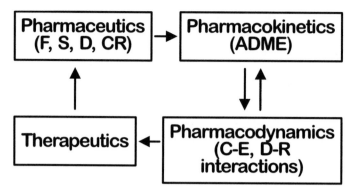

FIGURE 12.1.   Relationship among pharmaceutic (formulation, stability, dissolution, and controlled release), pharmacokinetic (absorption, distribution, metabolism, and elimination), and pharmacodynamic (concentration-effect relationship, drug-receptor interactions) processes in drug development and clinical therapy.

DRUG DISPOSITION MODELING STRATEGIES AND THEIR LIMITATIONS

Separate pharmacokinetic and pharmacodynamic studies have advantages and limitations. A defined relationship between drug concentration in biological fluids and therapeutic effect is a fundamental tenet for applying pharmacokinetic principles to optimize drug therapy. With the availability of sophisticated *in vitro* bioassay systems, this relationship can often be directly modeled. Most pharmacokinetic studies are still conducted using traditional compartmental analysis of the plasma and/or urine drug concentration-time data as presented in Chapter 7. Blood and urine are easy to collect and thus have been extensively analyzed. All blood or plasma based approaches are limited by the inability to define the mechanistic links between blood and tissue concentrations and then between tissue concentrations and drug effect. In traditional pharmacokinetic analysis, one assumes that the biological system is a simplified "unit" or "black box," and drug disposition is usually assumed to be tissue nonspecific. Thus, as repeatedly stressed in Chapter 7, the pharmacokinetic compartments and estimated parameters do not have direct physiological meaning and thus are limited in their capacity to extrapolate across different animal species, physiological or pathological conditions, and circumstances of drug administration. In addition to the traditional pharmacokinetic methods used to quantify and predict drug concentrations, one could conduct labor-intensive tissue kinetic studies or physiological-based pharmacokinetic (PB-PK) modeling studies as developed in Chapter 10. Or one could use novel neural network computational methods that directly link concentrations and effects independent of any biological structure, an approach recently studied by our group. This later approach is fairly efficient at handling complex interactions that are based on both linear and nonlinear kinetics, although the models produced are devoid of any mechanistic context and blind the user to the nature of the mathematical linkages employed.

One must stress, however, that the ultimate purpose of drug administration is to achieve the desired therapeutic effect rather than to achieve and/or maintain certain drug concentrations in a specific body space. Only when drug effect can be directly predicted or assessed from drug concentrations, does pharmacokinetic analysis become applicable and meaningful. Alternatively, when the endpoint is the actual drug concentration in a tissue as measured by a regulatory agency, such as seen in food-animal tissue residue studies, pharmacokinetic analysis is the appropriate approach as the concentration itself is the phenomenological endpoint.

Although monitoring drug blood concentration is standard practice for designing drug dosage regimens, the extent to which drug concentration-effect relationships have been evaluated varies greatly among the commonly monitored therapeutic drugs. Drug concentration-effect relationships are usually complex and often population-dependent, requiring a critical assessment of the context within which pharmacokinetic principles can be rationally applied to evaluate and optimize therapy. Despite the strong theoretical basis and the sound rationale for applying pharmacokinetics to routine therapy, the process is not straightforward and may have considerable limitations under certain circumstances. For instance, it is very difficult to predict drug effect from the blood concentration-time profile if the pharmacokinetic profile at the target site is not "in phase" with blood because of unique organ perfusion, complex patterns of tissue binding and intracellular sequestration, or local metabolism at the target site. In fact, nonparallel blood-tissue profiles are commonly encountered. On the other hand, independent pharmacodynamic analysis focuses on the time course of drug effect and the dose-response relationship. A pharmacodynamic study is not sufficient to reveal the mechanisms of some observed phenomena and, accordingly, cannot provide the information necessary to improve drug therapy. In pharmacodynamic studies, the dynamic relationship and interactions between drug concentrations and therapeutic effects are usually ignored.

Due to the obvious limitations associated with separated pharmacokinetic and pharmacodynamic analyses, a simultaneous PK-PD modeling approach was established in the late 1970s. Since then, significant progress has been made in mathematical definition of pharmacodynamic effects, in quantitation of concentrations and effect and, finally, in developing enabling computerized modeling techniques. Drug-disposition kinetics quantitating the ADME processes must be closely linked to the biological effect process described by pharmacodynamic models. It is the PK-PD model that correlates the mass transfer embedded in pharmacokinetic models to drug effect. If the direct correlation between change in drug mass in a central pharmacokinetic compartment and drug-effect profile is uncertain, PK-PD modeling may be formulated to include peripheral tissue compartments and then integrate the drug mass transfer between different kinetic compartments with drug effect in the compartment of interest. This will be the focus of the PK-PD models to be developed.

As a note, to obtain the maximal data extrapolation capacity of both drug concentration and activity, PB-PK-PD modeling would be the optimal approach since the drug mass transfer, physiological process, mechanisms of drug action, and PK-PD interactions are all integrated into one modeling effort. These approaches also facilitate linking to pharmacodynamic data obtained from *in vitro* systems. Similarly, population models (see Chapter 14) can be used to describe the pharmacokinetic disposition of a drug across individuals and disease subgroups, and then be linked to pharmacodynamic data to create population-based PK-PD models.

The overall goal of this chapter is to introduce the basic principles, theoretical assumptions, general experimental requirements, and procedures for formulating integrated PK-PD models. It is assumed that the reader is now familiar with the basic principles of pharmacokinetics embodied in earlier chapters. The models will be illustrated with studies conducted by one of the authors (GLQ) using central nervous system drugs in animals. Recent advances and research directions in this area will also be briefly introduced.

PHARMACODYNAMICS: THE CONCENTRATION-RESPONSE RELATIONSHIP

Theoretically, a drug's effect-time profile is governed by its input function (route, dosage, and rate), pharmacokinetic and pharmacodynamic properties. However, many additional factors (e.g., receptor sensitivities, pathophysiological state, poorly defined or measured clinical endpoints, formation of active metabolites, and insensitive and/or nonspecific

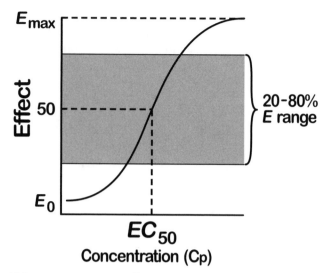

FIGURE 12.2.   Sigmoidal concentration versus effect (*Cp-E*) relationship. E_0 is the baseline effect at time zero, E_{max} is the maximum effect, and EC_{50} is the concentration corresponding to a half-maximal response.

analytical methods) can influence the correlation of effect with blood concentration. Prior to the 1960s, studies were focused on exploring theoretical aspects of dose-response relationships and only later followed by actual experimental investigations.

For drugs described by a one-compartment pharmacokinetic model, it was recognized that the log *Cp-E* relationship (plasma concentration versus effect) was linear within the 20 to 80% maximal effect (E_{max}) range, although a sigmoid model could describe the entire curve. The sigmoidal *Cp-E* relationship derives from the basic pharmacology of drug interaction with receptors, which is a saturable process. This is illustrated in Figure 12.2, which has the characteristic shape of any basic dose-response relationship. This type of curve is characterized by a lower tail at E_0, an upper tail or plateau at E_{max}, and the central point reflecting the half-maximal response (E_{50}), which occurs at the concentration defined as EC_{50}. Most pharmacodynamic models restrain their inference space (recall Chapter 1, Figure 1.2) to the linear portion of this curve and transform the data to obtain appropriate parameter estimates. The more complex sigmoidal models describe the entire *Cp-E* relationship for all concentrations and levels of response (E). Figure 12.2 should be referred to as the models discussed below are presented.

The underlying assumptions for this dose-response relation is that (1) drug effect can be described as a function of drug amount, (2) no active metabolite is produced, and (3) drug elimination follows first-order kinetics. In a one-compartment model where drug effect parallels plasma concentrations (body behaves as a single homogeneous compartment), the simple *Cp-E* equations below are sufficient to fully develop a PK-PD model. However, for multicompartment model drugs, this rule is applicable only when the drug target site is located in the central compartment. If drug effect is plotted against total drug amount in the body instead of that in the central compartment, the dose-response relationship often still can be quantified using the rule applicable for a one-compartment drug. To quantify various dose-effect relationships, many pharmacodynamic models have been defined and are broadly classified into two major categories: linear and nonlinear. They differ only in the need to linearize the observed *Cp-E* relationship.

Linear Pharmacodynamic Models.   The basic concentration-effect (*Cp-E*) model can be expressed as

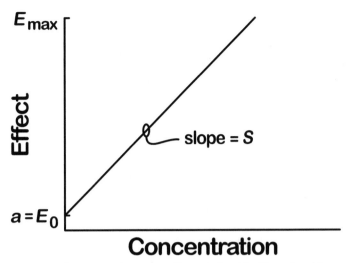

FIGURE 12.3.   Linearization of concentration-versus-effect relationship. Note that this approach is often applicable only within the linear (20 to 80% E_{max}) range of the dose-response relationship shown in Figure 12.2.

$$E = a + S\ Cp \tag{12.1}$$

where Cp is the drug concentration in plasma, (a) represents the baseline response at zero concentration before dosing, and S is the linear regression coefficient or slope of the dose-effect straight-line (Figure 12.3). Note that this equation is written in the now all-too-familiar slope-intercept form ($Y = b + mX$), whose solution is similar to that presented in Chapter 7 for solving pharmacokinetic equations. A negative slope can be employed if the drug has an inhibitory effect. Although this linear pharmacodynamic model is simple and easy to use, it is unsuitable for accurately predicting the baseline effect at time zero ($E_0 =$ intercept term a) since E_0 is not predicted by back extrapolating the linear segment of the sigmoidal curve in Figure 12.2. Similarly, E_{max} cannot be estimated because the drug effect would be infinite with a linear extrapolation, a biologically implausible scenario.

Similarly, the log Cp-E model can be formulated as

$$E = a + S\ \ln\ Cp \tag{12.2}$$

The only difference between this and the Cp-E model is that log concentration is used in an attempt to linearize the Cp-E plot (again note the similarity to the technique used throughout Chapter 7 to linearize exponential equations). Although the limitations of the Cp-E model are still present, this model is more common in pharmacodynamic studies. For most drugs encountered in medical practice, this model is applicable at least within the 20 to 80% E_{max} range. However, precautions must be taken when using this model beyond this range since, theoretically, the log Cp-E linear model would overestimate drug effects above 80% E_{max} and underestimate effects below 20% E_{max}. This is the basic limitation of extrapolating any model as originally discussed in Chapter 1. Classic examples of drugs described by this model are warfarin and thiopental.

Equation 12.3 presents a multiple linear regression model as

$$E = a + S_1 X_1 + S_2 X_2 + K + S_n X_n \tag{12.3}$$

where S_is are partial regression coefficients. The multiple linear regression model can account for fractional contributions of the drug or its active metabolite(s) in various tissues, body fluids, or pharmacokinetic compartments or of the sum of active components (parent drug, metabolites, co-dosed drugs) in a single compartment to the total effect. The significance of each compartment's or compound's contribution to the total observed effect may be determined by applying statistical tests on the corresponding partial regression coefficients $(S_1, S_2, \ldots, S_n)$. The model can be constructed as a full model by including all independent factors $(X_1, X_2, \ldots, X_n)$ or as a reduced model by omitting one or more X_i.

Nonlinear Pharmacodynamic Models. E_{max} and inhibitory E_{max} models can be defined respectively as

$$E = (E_{max} \ C)/(C + EC_{50})$$ (12.4)

$$E = E_0 - (E_{max} \ C)/(C + EC_{50})$$ (12.5)

where E_{max} is the maximal effect after dosing, E_0 is the baseline effect at time zero, C and EC_{50} are the concentrations at the target site and the drug concentration at steady-state to produce half E_{max}, respectively (see Figure 12.2). These two nonlinear pharmacodynamic models are widely used as they extend the data analysis with confidence beyond the 20 to 80% effect range by using equations that describe the Cp-E profile more accurately.

Sigmoid E_{max} and inhibitory sigmoid E_{max} models are defined, respectively, as

$$E = (E_{max} \ C^{\gamma})/(C^{\gamma} + EC_{50}{}^{\gamma})$$ (12.6)

$$E = E_0 - (E_{max} \ C^{\gamma})/(C^{\gamma} + EC_{50}{}^{\gamma})$$ (12.7)

The power function γ (first encountered in Chapter 7, equation 7.59) has been introduced into the E_{max} and inhibitory E_{max} models to more precisely derive the sigmoidal pharmacodynamic models. γ is a unitless parameter, which determines the slope of the sigmoid C-E curve and is related to the receptor-drug binding ratio. E_{max}, E_0, C, and EC_{50} are as defined in equations 12.4 and 12.5 and depicted in Figure 12.2. The only difference between these two models is the nature of drug effect (either stimulating or inhibitory) as reflected by the inclusion of the E_0 term in equation 12.7, for inhibitory effect modeling. These two pharmacodynamic models are often encountered in the literature and are very useful to predict E_0 and E_{max} compared to linear pharmacodynamic models. All of these models are directly applicable to the analysis of *in vitro* bioassay data.

The drug concentration C used in the *in vivo* pharmacodynamic models above is calculated as

$$C = (Ke_0 A_e)/(K_{je} \ V_j)$$ (12.8)

where V_j is the volume of the driving pharmacokinetic compartment to which the E-Comp has been linked, A_e is the amount of drug in the E-Comp, Ke_0 is the elimination rate constant, and K_{je} is the rate constant linking compartment j and the E-Comp. This approach will be developed shortly.

Equations 12.6 and 12.7 are better known as the Hill equation, which was first formulated in 1910 for studying the O_2 and hemoglobin association-dissociation process and subsequently used for quantifying more complex binding processes, such as enzyme/receptor-substrate (drug, hormone, etc.) binding. As early as 1968, Wagner and his coworkers suggested use of the Hill equation to describe the drug C-E relationship. Sheiner showed that Hill's equation was useful in PK-PD studies based on both theoretical and practical evidence and could be used to define the Michaelis-Menten relationship

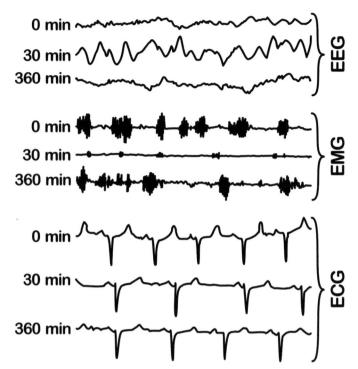

FIGURE 12.4.   Xylazole effects (2.5 mg/kg, IM) on EEG, EMG, and ECG in healthy adult sheep showing the baseline response (~0 min), E_{max} (~30 min), and the recovered response (~360 min).

as long as the parameters were properly selected. Chapter 9 fully discusses the derivation and use of Michaelis-Menten kinetics as applied to drug metabolism. Most physiological and pharmacological relationships between drug amount and biological effect can be described by a sigmoid curve, which is defined by the Hill equation. A threshold effect level can also be calculated using this model. In pharmacodynamic and PK-PD modeling studies of a large number of drugs, the Hill equation has been successfully employed. It is often used to quantitate *in vitro* bioassay results and has been used by the author to predict pharmacodynamic effects in skin by linking it to the pharmacokinetic model in Figure 10.5 (see Chapter 10). The drugs whose dose-effect curves can be determined by it include antiarrhythmic drugs, the anticonvulsant drug oxazepam, the muscle relaxants d-tubocurarine and alcuronium, the diuretic bumetanide, the anticoagulant warfarin, the analgesics methadone and meperidine, the animal sedative xylazole, and atropine. As the most important pharmacodynamic model, the Hill equation was also used in the theoretical formulation of a nonparametric PK-PD modeling approach. An analysis using the Hill equation will be addressed using meperidine later in this chapter.

The inhibitory sigmoid E_{max} model is similar to the Hill equation but more suitable to the pharmacodynamic analysis of an inhibitory effect without requiring any data transformation. This model has been widely used in the pharmacodynamic studies of many drugs with inhibitory effects such as the nondepolarizing neuromuscular blocking agent's muscle relaxation effect and thiopental, fentanyl, alfentanil, and ketamine (and its enantiomers) effects on the electroencephalogram (EEG).

One of the authors has used this model in the PK-PD analysis of xylazole to predict a number of therapeutic and side effects in sheep (Figure 12.4) using the EEG, electromyelogram (EMG) and electrocardiogram (ECG) as effect measurements. However, if the inhibitory effect data are instead transformed into fractional effects prior to conducting

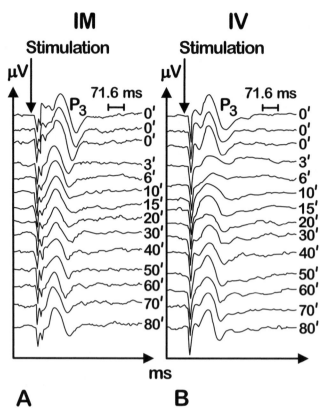

FIGURE 12.5.   Meperidine (5 mg/kg, IM or IV) effects on the P_3 wave of cerebral evoked potentials (CEP-P3) in adult postoperative goats at different times postdosing. The P_3 area reduction was used as a quantitative measurement of analgesic effect of meperidine.

PK-PD modeling, the E_0 term can be omitted. This model is then identical to the Hill equation. This approach gives one the flexibility to use modeling software in which the inhibitory sigmoid E_{max} model is not provided. For example, the meperidine analgesic effect can be indirectly quantified by using cerebral evoked potential P_3 wave (CEP-P3) area reduction as illustrated in Figure 12.5. The stronger the analgesic effect is, the smaller the CEP-P3 wave area is. If the CEP-P3 area data for all the time points i (A_i) is transformed into a percentage of baseline value (effect measurement at time zero [A_0]), the new set of % effect (E_i) may be used in a sigmoid E_{max} model instead of a inhibitory sigmoid E_{max} model as

$$E_i = ((E_0 - E_i) / E_0) \, 100\% \qquad (12.9)$$

Several other PD models are also useful under certain conditions. For instance, the *β-function* is suitable for describing convex *C-E* curves. The *logistic function,* based on the Hill equation, and the *Langmuir equation* (hyperbolic function) are also useful under certain circumstances. The interested reader should consult the literature and more advanced texts to implement these approaches.

In summary, the advantages of linear pharmacodynamic models are simplicity in the experimentation, modeling, and parameter calculation and wide application in quantitation of the linear segment of *C-E* curves (see Figures 12.2 and 12.3). However, a disadvantage of the linear models is that any extrapolation beyond the experimental observation is questionable and may not be reliable. Furthermore, for some drugs, the desirable therapeutic effect may be less or greater than the 20 to 80% limits. Therefore, it is often

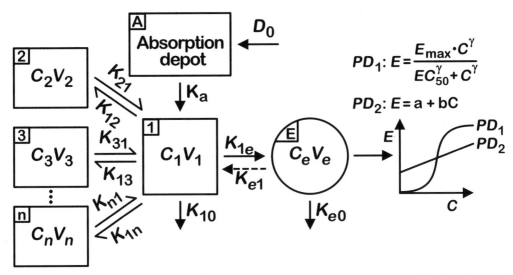

FIGURE 12.6. Generalized simultaneous PK-PD model. An effector compartment was linked to the central pharmacokinetic compartment of an n-compartment model. The relationship between drug amount in the effector compartment ($C_eV_e = A_e$) and the observed effect (E) was defined by selected pharmacodynamic model(s).

essential to formulate nonlinear pharmacodynamic models. These same limitations were faced when constructing pharmacokinetic models in Chapters 7 and 8 when concentrations were beyond the range of first-order relationships. Model selection is primarily based on the nature of drug activity and the shape of the E-Cp curve with consideration of dosage effects. The most common and useful pharmacodynamic models are the sigmoid E_{max} model and the log Cp-E model. The sigmoid E_{max} model is especially important since it may provide additional information about the drug-receptor binding ratio and the sensitivity of an individual to the drug.

INTEGRATED PK-PD MODELING: APPROACHES AND IMPLEMENTATION

The formal introduction of simultaneous PK-PD modeling was first accomplished by Sheiner and colleagues (1979), who recognized that in the traditional pharmacodynamic analysis discussed above, the correlation between drug concentration in the blood and observed effect is assumed to occur in a time-locked fashion. It is when the effect-time profile doesn't parallel the concentration-time profile that the more complex simultaneous PK-PD models described below are required. Traditional pharmacokinetics also focus on mass transport of drug and create models that are often insensitive to the negligible amounts of drug (relative to other compartments) that may cause an effect at the target site (recall discussion of Figure 2.1, Chapter 2). Similarly, these active concentrations may have a minimal impact on the determination of the value of ADME parameters. In PK-PD models, it becomes necessary to identify the target site (so-called biophase) as an E-Comp and distinguish it from the normal pharmacokinetic compartments so that the concentration-time profile in the E-Comp can be correlated to drug effect.

These concepts can be appreciated from the generalized PK-PD model depicted in Figure 12.6. The left half of this model is identical to the multicompartment models previously discussed, such as those depicted in Figures 7.20 and 7.21 (see Chapter 7), while the right-half effect component is an extension of the basic pharmacodynamic model in Figure 12.2. This data could initially be obtained from an *in vitro* assay system, which essentially is an experimental model of the biophase. The assumptions inherent to the pharmacokinetic components are the same as those presented in Chapter 7 and should be reviewed before progressing further in this discussion. The important concept to consider is the bridging between the kinetic and effect compartment, which is embodied in K_{1e}, the distribution rate constant of the active moiety (drug or metabolite) into the relative effect compartment being modeled.

This biophase or effect-compartment does not necessarily have any specific anatomical reality since depending on the drug in question, it may reside in multiple tissues and thus also have input from multiple compartments. The rate constant K_{1e} reflects barriers encountered as the active moiety reaches its specific receptor and is a function of anatomical location, rate of blood perfusion, and tissue permeabilities. If the biophase distribution process is fast relative to elimination and drug distribution into other pharmacokinetic compartments, the effect compartment is in rapid equilibrium with Cp, and therefore the determined Cp can serve as a good indicator of concentration at the target site and thus effect (E). However, if the redistribution (K_{e1}) from the biophase back into the plasma compartment is a slow process compared to other rate constants, the biophase is not in equilibrium with the systemic compartment. The Ce-T profile would then not be reflected by the Cp-T data. Suggesting a different compartment may work better.

There are two primary methods employed in PK-PD modeling: parametric and nonparametric. In the parametric approach, there are specific structural requirements for both pharmacokinetic and pharmacodynamic models. In the nonparametric analysis, the structure of neither the pharmacokinetic nor pharmacodynamic models needs to be specified. The reader must not confuse the terms parametric and nonparametric used in PK-PD modeling with the same terms applied to population pharmacokinetic modeling presented in Chapter 14, as the latter relates to whether or not specific statistical variance models are being defined in an analysis.

In general, integrated PK-PD analysis may be required when (1) the time course of the drug effect does not parallel the blood concentration-time profile; (2) a metabolite contributes to the total pharmacodynamic response; (3) one compound has multiple activities, and the sites of action have different kinetic characteristics; (4) a candidate drug has good pharmacodynamic but complex pharmacokinetic properties; (5) pharmacokinetics of the drug at the target site are not identical to that of the central compartment, (6) special tissue distribution/binding, blood concentration-dependent protein binding, and protein binding-dependent drug effects are present; (7) biological systems (animal or human) develop tolerance and sensitization to a drug; or (8) a mechanistic explanation is needed to explore the reason for unexpected changes in therapeutic effect seen under certain pathological conditions. There are obviously other circumstances in which PK-PD modeling would be useful, but it is usually required only when there is no simple relation between an observed C-T profile and drug effect.

Synchronization of Concentration-Effect Relationships and the Concept of Hysteresis. If the *C-T* and *C-E* profiles were perfectly in phase, simple and independent pharmacodynamic and pharmacokinetic analyses could be performed. The target site or biophase could be substituted by the blood *C-T* profile in any of the pharmacodynamic models presented earlier (equations 12.1 through 12.9) in order to avoid a complex simultaneous PK-PD modeling exercise. The complexity arises when the concentrations are not synchronized with the observed effects. For example, the peak of the *C-T* profile occurs at 1 hour, while the maximum observed effect is seen at 3 hours; or the concentrations deplete by 24 hours, but the effect persists for 36 hours. *In these cases, the same magnitude of effect is not always seen with the same drug concentration.* This phenomenon is termed *hysteresis*. In these situations, PK-PD modeling may be required. Hysteresis is depicted in Figure 12.7 which shows the relationship between plasma concentration, onset and

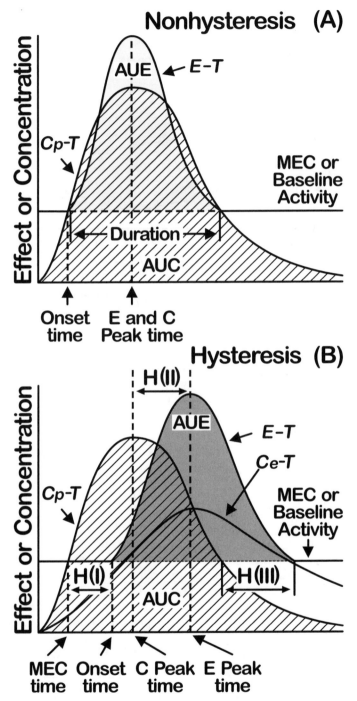

FIGURE 12.7. Relationship among blood concentration, minimal effective concentration (MEC), and drug effect. (A) Effect can (hysteresis not present) or (B) effect cannot (hysteresis present) be correlated to the plasma concentration (Cp) in terms of onset time, peaking time, and duration. H(I), H(II) and H(III) quantitate the magnitude of the hysteresis effect.

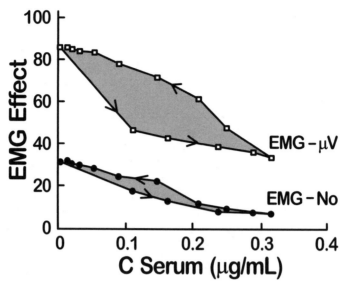

FIGURE 12.8.   Classical hysteresis plots from xylazole studies (2.5 mg/kg, IM) in healthy adult sheep. Xylazole effects on electromyogram (EMG) amplitude (μV; □) and activity (# peaks/min; •) were plotted against drug concentration in serum (postdosing time) to illustrate a counterclockwise hysteresis loop.

duration of drug effect. In the case of nonhysteresis (Figure 12.7A), blood concentration exactly predicts effect in terms of time as the Cp-T and E-T profiles overlap, allowing independent pharmacokinetic and pharmacodynamic models to be utilized. However, if they are out of phase (Figure 12.4 B), plasma concentration does not reflect the effect profile, and hysteresis is present. Times of peak concentration and effect are different. *The key factor that necessitates simultaneous PK-PD modeling is the presence of hysteresis in Cp-T and E-T profiles.*

The magnitude of this shift can be calculated by determining the degree of hysteresis at different time points. In Figure 12.7B, H (I) is the difference between the effect onset time and the minimum effective blood concentration, H (II) is the time difference between peak effect and the maximum blood concentration, and H (III) is the time difference between loss of effect and the time minimum effective concentration is reached at the end of a dosage regimen. The Cp-T and E-T data can also be used to derive a Ce-T profile that more closely reflects the true pharmacodynamic relationship.

This concept may be illustrated in Figure 12.8, which is a classical hysteresis plot generated from the inhibitory effect of xylazole on EMG in sheep introduced in Figure 12.4. The easiest method to assess if hysteresis is present is to plot the Cp-E data as a function of postdosing time to determine how significant the so-called hysteresis loop is. The data points are connected by arrows with increasing times. The "loop area" and "direction of the loop formation" with time provides useful information about the "depth/shallowness" of the effect compartment. In this example, maximal EMG activity is seen in the absence of drug, thus low Cp levels correlate to higher EMG effect responses. The EMG amplitude (μV) plot starts at approximately 85% effect and drops on the lower curve as concentrations increase. At Cp_{max} (approximately 0.32 μg/mL), the EMG effect is 40%. As concentrations again decrease postpeak in the depletion phase, the recovery in EMG is more rapid, as seen by the upper return component of the C-E plot. This is a counterclockwise hysteresis loop. The same pattern is seen in the EMG activity-frequency (# peaks/min) plot.

A counterclockwise hysteresis loop in a Cp-E plot suggests that the effect compartment is "deeper" (slower distribution rate constants, as defined in Chapter 7) than the plasma

Tolerance - response to given concentration of drug is reduced. EC₅₀ increases.
Potency - relation between a drug's mass and its effect

12 • Simultaneous Pharmacokinetic–Pharmacodynamic Modeling   **227**
Efficacy - related to the maximal effect a drug can ever have.

or central compartment and formation of drug tolerance may be expected. A counter-clockwise hysteresis loop is often observed after intravenous (IV) administration of a drug, although it may also be seen with other dosing methods depending on absorption and target tissue distribution kinetics. A clockwise loop suggests a shallow effect compartment. In constructing such plots, every effort should be made to collect simultaneous PK (plasma) and PD (effect) samples to facilitate the determination of the hysteresis loop and the construction of an appropriate PK-PD model. In addition, one may also plot the effect data against various tissue (peripheral) compartments of a multicompartment model to better determine the kinetic relationship between drug target site and the relevant pharmacokinetic compartment, whereby the appropriate compartment is selected as that which has the smallest degree of hysteresis.

As discussed above, different peaking times of the Cp-T and E-T curves strongly suggest the existence of a hysteresis loop. As a matter of fact, almost every drug possesses some degree of hysteresis between its blood concentration and effect with nonparallelism of concentration and effect curves in one or several pharmacokinetic compartments common. The impacts of the site of blood sampling (vein versus artery), the dosing rate, and the route of administration must be taken into account when evaluating this phenomenon. For potent drugs, the determination of Cp-E hysteresis may be especially important to evaluate the need for a loading dose (see Chapter 11) and the determination of the minimum effective blood concentration.

Approaches to PK-PD Model Construction.   Once the pharmacokinetic models are well defined and appropriate pharmacodynamic end points have been determined, it is possible to combine these into a simultaneous PK-PD model in which an effect compartment is linked to the pharmacokinetic model. The effect compartment then drives the form of the pharmacodynamic equation needed.

In PK-PD model formulation, three major components have to be considered: (1) the structure of the pharmacokinetic model, (2) selection of the pharmacodynamic model, and (3) selection of a mechanistic PK-PD link. Chapters 7 and 9 should be consulted to select the appropriate structure (first-order or zero-order) of the pharmacokinetic model and definition of intercompartmental transfer rate constants. This analysis may be done independent of the pharmacodynamic modeling and is identical to modeling any data using pharmacokinetic techniques. The selection of the pharmacodynamic model is based on the nature of the appropriate concentration-response relationship (e.g., Cp-E curve) that can be determined using various plotting methods, such as linear Cp-E (equations 12.1 and 12.3), log Cp-E (equation 12.2), or nonlinear models (equations 12.4 and 12.5). The nature of the drug effect (e.g., simulating or inhibitory) should be determined.

The critical step is now to properly integrate the selected pharmacodynamic model with the pharmacokinetic model; i.e., to select correct PK-PD linkage(s). Which pharmacokinetic compartment(s) is "closest" to the observed effect (minimum hysteresis), and how should it be linked to the proposed effect compartment (linear or nonlinear, constant or time/concentration-dependent rates)? Are there PD-PK feedback control loops that should be included in the model?

Parametric approach.   The parametric approach to PK-PD modeling is best represented by the Sheiner model. This method requires preconstructed pharmacokinetic and pharmacodynamic models. In general, the biophase compartment is assumed to be kinetically homogenous; i.e., the concentration of active moiety is uniformly distributed, and the drug-receptor interaction is instantaneous and governed by the law of mass action. Finally, the dose-response relationship is time-independent.

The general assumptions for PK-PD modeling are as follows: (1) Pharmacokinetic parameters are independent of pharmacodynamic processes (insignificant PD-PK interactions), and the E-compartment is small enough to not have a significant impact on drug disposition; (2) input and output from the E-compartment follows first-order kinetics, and the E-compartment has a one-way connection with the relevant driving pharmacokinetic compartment (PK $\Rightarrow$ E-compartment only); and (3) the relationship between drug concentration in the biophase and the observed effect (*Ce-E*) is quantifiable (linearly or nonlinearly) to enable selection of an appropriate effect model. However, if pharmacodynamic events exert feedback control over the pharmacokinetic processes (e.g., cytokine release, toxicity), if the pharmacokinetic model shows nonlinearity, or if the *C-E* relationship is time- or concentration-dependent, this approach may be inappropriate. A major limitation of these models occurs when there is an irreversible interaction between the drug and receptor or when a threshold for activity is present, such as in models used to predict carcinogenesis and, in some cases, antimicrobial activity. The back extrapolation from the linear portion, or even the lower tail, of the sigmoidal *E-T* relationship may be problematic. Stochastic techniques have been applied to this problem. Alternatively, a threshold concentration (C_{thresh}) may be defined where at $C_t < C_{thresh}$, E is assumed to be zero. At $C_t > C_{thresh}$, E is then expressed according to the relevant *C-E* model. For antimicrobials, C_{thresh} could be defined as MIC.

A PK-PD model can be constructed as follows. Select the appropriate pharmacokinetic and pharmacodynamic models. Link the E-comp to the jth pharmacokinetic compartment using a unidirectional first-order rate constant K_{je} (in most cases $j = 1$). Quantitate the hypothetical amount of drug in the E-Comp being eliminated (A_e) using another first-order rate constant (K_{e0}) from the proposed E-Comp. Correlate A_e to the observed effect (pharmacodynamic output) via a selected pharmacodynamic model. *Recall that since the target site is often very small compared to the whole body's volume, the absolute mass transfer of drug into and out of the E-compartment will not change the overall pharmacokinetic disposition of the drug.* Since K_{je} is often much smaller than other pharmacokinetic mass transfer rate constants, the accuracy of the K_{je} estimation is not critical to the final PK-PD analysis. In fact, K_{je} often does not require an independent estimation. The pharmacokinetic and pharmacodynamic models are linked together by a biophase or E-compartment to establish an integrated PK-PD model structure, as illustrated in Figure 12.6.

Among all of the rate constants in the PK-PD model, K_{e0} is the most important. It is related to blood perfusion and rate of diffusion to target tissue, the target tissue/blood partition coefficient, the rates of formation and dissociation of the drug-receptor complex, and characteristics of the time course of drug effect. K_{e0} is also useful in clarifying the relationship between the effect compartment and other pharmacokinetic compartments. For example, theoretically, if K_{e0} is much larger than all the other rate constants linking compartments, the kinetics in the effect compartment will be the same as in the central compartment. In this case, drug effect can be directly determined by measuring plasma concentrations. If K_{e0} is close to K_{j1}, the kinetics in the effect compartment will instead parallel the jth pharmacokinetic compartment.

From the generalized PK-PD model presented in Figure 12.6, one can define the changing rate of drug in the E-compartment as $dA_e / dt = K_{1e} A_1 - K_{e0} A_e$, which on solution yields

$$A_e(t) = K_{1e} \sum_{j=1}^{n} \{[A_j / (k_{e0} - \alpha_j)][e^{-\alpha_j t} - e^{-k_{e0} t}]\} \tag{12.10}$$

This drug amount is a function of postdosing time in the E-compartment when the E-Comp is linked to the central pharmacokinetic compartment. $A_e(t)$ also is applicable to other PK-PD model configurations with various E-comp linking methods (peripheral compartments, urine), different pharmacokinetic models (1-, 2-, or 3-compartment model), or different

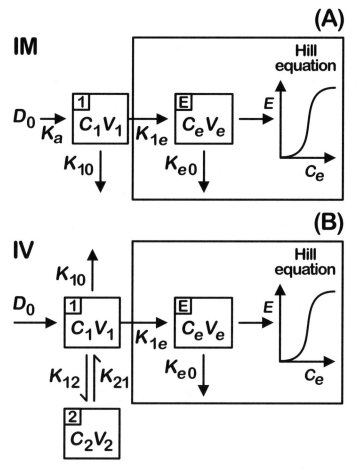

FIGURE 12.9. Meperidine PK-PD models after (A) IM and (B) IV dosing (5 mg/kg) in adult postoperative goats. A sigmoid E_{max} pharmacodynamic model was used to describe the relationship between drug concentration (C_e) at the target site (effector compartment) and analgesic effect expressed as CEP-P3 area reduction. (see text and Figure 12.5 for details).

TABLE 12.1.   PK-PD Parameters of Meperidine (5 mg/kg) in Goats (mean ± SD)

	γ	EC_{50} (μg/mL)	E_{max} (%)	K_{e0} (min^{-1})	$t_{1/2Ke0}$ (min)	AUE (min%)	r
IM	2.61 (0.30)	0.70* (0.08)	89.6 (3.9)	0.374* (0.064)	2.6*	2513 (294)	0.94 (0.01)
IV	2.37 (0.32)	0.41 (0.07)	85.9 (2.66)	0.112 (0.012)	7.3	2122 (249)	0.95 (0.01)

γ = Hill coefficient; $t_{1/2Ke0}$ = ln2/K_{e0}, half-life of equilibrium between drug plasma concentration and effect.
*$p < 0.05$.

routes of drug administration (IV bolus or infusion; extravascular dosing methods). Metabolite pharmacokinetic models as described in Chapter 9 may also be utilized.

Examples. PK-PD models have been successfully formulated with meperidine and xylazole in domestic animals. The PK-PD models are depicted in Figures 12.9 and 12.10, and the parameters resulting from these analyses are listed in Tables 12.1 and 12.2, respectively. $T_{1/2}(K_{e0})$ {= Ln_2 / K_{e0}} has been recognized as an important parameter that correlated to the degree of hysteresis between plasma concentration and drug effect. With meperidine, considerable hysteresis between Cp and effect was demonstrated for both the

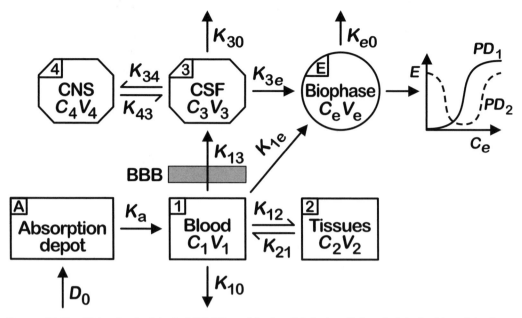

FIGURE 12.10.   Xylazole physiological PK-PD model after IM dosing (2.5 mg/kg) in healthy adult sheep. Blood-brain barrier, central nervous system tissue, and cerebrospinal fluid compartments were considered in this PK-PD model construction. Different pharmacodynamic models were applied in the data analysis depending on the nature of drug effects.

TABLE 12.2.   Xylazole (2.5 mg/kg, IM) PK-PD Parameters in Healthy Adult Sheep (mean, $n = 10$)

Effect	Parameter	PD Model	E_{max}	EC_{50} µg/mL	γ	K_{e0} min^{-1}	$T_{1/2}(K_{e0})$ min	AUE (min effect)
EEG	Frequency(Hz)	ISE	17.22	4.08	0.44	0.0217	32	4,936
	Amplitude(µV)	SE	21.63	0.53	3.41	0.0197	35	5,424
EMG	Activity(#/min)	ISE	30.16	1.22	1.31	0.0259	27	8,840
	Amplitude(µV)	ISE	84.95	2.94	0.60	0.0603	11	27,115
ECG	P-R int. (sec)	SE	0.139	0.26	1.19	0.0097	71	46

γ = Hill coefficient; $t_{1/2Ke0}$ = ln2/K_{e0}, half-life of equilibrium between drug plasma concentration and effect.
EEG = electroencephalogram; EMG = electromyogram; ECG = electrocardiogram; ISE = inhibitory sigmoid E_{max} model;
SE = sigmoid E_{max} model.

IM and IV routes; therefore, the analgesic effect could not be directly estimated solely using pharmacokinetic parameters such as $T_{1/2}$, $T_{1/2}$ (K_a), or T_{max}.

The Hill coefficient (γ) determines the steepness of the sigmoid concentration-effect curve and is related to the total number of drug molecules bound to each specific receptor. The mean γ values for the IM and IV experiments were 2.61 and 2.37, respectively, suggesting that the inhibitory effect of meperidine on CEP-P3 was most likely achieved through specific drug-receptor binding having a 2:1 or 3:1 molecular binding ratio.

Predicting the C-E Relationship.   Upon the determination of the $A_e(t)$ function in the PK-PD model, one may then be able to obtain the $C_e(t)$ function, which describes the kinetics of drug concentration in the E-comp by applying a steady-state approach. The $C_e(t)$ profile may then be incorporated into the selected pharmacodynamic model and the PK-PD model parameters determined by fitting the model to the observed *Cp-E-T* data. Once the PK-PD parameters are obtained, both the drug-concentration and the drug-effect profiles may be predicted and simulated. Figures 12.11 and 12.12 demonstrate good PK-PD

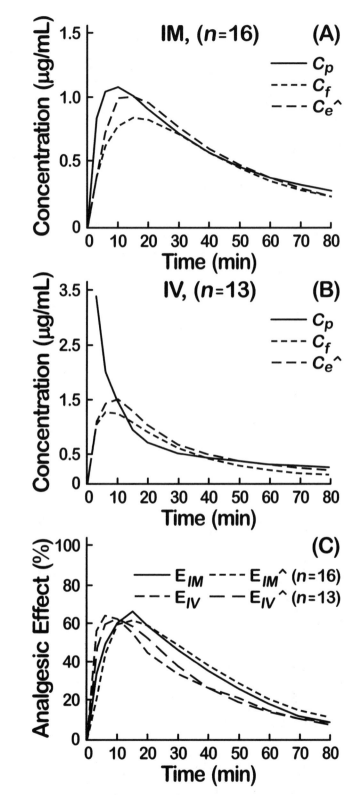

FIGURE 12.11. Meperidine concentration (A, B) and effect (C) prediction by PK-PD model after IM and IV dosing (5 mg/kg) in adult postoperative goats. C_p = experimentally determined plasma concentration; C_f = experimentally determined cerebrospinal fluid concentration; C_e^ = model predicted concentration in target site; E_{im} and E_{iv} are experimentally determined effects after IM and IV dosing, respectively; E_{im}^ and E_{iv}^ are model predicted effects after IM and IV dosing, respectively.

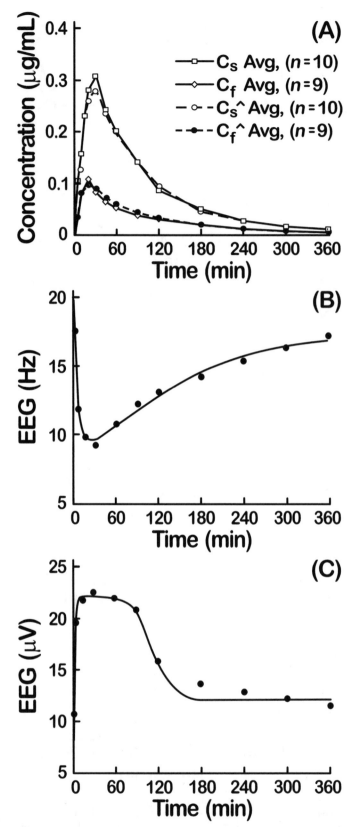

FIGURE 12.12. Prediction of xylazole concentrations (A: in plasma and cerebrospinal fluid) and EEG effects (B: frequency, C: amplitude) using a PK-PD model after IM dosing (2.5 mg/kg) in healthy adult sheep.

model predictions of both concentrations and effects for meperidine and xylazole in domestic animals.

Nonparametric PK-PD Modeling. This method requires that a specific pharmacokinetic model be linked to the E-Comp, but not to the pharmacodynamic model; i.e., no assumption or specification of a Ce-E relationship is required. In this method, an initial value of K_{e0} is arbitrarily assigned to govern drug elimination from the E-Comp, and the $C_e(t)$ profile is calculated. The $C_e(t)$ values are plotted against the corresponding observed effect data to examine the magnitude of the hysteresis loop. The final K_{e0} value is then optimized by continuous adjustment of K_{e0} until the hysteresis loop disappears (the area close to zero, H(I), H(II), and H(III) approaches zero). Other approaches also do not specify the structure of either the pharmacodynamic or the pharmacokinetic model with model parameters now calculated using computerized simulation based on the observed Cp–E-T data. The simulation results are then compared using predefined statistical criteria.

Computerized data fitting in any PK-PD analysis can be accomplished with various computer software packages. The approaches used are identical to that described in Chapter 13 except that effect data, in addition to concentration data from various matrices, are used as input, and a pharmacodynamic model is used to describe the effect relationship. In summary, the parametric PK-PD modeling approach is more established than, and has many advantages over, the nonparametric PK-PD analysis. However, the nonparametric approach requires fewer assumptions and has demonstrated applicability in many situations.

RATE CONSTANT DETERMINATION IN PK-PD MODELS

As presented in earlier chapters, the most reliable pharmacokinetic model is developed based upon data from a well-designed and carefully conducted IV bolus study with proper dosing, sampling, analytical, and statistical procedures. The intrinsic pharmacokinetic parameters governing drug distribution, metabolism, and excretion can be estimated without the confounding influence of complex input-absorption processes in perfusion/extravascular dosing studies. In a single-dose PK-PD study, bolus (instantaneous) IV injection and first-order IV infusion dosing methods can be used in sequence to control and identify the rate-limiting steps in the PK-PD modeling studies. In the case of a one-compartment open pharmacokinetic model ($n = 1$, Figure 12.6), the hypothetical amount of drug in the E-Comp can be described by the following equations depending on the input kinetics of the drug.
IV bolus dose model:

$$A_e = \frac{K_{1e}D_0}{K_{e0} - K_e}(e^{-K_e t} - e^{-K_{e0} t}) \tag{12.11}$$

Zero-order IV infusion model:

$$A_e = \frac{K_{1e}K_0}{K_e(K_{e0} - K_e)}(1 - e^{-K_e T})e^{-K_e t'} + \frac{K_{1e}K_0}{K_{e0}(K_e - K_{e0})}(1 - e^{-K_{e0} T})e^{-K_{e0} t'} \tag{12.12}$$

First-order input (IV infusion and other first-order absorption) models:

$$A_e = \frac{K_{1e}K_a D_0}{(K_e - K_a)(K_{e0} - K_a)}(e^{-K_a t}) + \frac{K_{1e}K_a D_0}{(K_a - K_e)(K_{e0} - K_e)}(e^{-K_e t})$$
$$+ \frac{K_{1e}K_a D_0}{(K_a - K_{e0})(K_e - K_{e0})}(e^{-K_{e0} t}) \tag{12.13}$$

where D_0 is the initial dose, K_e is elimination rate constant, K_{1e} and K_{e0} are first-order input and output rate constants for the E-Comp, respectively, K_0 is zero-order-input rate constant, K_a is first-order input-absorption rate constant to the pharmacokinetic model after first-order IV infusion or first-order absorption, t is postdosing time, T is duration of the zero-order infusion, and t' is time post-zero-order infusion. Therefore, $t = T + t'$ in the zero-order IV infusion studies.

As described in Chapter 7, the concentration-time profile of a one-compartment model is controlled by only one rate-limiting process, K_e, when the drug is introduced to the body by IV bolus injection or zero-order infusion. In contrast, the pharmacodynamic process is controlled by two rate-limiting processes, K_e and K_{e0}. When a first-order absorption process is involved in the pharmacokinetic model, an additional rate-limiting process of K_a is added. Under this circumstance, by varying the K_a, the rate-limiting process and/or controlling step may be isolated so as to separate the drug receptor kinetics from the central-peripheral compartment disposition. This conceptual approach has been elegantly applied in a study with verapamil in humans.

The input of a drug into the driving compartment (the pharmacokinetic compartment to which an E-Comp is linked) controls the concentration profile in this as well as in the E-Comp. The A_e-effect relationship (pharmacodynamic model) is not affected by drug-input rate in a single-dose study. Equations 12.11 through 12.13 can be used in the PK-PD modeling of a one-compartment model drug if a proper pharmacodynamic model has been defined. However, in a multiple dosing study, the pharmacodynamic model can be altered if the biological system develops tolerance or sensitization to the drug. This phenomenon has not been adequately considered in conventional pharmacokinetic studies. One of the advantages of mechanistically integrated PK-PD analysis is that drug tolerance and sensitization can be characterized.

An IV bolus study can be conducted to determine the intrinsic pharmacokinetics of the drug and its resulting pharmacodynamic profile. A first-order infusion rate can then be sequentially controlled within a range of fastest to slowest rates such that the pharmacodynamic parameters of the integrated PK-PD model can be isolated even if they would usually be concealed by the pharmacokinetic process associated with the integrated model. A PK-PD model initially established using single IV dose studies has to be tested by a different dosing route with either single and/or multiple doses. In the single-dose situation, the investigator should make an effort to cover the entire effect curve from baseline effect (E_0) to the maximal effect (E_{max}) expected during the multiple-dosing regimen evaluation.

A good PK-PD model should be able to accurately predict the pharmacokinetic and pharmacodynamic outputs of different dosage regimens in terms of dosing route and frequency. Even though an adequate fit to single-dose data is obtained, if an inappropriate model has been selected, the predicted and observed effects will often systematically diverge as multiple doses are administered. This approach is not universally applicable as an inappropriate model often cannot be distinguished from a model shift (model alteration during drug therapy due to sensitization or tolerance). (Recall the cases of enzyme induction presented in Chapter 9.) However, relevant information can be obtained for drugs with short duration of effect and multiple-dose protocols. If pharmacokinetics and pharmacodynamics are independent of dosing frequency, the multiple-dosing pharmacokinetic approach should be predictive of drug concentration and effect by applying the equations used from a single-dose study.

Time-dependent changes in both pharmacokinetic and pharmacodynamic parameters can be incorporated into the model equations to accommodate alterations that occur during repeated dosing. A cascade dosing approach can be used to significantly shorten the study time. This requires elaborate loading-dose schemes to rapidly achieve steady-state (e.g., computer-controlled infusion protocols as described for Figure 8.5 in Chapter 8). In addition, a tolerance model could be formulated incorporating time-dependent functions of a, S, K_{1e}, K_{e0}, EC_{50}, (and/or E_{max} (see equations 12.1 through 12.7) to subsequently adjust doses to optimize therapy with sufficient pharmacological effect and minimal toxicity; that is, to maintain drug concentrations within the so-called therapeutic window depicted in Figure 11.4 (see Chapter 11).

A PK-PD MODEL APPLIED TO SKIN

Throughout this text, we have illustrated the various pharmacokinetic approaches by modeling percutaneous absorption studies of drugs and pesticides in skin. To complete this topic, a pharmacodynamic model was linked to the pharmacokinetic model illustrated in Figure 10.5 (see Chapter 10). The goal was to generalize the drug-solvent interactions (two-component mixture) in this earlier model to any number of penetrating chemicals applied to skin as an n-component mixture. Each chemical's absorption profile is described according to a model similar to the right-hand part of Figure 10.5. However, now these "absorption units" are connected to each other by pharmacodynamic links. The model utilizes a modified Hill equation to simulate observed pharmacodynamic (vascular changes) and physicochemical (cytokine release) effects. The interchemical effects of this model are postulated as concentration-dependent at the effector site (E-Comp); that is, the extent of an effect is a function of the concentration of the effector compound at the sites of receptors (e.g., vascular epithelium) or target domains (e.g., stratum corneum intercellular matrix) of the affected tissue.

These interchemical effects can be simulated kinetically by modification of intercompartmental transfer rates for the affected unit as functions of concentrations of effector compounds in effector compartments of the effector unit (chemical). For example, (1) a vasodilator in a mixture could influence the absorption of all co-penetrating components by effectively increasing the transfer rates into and out of the dermis/vasculature compartments of affected units; (2) a surfactant could alter the surface tension of a dosed solution or cause epidermal irritation and cytokine release, and modify the penetrability of other components of a mixture, which could be represented by affecting evaporative loss, depot formation, and/or penetrating rates; and (3) a solvent could modify the barrier function of the stratum corneum by altering its lipid structure, thereby influencing the rate of penetration of co-penetrants, which is manifested in the model by a modification in the stratum corneum transfer rate previously incorporated in the model described for solvent effect in Figure 10.5 and described in equation 10.7 (see Chapter 10). The study involved parathion penetration and absorption dosed in a mixture with four other compounds: dimethylsulfoxide as solvent, $SnCl_2$ as a reducing agent, sodium lauryl sulfate as a surfactant, and methyl nicotinate as a vasodilator. This resulted in a model of five chemicals ($J = 5$, see below), each having the same multicompartment model structure.

Assuming intracompartmental instantaneous and homogeneous mixing, and using the principles in this and previous chapters, we defined the following modified Hill equation as

$$k_{isq} = k_{isq0} + \sum_{j \in J} \sum_{r \in R} \left(\frac{b_{jrisq} \bullet v_{isq}(m_{jr}) \bullet m_{jr}^{\ b}}{m_{jr}^{\ b} + K_{jr}} \right) \tag{12.14}$$

where k_{isq} is the rate describing transfer of the ith chemical from the sth compartment to the qth compartment;

   m_{jr} is the mass of compound j in compartment r;
   k_{isq0} is the initial rate; and

$$v_{isq}(m_{jr}) = m_{jr} - \theta_{jrisq0} \text{ for } \theta_{jrisq0} < m_{jr} \leq \theta_{jrisq1}$$
$$= \theta_{jrisq1} - \theta_{jrisq0} \text{ for } m_{jr} > \theta_{jrisq1}$$
$$= 0 \text{ for } m_{jr} \leq \theta_{jrisq0}$$

where θ_{jrisq0} is the lower threshold for m_{jrisq}'s influence on k_{isq};

θ_{jrisq1} is the upper threshold for m_{jrisq}'s influence on k_{isq};

K_{jr} is the Michaelis constant equivalent for m_{jr};

h is the Hill coefficient assigned to m_{jr}; and finally

b_{jrisq} is a proportionality constant.

The summation is over all compartments ($r \in R$), and all chemicals ($j \in J$), where R is the defined set of unit compartments and J is the defined set of chemicals. We refer to θ_{jrisq0} and θ_{jrisq1} as *effect* thresholds and b as the effect *potential* for a given interaction. The initial rate, k_{isq0}, is that estimated for chemical i alone (i.e., neat, without influences from other compounds). As a piecewise continuous function, $v(m_{jr})$ departs from the familiar constant v_{max} of nonlinear kinetics. This modification allows application of the expression to mass transfer rates. The lower effect threshold, θ_{jrisq0}, is defined as the minimal mass (m_{jr}) of compound j in compartment r that influences transfer of compound i from compartment s to compartment q, whereas the upper threshold, θ_{jrisq1}, is that mass beyond which negligible *additional* influence is exerted. The range for $v_{isq}(m_{jr})$ is thus $0 \leq v_{isq}(m_{jr}) \leq \theta_{jrisq1} - \theta_{jrisq0}$. K_{jr} is *not* the classic Michaelis-Menten constant of nonlinear kinetics but serves a similar functional purpose. The potential, b_{jrisq}, defines the sign and magnitude of the influence on the affected transfer rate. If the effect is to increase mass transfer, $b_{jrisq} > 0$, and conversely, if the effect is to decrease it, $b_{jrisq} < 0$.

This model was used to asses which components of the applied mixture significantly affected parathion disposition. The original manuscript should be consulted for additional details (Williams et al, 1996). It was used as a tool for designing future studies and probing how chemicals interact with each other when dosed as a mixture, and as preliminary structure for a risk assessment model.

SUMMARY

In conclusion, when the decision is reached to conduct a PK-PD analysis, the following steps should be considered when formulating the model. The pharmacokinetic profile of the drug should be first defined so that experiments that link concentrations (Cp) and effect (E) can be properly designed. The steps are as follows: (1) understand the general assumptions to both pharmacokinetic and pharmacodynamic models; (2) simultaneously and serially quantitate Cp and E; (3) determine and optimize the estimate of K_{e0} by hysteresis plotting; (4) optimize the pharmacodynamic model according to the nature of the effect and shape of the E-C response; (5) define PK-PD and PD-PD linkages and/or interactions, and then appropriately establish the relevant feedback control loops in the model; (6) formulate and verify the PK-PD model's experimental design and adequacy of data fitting, using appropriate statistical procedures (similar to that described in Chapter 13); and (7) use the model to obtain C-E-T data simulations and predictions. A major strength of these approaches is that *in vitro* models of drug action may be used to define the E-T relationship in the E-Comp or biophase, since these systems are often similar to the target site being modeled *in vivo*.

Although pharmacokinetic analysis is widely used as a supportive tool in pharmacological and toxicological studies, little attempt has been made to routinely conduct PK-PD modeling and to extrapolate the results to target species. However, increasing research and regulatory attention has been paid to a mechanistically integrated PK-PD modeling approach. PK-PD modeling can be used from early discovery of new drug leads through the clinical evaluation of an established therapeutic. Preclinical PK-PD studies are useful for validating pharmacological models and to bridge the gap between animals and humans by assessing safety in toxicological investigations. A major use of a PK-PD model is thus to simulate the doses that could be employed in early human or target animal clinical trials that are predicted to be safe and efficacious. Mechanistic PK-PD studies can be done during later clinical trials (phases II and III) to clarify potential impacts of physiological and pathological variables on drug efficiency and safety. The U.S. Food and Drug Administration has recommended applying PK-PD modeling early in the human drug-development processes to improve the efficiency of the process since these studies can provide a better understanding of the clinical pharmacology of the drug and facilitate the design of subsequent clinical trials. These approaches have not been widely used in comparative medicine; however, with the advent of software packages that facilitate model construction and analysis, their use could provide a more rational and mechanistic approach to therapeutics.

SUGGESTED READINGS

(The basic pharmacokinetic texts listed in the Selected Readings for Chapter 7 should be consulted for chapters on this subject)

Brier, M.E., and G.R. Aronoff. 1996. Application of neural networks to clinical pharmacology. *International Journal of Clinical Pharmacology and Therapeutics.* 34:510-514.

Colburn, W.A. 1981. Simultaneous pharmacokinetic and pharmacodynamic modeling. *Journal of Pharmacokinetics and Biopharmaceutics.* 9:367-388.

Colburn, W.A. 1988. Combined pharmacokinetic/pharmacodynamic (PK/PD) modeling. *Journal of Clinical Pharmacology.* 28:769-771.

D'Argenio, D.Z. 1993. *Advanced Methods of Pharmacokinetic and Pharmacodynamic Systems Analysis: Vol 2.* , New York: Plenum Press.

Dayneka, N.L., V. Garg, and W.J. Jusko. 1993. Comparison of four basic models of indirect pharmacodynamic responses. *Journal of Pharmacokinetics and Biopharmaceutics.* 21:457-478.

Derendorf, H., and G. Hochhaus. 1995. *Handbook of Pharmacokinetic/Pharmacodynamic Correlation.* Boca Raton, FL.: CRC Press.

Foreman, J.C., and T. Johansen. 1996. *Textbook of Receptor Pharmacology.* Boca Raton, FL: CRC Press.

Fuseau, E., and L.B. Sheiner. 1984. Simultaneous modeling of pharmacokinetics and pharmacodynamics with a non-parametric pharmacodynamic model. *Clinical Pharmacology and Therapeutics.* 35:733-741.

Ganzinger, U., and K. Neumann. 1992. Quantification of tissue distribution of antibiotics by kinetic hysteresis analysis. *European Journal of Clinical Pharmacology.* 43:517-522.

Gehring, P.J., P.G. Watanabe, and C.N. Park. 1978. Resolution of dose-response toxicity data for chemicals requiring metabolic activation: Example—vinyl chloride. *Toxicology and Applied Pharmacology.* 44:581-591.

Holford, N.H., and L.B. Sheiner. 1982. Kinetics of pharmacologic response. *Pharmacology and Therapeutics.* 16:143-166.

Mandema, J.W., and D.R. Stanski. 1996. Population pharmacodynamic model for ketorolac analgesia. *Clinical Pharmacology and Therapeutics.* 60:619-635.

Peck, C.C., W.H. Barr, L.Z. Benet, J. Collins, R.E. Desjardins, D.E. Furst, J.G. Harter, G. Levy, T. Ludden, J.H. Rodman, L. Sanathanan, J.J. Schentag, V.P. Shah, L.B. Sheiner, J.P. Skelly, D.R. Stanski, R.J. Temple, C.T. Viswanathan, J. Weissinger, and A. Yacobi. 1994. Opportunities for integration of pharmacokinetics, pharmacodynamics, and toxicokinetics in rational drug development. *Journal of Clinical Pharmacology.* 34:111-119.

Qiao, G.L., and K.F. Fung. 1993. Pharmacokinetic-pharmacodynamic modeling of meperidine in goats (I): Pharmacokinetics. *Journal of Veterinary Pharmacology and Therapeutics.* 16:426-437.

Qiao, G.L., and K.F. Fung. 1994. Pharmacokinetic-pharmacodynamic modeling of meperidine in goats (II): Modeling. *Journal of Veterinary Pharmacology and Therapeutics.* 17:127-134.

Sheiner, L.B., D. R. Stanski, S. Vozeh, R.D. Miller, and J. Ham. 1979. Simultaneous modeling of pharmacokinetics and pharmacodynamics: Application to d-tubocurarine. *Clinical Pharmacology and Therapeutics.* 25:358-371.

Smith, R.B., P.D. Kroboyh, and R.P. Juhl. 1988. *Pharmacokinetics and Pharmacodynamics: Vol. 2. Current Problems and Potential Solutions.* Cincinnati, OH: HW Books.

Stanski, D.R., J. Ham, R.D. Miller, and L.B. Sheiner. 1979. Pharmacokinetics and pharmacodynamics of d-tubocurarine during nitrous oxide-narcotic and halothane anesthesia in man. *Anesthesiology.* 51:235-241.

Unadkat, J.D., F. Bartha, and L.B. Sheiner. 1986. Simultaneous modeling of pharmacokinetics and pharmacodynamics with non-parametric kinetic and dynamic models. *Clinical Pharmacology and Therapeutics.* 40:86-93.

Veng-Pedersen, P., J.W. Mandema, and M. Danhof. 1991. A systems approach to pharmacodynamics. III. An algorithm and computer program, COLAPS, for pharmacodynamic modeling. *Journal of Pharmaceutical Sciences.* 80:488-495.

Williams, P.L., D. Thompson, G.L. Qiao, N.A. Monteiro-Riviere, R.E. Baynes, and J.E. Riviere. 1996. The use of mechanistically defined chemical mixtures (MDCM) to assess mixture component effects on the percutaneous absorption and cutaneous disposition of topically exposed chemicals. II. Development of a general dermatopharmacokinetic model for use in risk assessment. *Toxicology and Applied Pharmacology.* 141:487-496.

13

Study Design and Data Analysis

Mastery and comprehension of curve-fitting principles may be one of the most neglected areas in pharmacokinetics. It is at this stage that the quality of the analysis is in full control of the investigator. As can be appreciated from the discussion in earlier chapters, both compartmental and noncompartmental analyses require accurate curve-fitting for calculation of the parameters that describe the C-T profile, namely the slopes λ_n and intercepts A_n. Errors in this stage of the process may produce parameter estimates that are wrong simply because the data were improperly analyzed and not because the underlying model was incorrectly specified. There are a number of basic statistical principles that must be followed in any curve-fitting analysis. The reader is encouraged to consult a statistics text for a complete presentation of these principles and techniques. This chapter will introduce some basic concepts since it is essential to have an intuitive grasp of this process before analyzing data using automated software.

INTRODUCTION TO STATISTICAL CONCEPTS

The problem to be considered is how to fit a pharmacokinetic model to the experimental data. How does one judge that the fit is correct? If a drug is reasonably well "behaved," then the curve-fitting process should be relatively easy. For illustrative purposes, we will consider a drug with linear pharmacokinetic properties. The task then is to select the proper model (e.g., one-, two-, or three-exponential equation). Numerous commercial statistical and pharmacokinetic packages are used, which all share common attributes. The principles will be presented, and then a number of packages available at the time of writing will be illustrated.

The first step in understanding this process is to rewrite the basic monoexponential pharmacokinetic equation [the model to be fitted] to include statistical error components:

$$C_t = [A_1 \, e^{-\lambda_1 t}] + \mu_t + \varepsilon_t \tag{13.1}$$

where μ_t is unexplained variation in C_t due to lack of model fit (model misspecification) or bias, and ε_t is unexplained variation due to random error. Even if the monoexponential equation represents the optimal model to describe these data ($\mu_t = 0$), there always will be a random error component due to experimental (e.g., sample timing, analytical error) or in-

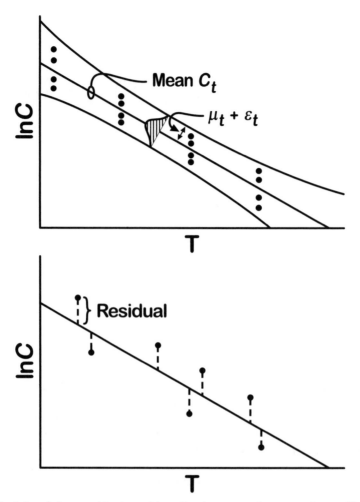

FIGURE 13.1.   Statistics of pharmacokinetic model-predicted concentration versus time profile. The mean predicted concentration at any time (t) is C_t. Actual data points are (•). Top panel: Variance envelope characterized by $\mu_t + \varepsilon_t$ defined by the nature of its frequency distribution. Bottom panel: Definition of the residual as the vertical difference between the observed and model-predicted concentration. The square of this distance is added for all data points to obtain the sums of squares, which is minimized in a regression program.

traindividual variation. Thus, any regression analysis will always have a degree of uncertainty, and the predictions will thus be bounded in a confidence interval that is largely defined by the magnitude of $\mu + \varepsilon$. This prediction envelope, defined by the actual statistical distribution of the error components, is illustrated in the top panel of Figure 13.1.

One must realize that, regardless of the complexity of the model to be fitted in equation 13.1, the identical regression process is utilized to minimize the error components. Some programs fit the exponential equations using techniques of nonlinear regression analysis, while other simpler programs linearize the exponential equations by logarithmic transformation to fit the equation in the slope-intercept form by simple linear regression (recall discussions in Chapter 7). All of the models presented earlier in this text may be fit to data using some implementation of statistical regression. One should recall from Chapter 10 that these approaches are conceptually different from those employed in physiologically based pharmacokinetics (PBPK) modeling, in which the goodness of fit to the C-T data alone is not the primary constraint involved in model selection.

As will be presented in Chapter 14, population pharmacokinetic approaches essentially attempt to correlate the interindividual component of error with observable clinical parameters (termed concomitant variables), thereby improving the model-explained variation and reducing the true random error ε. Some models even remove analytical error from this term. If the statistical distribution of ε can be mathematically defined, then the overall regression analysis can be improved even further. Our focus in this chapter is on the errors resulting from the model prediction in one individual and thus the error terms μ and ε are primarily related to the curve-fitting procedure. Different terminology will be employed in Chapter 14 as the aim of the modeling is different. However, conceptually, the problem is the same except that now, in addition to μ and ε, interindividual variance components will be included.

CURVE-FITTING

In all software packages, the computer will attempt to fit the data to a number of different models, using a wide variety of statistical algorithms, and calculate various indices of *goodness of fit*. Pharmacokinetic curve-fitting involves the use of regression techniques to fit a mathematical model to experimental data. By definition, experimental data represent a sample of the population, and in any regression program, a computer is attempting to minimize the fitting error (related to μ and ε), which is based on comparing values of residuals. The residual is defined as

$$\text{Residual} = \text{Observed} - \text{Predicted} \tag{13.2}$$

which for a biexponential model is

$$\text{Residual} = \text{Observed} - (A_1 e^{-\lambda_1 t} + A_2 e^{-\lambda_2 t}) \tag{13.3}$$

As can be seen in the bottom panel of Figure 13.1, the residual is the vertical difference between the value at time t predicted by the model and the actual experimental data point observed in the sample. The goal in a regression analysis is to reduce the overall magnitude of these residuals. The computer accomplishes this by minimizing a term called the residual sums of squares (SS), defined as

$$SS = \sum (\text{Residual})^2 \tag{13.4}$$

Regression analysis attempts to partition the SS in an experimental sample into components that can be explained by the model and the residual which cannot. Based on the basic statistical model in equation 13.1, this residual SS is actually composed of two components—an SS due to bias or lack of model fit and an SS due to random error. The concept that must be understood in regression analysis is that a model will explain a certain amount of variation in the experimental data. A superior model will explain more of the variation. The unexplained component of the variation (quantitated as the SS) will be due to bias and random error. The analysis attempts to reduce or eliminate the bias or lack of fit component. There will always be a random error component, which then defines the inherent variability in the data and the nature of the prediction envelope. This random error component is then used to test the model for statistical significance and define confidence limits for the model predictions.

In statistics, the goodness of fit of a regression analysis is often assessed by the value of the correlation coefficient, R, where

$$R = f(\sum \text{residual} / \sqrt{SS}) \tag{13.5}$$

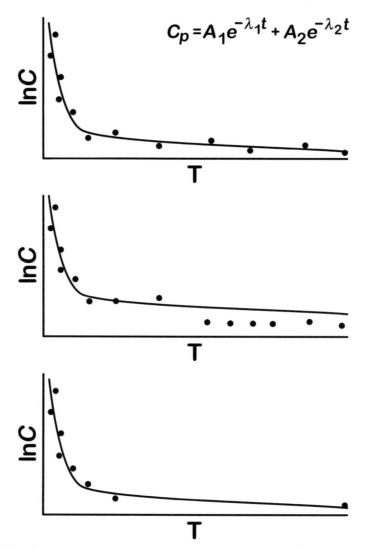

FIGURE 13.2.   Three biexponential plasma concentration versus time curves. Top panel: an excellent fit between observed and predicted concentrations, Middle panel: overprediction of terminal-phase concentrations, Bottom panel: an unbalanced experiment with sparse data in the terminal phase.

A perfect correlation has a value of $R = 1$. A more useful parameter is the coefficient of determination (R^2), which by definition is the fraction of the total variation of the data that can be explained by the fitted model. As can be seen, R and R^2 are very dependent upon the absolute magnitude of the SS and thus are completely influenced by the earlier and greater concentrations. All regression techniques operate by iteratively minimizing SS; that is, by computing different estimates of, say, A's and λ's in a model until the lowest value of SS occurs. When this occurs, statistics such as R will approach their optimal value.

Consider the influence of the early (high concentrations) versus late (low concentrations) time points of a kinetic experiment on SS. Assume that the prediction is off by 10% and the concentration data range from 20 µg/mL at 10 minutes to 0.1 µg/mL at 24 hours. The program will try to improve the fit of the early time point since it is trying to minimize the SS generated by an error in the 20 µg/mL sample. More progress is achieved reducing the *SS* contribution from the earlier time points than the later ones since the concentrations (and hence residuals) vary by a factor of 200.

One of the most powerful approaches to assess goodness of fit is to graphically examine the model-predicted versus observed data to ensure that the selected model is realistic. Numerical approaches often obscure this basic comparison. Figure 13.2 shows several examples of actual versus predicted data generated from a two-compartment open model. The ideal fit is depicted in the top panel. The middle panel shows a terminal phase that overestimates most of the data points. This may have resulted because the minimization of *SS* was completely determined by the residuals of the earlier time points, as discussed above. Statistical parameters such as R^2 for this fit may be very good since both of these procedures would be heavily influenced by the good curve-fit to the higher concentrations.

The fit in the middle panel of Figure 13.2 could be corrected by weighting the regression analysis (and hence the *SS* for each data point) by $1 / Cp$ or $1 / (Cp)^2$ to give equal consideration to the lower concentrations. Practically, $1 / (Cp)^2$ is often used if concentrations vary over a few orders of magnitude. Recalling the concentration and time ranges presented in Table 7.3 (see Chapter 7), this approach is critical when fitting three or more exponential terms to data.

The selection of the weight is properly determined by the variance structure of the data, which is determined by the variability due to analytical, physiological, and intra-individual factors (e.g., determinants $\mu + \varepsilon$). The need for this can be appreciated by examining the data in the monoexponential C-T profile in Figure 13.3. In the top panel, the data points have homogeneous variance (homoscedacticity), and a weighting scheme may not be necessary as it is for nonhomogeneous variance. Weighting may still be required, however, to compensate for the range of concentrations. In the bottom panel, the variance is much greater at lower than higher concentrations (heteroscedacticity), and the points should be weighted by 1/variance to minimize this highly variable data from overinfluencing the final fit. The optimal approach is to select an appropriate weighting scheme to compensate for this nonhomogeneous variance structure. Depending on the nature of the pharmacokinetic model being estimated, data with nonhomogeneous variance may adversely affect the values of the parameter estimates.

This scenario is encountered in settings in which analytical methods are pushed to their limit of detection, and lower, more variable, concentrations will have undue influence on the model selected. If there is a problem with assay sensitivity, a "bottoming out" of the C-T profile is typically seen. The statistics of this curve-fit may be excellent as all points are predicted from this model; however, the cause of the flattening is analytical and not biological. This is often seen in veterinary medicine when withdrawal times are studied (the focus of Chapter 17). One possible solution is to just consider the early time points where the model and data appear to be good. However, if this is done, the model will only be good at predicting concentrations at early times, the inference space for this experiment (recall discussion of Figure 1.2 in Chapter 1).

These weighting processes result in generation of weighted sums of squares (*WSS*), which are then employed in all subsequent statistical comparisons. Numerous approaches to generate *WSS* have been reported, and options for their selection are embedded in various software packages. More sophisticated approaches directly model the observed variance's statistical properties (e.g., normal or log-normal distributions) in the regression program, a process termed the extended least-squares method. The final weighting strategy is dependent upon the range of concentrations as well as the actual variability of the data. Chapter 14 should be consulted for a more in-depth discussion of these techniques. *It is important to note that when different models are evaluated for goodness of fit using these criteria, the same weighting schemes must be employed when making comparisons.*

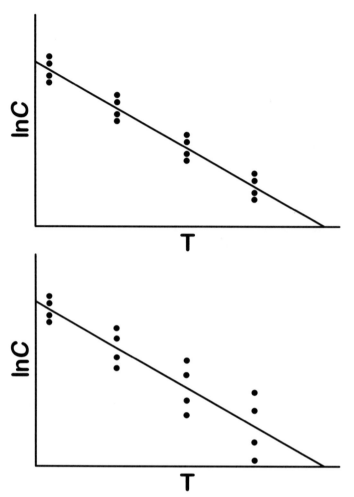

FIGURE 13.3.   A monoexponential model showing data with homogeneous variance (top panel) and one demonstrating heteroscedacticity (bottom panel). The latter is typical of data in which analytical variability increases at lower concentrations.

Another common problem is illustrated in the bottom panel of Figure 13.2, where there are no data in the final phase (only one point), which suggests that the estimate of the terminal phase is tenuous at best. This is typical of unbalanced experimental designs, where again the SS will be completely dominated by the points of the early phases. A similar situation can occur if the distribution phase has only a few data points.

Residual Plots.   Lack of model fit to the data can best be appreciated by examining a plot of residuals, a function present in most statistical programs. The predicted values in a residual plot are the horizontal line representing a perfect fit (residual = 0), while the actual residuals are plotted. As seen in the top graph of Figure 13.4, a good fit would indicate no bias in the residuals, which suggests the model neither overpredicts nor underpredicts the actual data throughout the course of an experiment. The middle panel is a plot of the example above, where the model misses the terminal phases, with the last six points having residuals below predictions. In the lower panel, a two-compartment model was used to predict a true three-compartment drug. In this case, the model first underpredicts then overpredicts, and then underpredicts the actual data. Such a plot requires

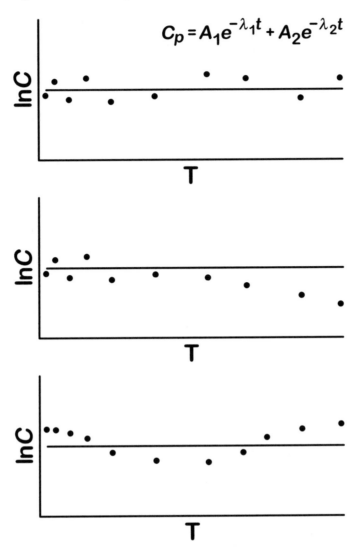

FIGURE 13.4. Residual plots resulting from a two-exponential pharmacokinetic model. Top panel: A well-balanced model with random residuals. Middle panel: Residuals indicate lack of model fit at late time points. Bottom panel: Residuals suggest that a three-exponential equation may better describe the data.

that a new model be considered. A good fit is characterized by a random pattern of residuals, which demonstrates that in general, the model is not biased.

As can be appreciated, there is a tremendous amount of information embedded in the residuals since they actually are plots reflecting μ and ε. Residual plots are often calculated using the WSS to more accurately present the goodness of fit obtained. Most software packages have the capacity to generate residual plots and calculate statistical indices quantitating their goodness of fit and their statistical distributions. For example, a nonbiased model ($\mu \to 0$) will have no pattern in residuals since they reflect the random error term ε. Thus they should alternate between plus and minus values, and their magnitude should reflect the normal Gaussian distribution of a true random error. This is seen in the top panel of Figure 13.4, where there are eight runs of plus or minus residuals. If however, the residuals have long runs before the residual sign changes (e.g., middle panel, five runs, and bottom panel, three runs, of Figure 13.4), then there is bias present (μ) and the model is not optimal. A large number of runs thus indicates a better model fit. Statistical tests for randomness of residuals, kurtosis, skewing, constancy of variance, and normality of residuals are included in many pharmacokinetic packages. Similarly, outliers can be easily detected in residual plots and eliminated with a known degree of statistical confidence. These assessments give the user a better idea of model fit.

Statistical Parameters.   Various statistical estimates of goodness of fit are used to quantitate the graphical impressions above. Automated pharmacokinetic packages will report out one or all of these statistics. These include R, R^2, estimated parameter coefficient of variations (*CV*, defined as parameter mean/standard error), the *F* test on a model's ability to reduce the *WSS*, and various criteria used to determine whether the simplest model is sufficient to fit the data (e.g., Aikake's Information Criterion, or AIC; Schwarz's criterion, or SC). The *CV* of the estimated parameters is a very robust indicator of the adequacy of the model parameter estimation since the standard error of any parameter estimate is related to the magnitude of the unexplained variation within an individual (μ and ε). The optimal model that truly describes the disposition of the drug will have a smaller *CV*.

The *F* test is used to judge the statistical significance of the value of R^2. It is widely used in analysis of variance and is a comparison of *SS* (or *WSS*) between two competing models that take into account the difference in the reduction in *SS* between the models based on the degrees of freedom (*df*). Note that this will parallel the reduction in the *extended least squares objective function* used in population pharmacokinetic models in Chapter 14. Degrees of freedom are defined as the number of data points analyzed minus the number of parameters estimated. For a monoexponential model with 10 C-T points and two parameters being estimated (A, λ), the df_{mono} would be 8. For a biexponential model being fitted to the same 10 data points, df_{bi} would equal 6. The greater the degrees of freedom, the more precise the analysis. The *F* statistic is calculated as

$$F(\Delta df, df_{bi}) = \{(SS_{mono} - SS_{bi}) / SS_{bi}\} \{df_{bi} / (df_{mono} - df_{bi})\} \tag{13.6}$$

The subscripts mono and bi refer to the models being compared. In the example described, $\Delta df = 2$, and thus the appropriate *F* statistic is $F(2,6)$. The value of the calculated *F* is now compared to a table of *F* statistics (computed directly in most software packages) for different levels of statistical significance ($\alpha = 0.05$ traditionally used). If the calculated *F* is greater than the reference *F*, then the biexponential model has resulted in a statistically significant reduction in *SS* and is a preferred model. In contrast, if the calculated *F* is less than the reference *F*, then the simpler model should be used.

Both the R^2 and *F* tests, which are based on *SS*, are fairly insensitive to lack of fit for lower concentrations, and thus a weighting scheme must often be employed and then these statistics calculated using *WSS* values. The *F* test may be used to compare any two models as long as the weighting schemes are identical in both. As can be appreciated from a consideration of degrees of freedom, the more data points in the analysis, the more sensitive the discrimination between models will be.

The *AIC* and *SC* are estimates of how complex a model needs to be (e.g., number of exponential phases) in order to optimally fit the models to the data. For an experiment with n C-T data points that estimates p parameters (*df* would now equal $n - p$),

$$AIC = n(\ln WSS) + 2p \tag{13.7}$$

$$SC = n(\ln WSS) + p (\ln n) \tag{13.8}$$

The model with the lowest value of either *AIC* or *SC* is the better model.

We have illustrated these techniques using simple monoexponential and biexponential models. There are numerous other techniques based on correlation matrices and other statistical metrics (e.g., Eigen value of the variance-covariance matrix) that may be used to explore complex multiparameter models. Although mathematically more complex to compute, the same indices described above may also be generated for any of the models described in previous chapters. The differences between *AIC* and *SC* in differentiating models will be based on the relative sizes of n and p that are the *df* in the experiment. If the purpose is to discriminate models, then the experiment must be designed to have a large *df* to accurately compute discriminating statistics and define mathematical identifiability. In other words, there must be enough data collected to have sufficient degrees of freedom to be able to define a model. An experiment conducted with four time points cannot be used to fit a three-compartment model to the data!

Often times, all four criteria (F test, R or R^2, *AIC*, and *SC*) select the best model. In other cases, especially when the degrees of freedom are low because of either too few data points or too many parameters being estimated, the results are not clear-cut. This author would strongly advise against relying on any one parameter. A final model should be selected based on an examination of all data viewed in the context of how the model will be applied.

Finally, we have only addressed the analysis of concentration-time profiles. Identical approaches are used when multiple matrices are sampled and concentrations in plasma, urine, and peripheral tissue versus time are modeled. An example is the parathion models depicted in Figures 7.24 and 7.25 (see Chapter 7). In these cases, the reduction in degrees of freedom introduced by the addition of compartments is offset by the increased number of observations obtained by analyzing more matrices and metabolites. Similar logic applies to modeling concentration data and effect compartments, as presented in Chapter 12. Residual plots for "predicted versus observed concentration" in all these matrices or "predicted versus observed effect" can be examined and statistics calculated to obtain the best fit to all of the data. The only real difference is that more complex models are specified in the input to the programs, making selection of the proper models a critical step, especially when nonlinear data are to be studied. The fit to multiple residual plots must be simultaneously assessed. In PKPD models, it is important to start with the optimal and simplest pharmacokinetic model that adequately describes the data to ensure that, after linking to a pharmacodynamic model, all variation in the concentration versus time data is adequately predicted by the pharmacokinetic model.

COMPUTER CURVE-FITTING EXAMPLES

These nuances of curve-fitting are best illustrated by example. The data listed in Table 13.1 are observed values obtained in the author's laboratory after an intravenous dose of 20 mg/kg of the antibiotic doxycycline to four preruminant calves. Concentrations were quantitated for total plasma doxycycline using a high-performance liquid chromatographic assay, validated with mass spectrometry, as being specific for unchanged parent drug (Riond et al, 1989). These data were then analyzed using six different commercially available software packages by scientists familiar and experienced with their use (see Table 13.2).

The results of these analyses are tabulated in Table 13.3 and output graphically presented for Win-Nonlin in Figure 13.5, SAAM II in Figure 13.6, SCIENTIST in Figure 13.7, PKAnalyst in Figure 13.8, and P-Pharm in Figure 13.9. As can be appreciated from examining the C-T profiles, the curve-fits were excellent. The parameters estimated using all five programs generally converged on similar values for A_2, λ_2, Cl, Vd_{ss} and mean residence time (MRT). The discrepancies were noted in the estimation of A_1 and λ_1,

TABLE 13.1. Sample Data Set Used as Input in Pharmacokinetic Software Packages (Doxycycline Plasma Concentration in µg/mL After an Intravenous Dose of 20 mg/kg)

Time (hours)	Animal 1	Animal 2	Animal 3	Animal 4
0.08	32.5	27.0	25.8	23.4
0.17	28.0	21.2	24.8	18.7
0.25	25.9	19.5	21.6	18.1
0.33	26.1	18.6	21.1	18.6
0.42	25.0	18.2	19.6	17.1
0.50	23.2	8.2	20.1	16.2
1.00	20.2	17.8	15.8	15.9
2.00	15.2	15.2	14.1	12.5
3.00	12.2	15.9	13.4	11.9
4.00	10.3	12.0	12.5	12.4
10.0	5.3	8.6	11.0	10.2
17.0	7.0	5.8	6.8	6.1
22.0	2.9	6.1	4.9	5.6
28.0	4.0	4.0	3.6	3.9
34.0	2.2	2.8	2.4	2.7
41.0	1.8	1.6	1.3	1.8
46.0	1.4	1.5	1.0	1.4
58.0	0.9	1.2	0.7	0.8
70.0	0.7	1.0	0.6	0.6

TABLE 13.2. Pharmacokinetic Software Packages Used and Scientists Who Analyzed the Data in Table 13.1

Scientist	Affiliation	Software Package
Dr. Jim Caputo	Pharmacia-UpJohn, Inc.	SCIENTIST (Micromath, Inc.)
		SAS-NLIN (SAS Institute, Inc.)
Dr. Arthur Craigmill	University California, Davis	PKAnalyst (Micromath, Inc.)
Dr. Gary Koritz	University Illinois, Urbana	P-Pharm (Simed, Inc.)
Dr. Mark Papich	North Carolina State University	SAAM II (NVI)
Dr. Guilin Qiao	North Carolina State University	Win-Nonlin (Scientific Consulting, Inc.)

reflecting the distribution phase of the C-T profile for these animals. This was primarily due to the contribution of animal 1, which had abnormal distribution characteristics compared to the other three animals in the study. This is due to *interindividual* differences in drug disposition since all six software programs fit this animal the same. Note that despite the differences in the early distribution phase, Cl, Vd_{ss}, and MRT were very tightly estimated. Included in this analysis is also a population pharmacokinetic approach (P-Pharm, see Figure 13.9), which fit the model simultaneously to all four animals. Note that for all parameters, this approach provided the "tightest" estimates. This approach will be dealt with in greater detail in the next chapter.

Estimation of distribution parameters is always fraught with difficulty since the concentrations are high and the sample times very short. Errors in the time of sample collection will have a major impact on the parameters obtained. For example, the first sample collected was at 5 minutes (0.08 hours). If the collection times were off by one minute, this would be an error of 20%. In contrast, if the timing were off by one minute for the 48-hour sample, the error would only be 0.03%! In fact, at later time points, timing errors of 10 to 15 minutes have little effect on the analysis (0.3% error at 48 hours). To

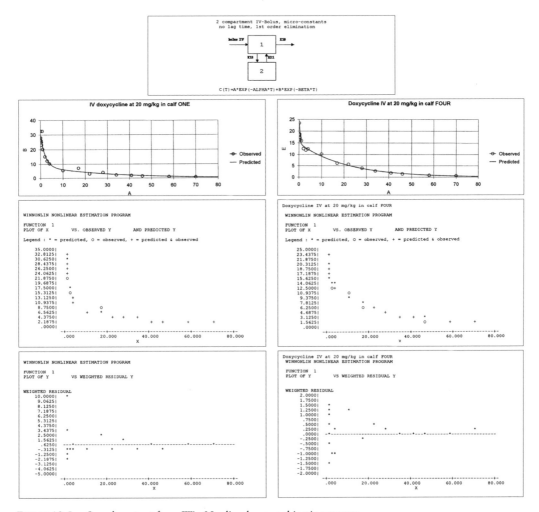

FIGURE 13.5.   Sample output from Win-Nonlin pharmacokinetic program.

minimize these errors, one should record the actual time that the blood sample was collected and use this in the data analysis. Similarly, in a large animal, the blood circulation time becomes important as the drug might not have been uniformly distributed throughout the body.

Table 13.4 lists the intercompartmental microconstants determined from these data analyses (Chapter 7, Figure 7.15) using a selection of three software packages. The values of Vd_{ss} and Cl can be obtained from Table 13.3. One can appreciate that the estimates of the elimination rate constant K_{10}, Vd, and Cl are relatively stable; however, the intercompartmental constants (K_{12} and K_{21}) differ greatly both between individuals within a software package and between packages. This is even a clearer illustration of the problems encountered in modeling distribution, and situations such as this are often cited as arguments against the use of compartmental models to describe drug disposition.

All of the software reported out regression statistics that confirmed the adequacy of an open two-compartment model to fit these data. R^2 values were greater than 0.98, F values (and similar statistics) indicated a significant fit, and residual statistics were generally acceptable. No analyst weighted the data, although some programs reported out a very slight tendency toward heteroscedacticity in the residuals, which would suggest weighting

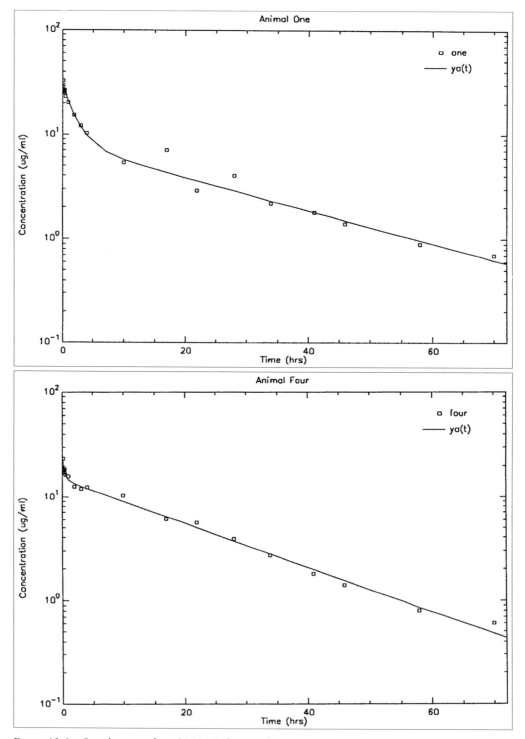

FIGURE 13.6. Sample output from SAAM-II pharmacokinetic program.

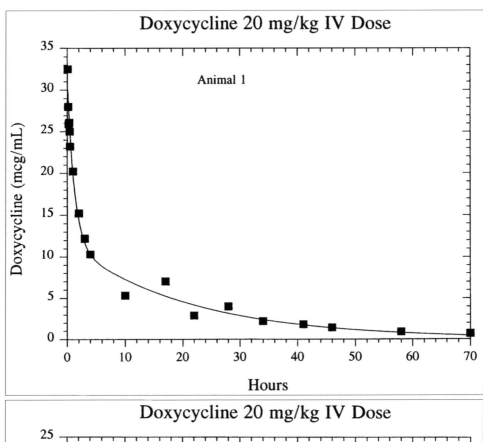

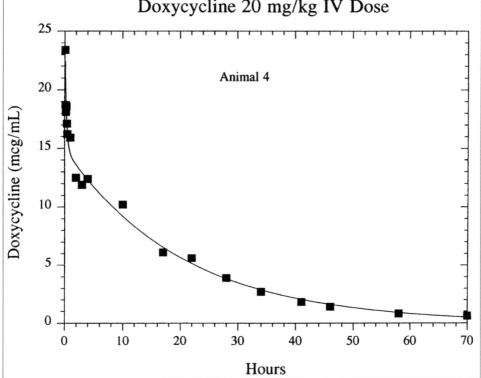

Figure 13.7.   Sample output from SCIENTIST pharmacokinetic program.

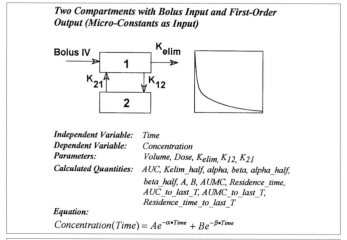

Independent Variable: Time
Dependent Variable: Concentration
Parameters: Volume, Dose, K_{elim}, K_{12}, K_{21}
Calculated Quantities: AUC, Kelim_half, alpha, beta, alpha_half, beta_half, A, B, AUMC, Residence_time, AUC_to_last_T, AUMC_to_last_T, Residence_time_to_last_T

Equation:

$$Concentration(Time) = Ae^{-\alpha \cdot Time} + Be^{-\beta \cdot Time}$$

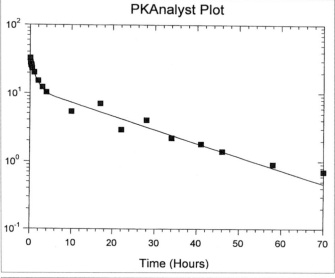

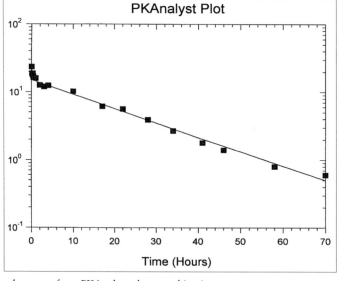

FIGURE 13.8.   Sample output from PKAnalyst pharmacokinetic program.

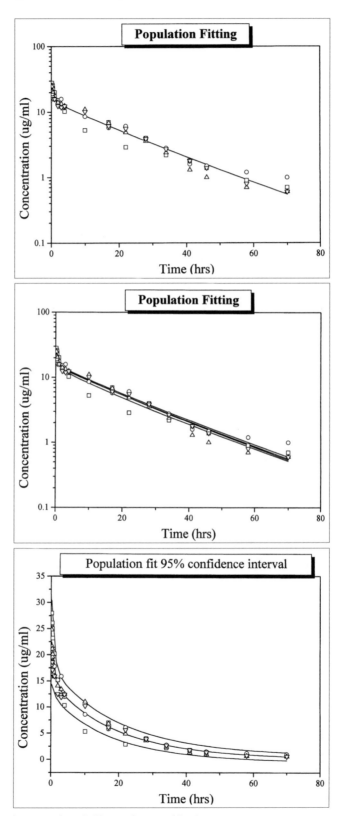

FIGURE 13.9.   Sample output from P-Pharm pharmacokinetic program.

TABLE 13.3. Pharmacokinetic Parameters (Mean + SD) Estimated Using Different Software Packages

Software	A_1 (μg/mL)	A_2 (μg/mL)	λ_1 (h⁻¹)	λ_2 (h⁻¹)	Cl (L/h-kg)	Vd_{ss} (L/kg)	MRT (h)
Win-Nonlin[1]	15.96 ±5.73	14.20 ±4.21	3.92 ±3.73	0.048 ± 0.010	0.066 ± 0.002	1.34 ± 0.28	20.4 ± 3.6
SAAM II[2]	14.30 ±5.28	13.7 ±3.90	2.78 ±2.02	0.048 ± 0.009	0.069 ± 0.005	1.38 ± 0.28	–
SCIENTIST[3]	15.34 ±4.80	15.02 ±2.68	4.04 ±3.66	0.051 ± 0.006	0.067 ± 0.004	1.27 ± 0.15	19.0 ±1.6
SASNLIN	15.2 ±4.82	15.03 ±2.61	3.94 ±3.61	0.051 ± 0.006	0.067 ± 0.004	1.27 ± 0.15	19.0 ±1.6
PKAnalyst[4]	15.34 ±4.80	15.02 ±0.67	4.04 ±3.66	0.051 ± 0.006	0.067 ± 0.004	1.28 ± 0.15	19.0 ±1.6
P-Pharm[5]	11.40 ±5.37	13.35 ±2.48	1.31 ±1.17	0.046 ± 0.057	–	–	–
P-Pharm Population	10.16 ±4.78	13.73 ±1.23	0.95 ±0.49	0.047 ± 0.003	–	–	–

[1]See Figure 13.5; [2] See Figure 13.6; [3] See Figure 13.7; [4] See Figure 13.8; [5] See Figure 13.9

TABLE 13.4. Two-Compartment Pharmacokinetic Micro-Constants (Mean + SD) Estimated Using Different Software Packages

Software	K_{10} (h⁻¹)	K_{12} (h⁻¹)	K_{21} (h⁻¹)	Vc (L/kg)
Win-Nonlin	0.099 ± 0.018	1.82 ± 1.93	2.05 ± 1.82	0.676 ± 0.107
SAAM II	0.096 ± 0.014	1.18 ± 0.92	1.56 ± 1.14	0.719 ± 0.088
SCIENTIST	0.106 ± 0.022	2.18 ± 2.22	2.36 ± 2.09	0.644 ± 0.061

to be appropriate. Some contributors attempted to fit a three-compartment model to the data, although R^2 did not improve and the *AIC* was lower with the two-compartment model.

In conclusion, regardless of the software package used, the sample data were adequately analyzed by all investigators. There are no platonic absolute values for these parameters since Table 13.3 clearly shows that the estimates are somewhat dependent upon the software. Thus, differences in parameters of, say, 10% are biologically meaningless since they fall well into the noise associated with the regression procedures. For two animals or two drugs to have different pharmacokinetic properties, parameter values must be different by values of a few coefficients of variation to be biologically important.

GENERAL CONCEPTS

To complete this discussion, I will present a personal overview of important principles of experimental design and curve-fitting in the form of several rules of thumb. These should be viewed as suggestions for improving the analysis of experimental data.

Independent of what type of pharmacokinetic modeling approach is to be applied, there are a few general guidelines that always should be followed, yet are often ignored, based on the author's review of numerous manuscripts in this field. These include the following:

1. Before beginning any study, it is always prudent to conduct a small pilot trial to determine what the serum C-T profile looks like. This ensures that the concentrations produced by the dose administered are in the proper range for the assay. Concentrations should always be significantly above the sensitivity of the assay, otherwise the terminal concentration profile tends to "flatten out," which erroneously suggests a long terminal $T_{1/2}$. Pilot studies are best conducted by taking samples at increasing time intervals to determine how long drug concentrations persist. To get an accurate estimate of a terminal half-life, one needs an experimental duration at least 3 to 5 times the actual $T_{1/2}$. Recall from Chapter 7 that in five $T_{1/2}$s, 97% of that exponential phase governed by the process is over. Depending on assay methods used, this strategy also allows one to plan for appropriate dilutions. Finally, a pilot study begins the process of model selection since, when the data are plotted on Cartesian and semilogarithmic scales, linearity may be easily assessed (see Chapter 7, Figures 7.1 and 7.2, and Chapter 9, Figure 9.3) and, if appropriate, the number of exponential phases in a linear C-T profile can often be estimated. Finally, it is important to remember that when conducting an intravenous pharmacokinetic study, one must administer the drug in a different cannula from that used to collect blood samples; otherwise, residual drug left over from the high concentration injection will contaminate samples. On this point, one must also remember to discard the initial fill-volume of any catheter to ensure that solution in the catheter for anticoagulation purposes will not dilute the actual sample.

2. At this point it is important to verify that the analytical assay used is appropriate and sensitive enough for the serum concentrations observed. It is better to conduct a few pilot studies to get the concentrations in a range optimal for assay than to do a complete study only to discover that they are out of range. Unfortunately, this occurs too often. This step also helps one select the volume of blood samples needed in the final experiment. The specificity of the assay should be defined. Are any metabolites present? Does the assay measure total or free drug concentrations?

3. The next phase is to determine how many samples are needed and when should they be taken. Ideally, an orthogonal sampling schedule should be selected whereby samples are spaced at increasing time intervals, making the number of samples per exponential phase balanced (e.g., equal number of time points per phase to avoid bias in fitting any

one model component). Of course, this assumes that a log-linear C-T profile has been identified in the pilot study. The reason behind this logic is evident from our discussion of the curve-stripping procedure (Chapter 7, Figure 7.16) since essentially one is estimating the intercepts (A_n) and exponents (λ_n) of a polyexponential equation. An unbalanced experimental design that results in too many samples in one phase will give more weight to that phase (all SS determined from that phase) and therefore bias the model. If, in the actual experiment, one finds that this has occurred, one might prefer to randomly delete samples from the data-rich phase to eliminate bias. The increasing time intervals between samples (every 5 minutes, then 15 minutes, then 30 minutes, then 1 hour, 2 hours, etc.) is always the best strategy to curve-fit exponential equations when the model (1, 2, or 3 terms) is not known since this results in an equally spaced spread of data when plotted on a semilog C-T plot. A 12–time-point study would be optimally designed as collecting samples at 5, 10, 15, 30, 45, 60, 90, 120, 180, 240, 360, and 480 minutes. A zero-time, predosing sample should always be collected.

In contrast, if the specific model is already defined for a species, and the goal of the study is to estimate the value of the parameters [intercepts (A_n) and slopes or exponents (λ_n)] for that model, then samples should be clustered within each exponential phase since one already knows where the phases are occurring. One avoids points in the inflection areas (times between phases where the curve bends) since depending on variability, they may be assigned to the wrong phase. If a two-compartment model fits the above data, samples in such a study might be best taken at 10, 15, 20, 60, 75, 90, 240, 275, 300, 400, 440, and 480 minutes. To design these experiments, studies must have already been conducted in the species of interest and a model defined. In most cases, the first scenario is operative and orthogonal design is best. The reader is referred to statistical texts on experimental design and optimal sampling strategies for a discussion of the differences between *model exploration* and *parameter estimation*. A final tool is to use model simulation software (e.g., ADAPT) and assign specific statistical properties to the preliminary model to select the optimal experimental design.

4. The number of animals used for the final experiment is dependent upon the purpose of the study and the variability in drug disposition between individual animals. Standard statistical texts may be consulted to determine sample size. It is important to remember that some of the derived pharmacokinetic parameters, such as $T_{1/2}$ are not normally distributed, requiring transformations to be performed (e.g., use log-normal or harmonic $T_{1/2}$, median, or mode instead of mean) before statistical analysis. A broad examination of the comparative pharmacokinetic literature suggests that the typical size of an intravenous-dose pharmacokinetic trial for a drug with normal variability in the population is approximately 4 to 6 animals.

The statistical aspects of interindividual and intraindividual variability will be extensively discussed in the next chapter, on population pharmacokinetic techniques. At this point, it is important to realize that any individual data point has many components of variability, including those attributed to the assay; to sample timing; to within-individual changes in drug disposition; to between-individual differences in underlying age, physiology, environment or disease states; and to an unexplained component identified as random error. The magnitude of this variability influences the sample size (number of time points and number of replicates) required to adequately fit a mathematical model to the data.

5. An allometric scaling technique could be used to arrive at the initial dose for the pilot study, assuming that a species' clearance and volume of distribution are proportional to its metabolic rate or body surface area. For example, assume that a kinetic study had already been conducted in species A at x mg/kg. You know that this dose is at least safe for use in species A. You want to know the initial dose y to use for your kinetic study in species B. This could be estimated as follows:

$$y \ (\text{mg} / \text{kg}) = x \ (\text{mg} / \text{kg})[\text{Body Weight}_A / \text{Body Weight}_B]^{.25} \qquad (13.9)$$

The background and development of this approach is fully described in the chapter on interspecies extrapolations (see equation 16.3 in Chapter 16). In this case, a small animal would receive a larger dose on a per-weight basis, which would ensure that drug concentrations persist for sufficient times to get a good estimate of $T_{1/2}$. If a larger animal was to be studied, the dose would be reduced to ensure that one was not now overdosing the animal. If a comparative pharmacokinetic study had already been done, as described in Chapter 16, then the specific allometric exponent for that drug could be used. Of course, some drugs (especially those metabolized) do not scale, and thus this technique may not work, a situation that could result in toxicity if one was going from a large to a small animal. *This must be considered only as an initial approach to designing a pilot trial in the absence of any better data and must be tempered by any available knowledge of the pharmacology of the drug being studied.*

SELECTED READINGS

Any basic text in statistics or regression should be consulted for a refresher on many of the topics covered in this chapter. An excellent source of information on curve-fitting can be found in the manuals accompanying many automated pharmacokinetic software packages. Finally, the Selected Readings in Chapter 14 contain excellent sources on the statistics of variability in pharmacokinetic studies.

Albert, K.S. 1980. *Drug Absorption and Disposition: Statistical Considerations.* Washington, D.C.: American Pharmaceutical Association.

Chatterjee, S., and B. Price. 1977. *Regression Analysis by Example.* New York: John Wiley & Sons.

Daniel, C., and F.S. Wood. 1980. *Fitting Equations to Data: Computer Analysis of Multifactor Data,* 2ed. New York: John Wiley & Sons.

D'Argenio, D.Z. 1981. Optimal sampling times for pharmacokinetic experiments. *Journal of Pharmacokinetics and Biopharmaceutics.* 9:739-756.

Gabrielsson, J., and D. Weiner. 1997. *Pharmacokinetic and Pharmacodynamic Data Analysis: Concepts and Applications,* 2d ed. Stockholm: Swedish Pharmaceutical Society Press.

Graves, D.A., C.S. Locke, K.T. Muir, and R.P. Miller. 1989. The influence of assay variability on pharmacokinetic parameter estimation. *Journal of Pharmacokinetics and Biopharmaceutics.* 17:571-592.

Holt, J.D., and W.D. Black. 1983. On the transformation technique in pharmacokinetic curve fitting. *Journal of Pharmacokinetics and Biopharmaceutics.* 11:183-187.

Lacey, L., and A. Dunne. 1984. The design of pharmacokinetic experiments for model discrimination. *Journal of Pharmacokinetics and Biopharmaceutics.* 12:351-365.

Riond, J.L., Hedeen K.M., Tyczkowska K., and J.E. Riviere. 1989. Determination of doxycycline in bovine tissues and body fluids by liquid chromatography using photodiode array ultraviolet-visible detection. *Journal of Pharmaceutical Sciences.* 78:44-47.

Schwilden, H., J. Honerkamp, J., and C. Elster. 1993. Pharmacokinetic model identification and parameter estimation as an ill-posed problem. *European Journal of Clinical Pharmacology.* 45:545-550.

Sheiner, L.B. 1984. Analysis of pharmacokinetic data using parametric models. I. Regression models. *Journal of Pharmacokinetics and Biopharmaceutics.* 12:93-117.

Sheiner, L.B. 1985. Analysis of pharmacokinetic data using parametric models. II. Point estimates of an individual's parameters. *Journal of Pharmacokinetics and Biopharmaceutics.* 14:515-540.

Tod, M., C. Padoin, K. Louchahi, B. Moreau-Tod, O. Petitjean, and G. Perret. 1994. Application of optimal sampling theory to the determination of metacycline pharmacokinetic parameters: Effect of model misspecification. *Journal of Pharmacokinetics and Biopharmaceutics.* 22:129-146.

14

Population Pharmacokinetic Models and Bayesian Forecasting Applied to Clinical Pharmacokinetics

The goal of drug treatment in clinical medicine is to produce a therapeutic benefit in patients while reducing the incidence of side effects and adverse drug reactions and, in veterinary medicine, avoiding violative tissue residues (Figure 1.3, see Chapter 1). Therefore, simultaneously achieving an "effective" concentration at the site of action while maintaining an "ineffective" concentration at the toxic sites of action are of paramount importance. The physiological mechanisms that control the circulation and effect of drugs in human or animal patients (processes discussed in Chapters 2 through 6) function at a level related to the physiological and clinical condition of the patient. Up to this point in this text, we have assumed that these processes are constant within individuals and have constructed models based on mean parameters. However, in the last chapter on data analysis, it became obvious that there is significant variability present in estimated pharmacokinetic parameters due to within and between individual effects.

SOURCES OF VARIABILITY

For certain drugs and under different pathophysiological, environmental, genetic, and demographic conditions, large differences in the pharmacokinetic and/or pharmacodynamic profiles can be seen across individuals (biological variability). Other sources of unknown random variability in the concentration-time profiles and dose-effect relationships of drugs may also be present in patient populations (statistical variability). The latter may be of two kinds; namely, random interindividual variability (individual deviations from population average values according to a probability distribution) and intraindividual variability (day-to-day variation, measurement error, and model misspecification, also assumed to occur according to a probability distribution), as previously discussed in reference to equation 13.1.

An understanding of pharmacokinetic and pharmacodynamic variability, its sources, and its influence on drug disposition and effect, is basic for rational drug therapy in target populations. Pharmacokinetic variability refers to differences in blood concentrations over time for a specific dose across individuals. As discussed in Chapters 7 and 9, this can be the consequence of differences in volume of distribution, elimination (excretion and

Co-authored by Dr. Tomás Martín-Jiménez

metabolism), and rate and extent of absorption (bioavailability). Pharmacodynamic variability, as presented in Chapter 12, can be the consequence of differences in drug levels at the site of action (as inferred mostly from drug concentration in the biophase) or differences in the effect produced by a given drug concentration at the site of action (biophase, E-Compartment). Both components are important and should be taken into account when modeling the variability in the dose-effect relationships of drugs. Unfortunately, in many instances pharmacodynamic variability is neglected by assuming that most of the variability in the pharmacologic response to a drug is due to pharmacokinetics, an unwarranted assumption. In fact, the clinical implications of interindividual variability in pharmacokinetics cannot be fully understood without a proper knowledge of the nature and extent of variability in the relationship between blood concentration of the drug and pharmacologic effect.

THE STANDARD APPROACH

Traditional approaches to pharmacokinetic analysis cannot provide information that allows an adequate characterization of this variability, its sources, and its implications for drug therapy. As discussed earlier (see Chapters 7, 8, 9, 13), studies are conducted in small homogeneous populations (from 6 sometimes up to 30 individuals) according to a rigidly designed experimental protocol. Extensive sampling takes place (often more than 20 samples per individual), with the sampling schedule fixed and the same for each individual. Data analysis proceeds in two stages. In the first stage, the data from each individual are analyzed to obtain estimates of the individual pharmacokinetic parameters (e.g., the focus of Chapter 13). A fitting procedure, such as weighted or unweighted nonlinear regression, is used to estimate each individual's parameters. In the second stage, the individual parameter estimates are pooled to provide measures of central tendency (means) and variability (variances) for the population parameters. The association between pharmacokinetic parameters and demographic characteristics may then be assessed by independent regression techniques. This technique is termed the standard two-stage (STS) method.

Despite its straightforward nature and familiarity, the STS method presents serious limitations. The first is that intensive sampling may be required to properly determine basic features of disposition in individuals with similar physiological states. Due to this restriction, this approach can only be applied to well-defined patient subpopulations, (such as patients with renal dysfunction or within a particularly significant age range) and is not practical for the study of a population that may include a broad range of factors of potential relevance. Consequently, this method cannot be used to explore unknown relationships between population characteristics and pharmacokinetic/pharmacodynamic outcome because the variability in observed pharmacokinetic parameters becomes too great. Second, because the study population is usually small and highly homogeneous (and many times healthy), biased population parameter estimates may be obtained that are not representative of the target population. This is especially true for the estimates of interindividual and intraindividual variability. The STS method pools together both sources of variability in a unique estimate of interindividual variability. Because of this, the estimate is artificially inflated and often inadequate for valid statistical inferences. Moreover, estimates of intraindividual variability are difficult to obtain and almost never reported. Third, this type of study is quite costly, because many times it requires pathogen-free animals, special housing and confinement facilities, compliance with good laboratory practice standards, and assay of numerous samples. The strength of this approach is rooted in its experimental nature and the fact that sufficient data are gathered from every individual so that robust individual estimates are always possible.

In summary, with the STS method it is not always possible to use routine clinical data to assess the influence of biological sources of variability on the pharmacokinetic and pharmacodynamic behavior of drugs on target patient populations. Furthermore, the estimates of statistical variability of the pharmacokinetic and pharmacodynamic parameters provided by these methods are unrealistic since they gather all sources of residual variability (essentially, interindividual and intraindividual variability) into a common variance estimate, and do not explicitly identify the nature nor source of intraindividual variability.

In contrast, population approaches to assessing the variability in the therapeutic behavior of drugs allow for estimation of pharmacokinetic and pharmacodynamic parameters in target patient populations, accounting for the effect of concomitant pathophysiological, environmental, demographic, and genetic variables (biological variability). They also allow for an explicit estimation of the between-individual and within-individual variability in disposition or concentration-effect relationships (statistical variability).

PHARMACOKINETIC AND PHARMACODYNAMIC BIOLOGICAL VARIABILITY

It is well appreciated in pharmacology that identical doses may produce effects that vary markedly in nature, extent, and duration in different individuals. The pharmacokinetic and pharmacodynamic profiles of many drugs differ across different individuals in a population, even when the population consists only of healthy individuals with homogeneous characteristics (recall interindividual variability in doxycycline pharmacokinetic parameters tabulated in Table 13.3, see Chapter 13). Some of the sources of pharmacological variability have been very well studied (age, weight, disease, breed, etc.), and for some drugs meaningful correlations have been established between pathophysiological factors and altered pharmacokinetic and pharmacodynamic parameters. Evaluation of drugs during clinical trials quantitatively assesses the influence of these factors, termed *concomitants*, on the therapeutic response. This allows for the design of optimal dosage regimens for specific patients or subpopulations of patients (target populations). However, assessing the influence of concomitant factors on the *mean* response is not enough for proper dosage regimen design. Quantitative estimation of the *unexplained* part of the variability in the patient population that remains after accounting for these other factors is also essential. *Once the variability in the parameters is defined in terms of concomitant factors and the unexplained variability is quantitated, the expected variability in concentration and response within the patient population associated with a specific dosage regimen can be estimated.*

In this section, some of the aforementioned concomitant factors will be discussed. The next section will deal with the sources of unexplained variability and their estimation. Demographic, pathophysiological, environmental, genetic factors (such as age, weight, sex, enzymatic make-up), health status, and concurrent use of other drugs have been reported to influence the fate and effect of drugs administered for therapeutic purposes.

Age.   The age of an animal or human has been shown to affect the distribution and elimination of many drugs. It influences drug metabolism, excretion, distribution, and binding. In general, drug elimination seems to improve from birth to maturity and thereafter declines with advancing age. For certain drugs, younger individuals tend to exhibit larger volumes of distribution and lower protein binding and have a greater ratio of extracellular to intracellular water content. Distribution of drugs can also be altered because of the continuous replacement of lean body mass by fat and the decrease in total body water.

The variability in drug response associated with age is most significant in the very young and very old. Differences in drug metabolism between individuals of different ages are also remarkable. In general, drug metabolism enzyme capacity is lower in very young individuals than adults, particularly for phase II glucuronidation. Renal excretion tends to be less efficient in very young individuals despite the fact that their ratio of kidney to total body weight is double that of adults, a finding suggestive of the kidney's structural and physiological immaturity early in the life of most species. In general, the half-life of many drugs shows a remarkable trend to increase with advancing age due to a decrease in the rate of drug elimination and, for lipophilic drugs, the increase in percent body fat. Physiological functions such as cardiac output, glomerular filtration, and drug metabolism are reduced to varied degrees in the geriatric patient. Oral absorption is also affected by changes in gastrointestinal pH, surface area, motility, and blood flow that parallel age changes. In very young animals, intestinal absorption can be altered. In nursing calves, drug absorption following oral administration is often greater than in adults.

Considering all these changes, the probability of adult patients experiencing adverse drug effects seems to increase with age. This probability is further enhanced by the fact that the geriatric patient is more likely to be receiving medication to treat processes directly or indirectly related to the aging process.

Body Weight.   Most pharmacokinetic parameters are correlated to body mass. This specific relationship will be explored in Chapter 16 when allometry is presented. The apparent volume of distribution is dependent on body weight since the volumes of total body water and extracellular fluid are directly linked to weight, especially for drugs that are poorly bound to tissue. As mentioned above, differences in volume of distribution may be related to differences in the lean/fat body mass ratio between individuals with different body weights. The degree of lipophilicity of the drug under consideration will determine the extent of change in volume of distribution under these circumstances. In contrast, hydrophilic drugs will tend to correlate to volumes of the extracellular fluid compartments. Other organ functions may also be affected by weight.

Gender.   Differences in drug disposition between sexes are usually less important than the differences attributable to other physiological variables. One source is sex-related differences in the lean/fat mass ratio between females and males. These effects are drug dependent. In females, different levels of circulating hormones at varied stages of the reproductive cycle or status of lactation could influence the therapeutic behavior of certain drugs. Pregnancy has been associated with delayed gastric emptying and reduced gastrointestinal motility, which in turn may reduce drug absorption. Pregnancy increases the volume of distribution for many drugs due to increases in body mass, altered plasma protein concentrations, and changes in distribution of blood flow. We found significant differences in the disposition of ampicillin, with the mean peak serum ampicillin concentration in pregnant mares being 2.5 times lower than in nonpregnant mares. Similar findings have been reported for this drug in women. In the case of very lipophilic and weakly basic drugs, lactation may provide a primary route of excretion. The major gender-related differences in disposition relate to drugs metabolized by hepatic cytochrome P_{450} enzymes, whose function is correlated to sex steroids. Similarly, drugs that bind to sex-hormone binding proteins will have gender-specific disposition.

Genetics.   Differences in drug metabolism among individuals in a population may account for a large part of the observed therapeutic variability. Genetic factors contribute significantly to the intersubject variation in the metabolic clearance of certain drugs (see Chapter 6). Consequently, subpopulations of slow and fast acetylators, poor and extensive debrisoquine metabolizers, and slow and fast succinylcholine metabolizers have been

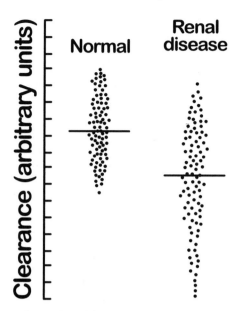

FIGURE 14.1.   Clearance in normal animals and those with renal disease illustrating how disease processes can change both the mean and variance of pharmacokinetic parameters in a population. When the interindividual variability is great, mean values are not representative of a large portion of the population, and individualized therapy may be required.

identified. Not all drugs show the same susceptibility to genetic differences; however, the potential for variability in drug disposition and effect due to this factor has to be taken into consideration. Genetic polymorphisms have been less extensively studied in veterinary medicine, although the presence of well-defined breed phenotypes would suggest that this may be a concern.

Disease.   Without a doubt, the factor that has the greatest potential for introducing variability in the pharmacokinetic and pharmacodynamic behavior of drugs is disease. The effects of renal disease will be presented in Chapter 15. Because of the central role of the liver in drug metabolism and excretion, hepatic disease has a major effect on drug disposition. Pathological conditions affecting other organs, such as the gastrointestinal tract, heart, and endocrine organs, may alter drug disposition and effect. We had shown that experimentally induced thyroid dysfunction in pigs changed renal glomerular filtration, which impacted on the clearance of gentamicin. Inflammation has been documented to alter drug protein binding and concentrations of binding proteins. Diabetes in humans is well known to alter antimicrobial drug disposition. This list could go on indefinitely; however, the point is well accepted that many disease states significantly alter drug disposition through a wide variety of pathophysiological mechanisms.

PHARMACOKINETIC AND PHARMACODYNAMIC STATISTICAL VARIABILITY

In general, disease processes may introduce changes not only in the mean values of the pharmacokinetic and pharmacodynamic parameters, but also in the nature of their population frequency distribution. Figure 14.1 illustrates this phenomenon based on our observations of gentamicin distribution in dogs, rats, and horses with renal disease. Changes in physiology due to the above factors modify the average value of clearance in the diseased population, as well as its interindividual variability, yet are not explained by the concomitant variable (fixed effect) that predicts the mean response. This remaining

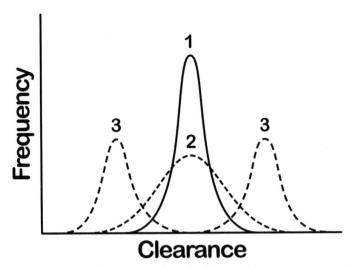

FIGURE 14.2.   Relationship between the average value of a pharmacokinetic parameter and its frequency distribution. For the three situations depicted, the mean clearance is constant, but the interindividual variability (and consequently the degree of uncertainty in dosage regimen determination) is wider for drug 2 than for drug 1. Drug 3 presents a population composed of two subgroups with different clearances (e.g., secondary to genetic polymorphisms or disease). In this case, it would be unlikely to find an individual in either subgroup with the average population mean. Knowledge of the probability distribution function of the parameters in a population is essential for proper dosage regimen design.

variability is random in nature and for modeling purposes will be characterized by virtue of the so-called *random effects*. The average value of a pharmacokinetic parameter does not provide enough information to develop rational dosage strategies in individuals.

This important concept is better illustrated in Figure 14.2, which represents the probability distributions of clearance for three hypothetical drugs. The three drugs depicted in this figure have a similar average value of clearance, but drug 2 exhibits larger interindividual variability than drug 1. This suggests that the level of uncertainty in individual predictions based on the average clearance will be larger for drug 2 than for drug 1. For drug 3, the situation is even more complicated, since the population is clearly represented by two separate subgroups. The population average value of clearance for this drug would not occur in any particular individual from either subgroup. These subgroups could represent populations of different ages or disease states and is typical of genetic polymorphisms in drug metabolism. A similar bimodal population was identified by our group with gentamicin in laboratory rats relative to their sensitivity to nephrotoxicity.

This simple figure illustrates how knowledge of the interindividual variability in population pharmacokinetic and/or pharmacodynamic parameters is essential, even after adjusting for the influence of concomitant variables (fixed effects) such as age or creatinine clearance as an indicator of renal disease. Different types of estimates of population pharmacokinetic and pharmacodynamic parameters are needed to characterize the remaining random interindividual variation that determines the nature of the frequency distributions in the examples presented. This relates to obtaining information about the probability distributions of deviations of individual pharmacokinetic and pharmacodynamic parameters from their population values. One also needs to know how these deviations correlate with one another. This information is provided by the variances and covariances of these probability distributions (random interindividual-effect parameters).

A second issue deals with the stability (reproducibility) of the observed outcome (blood concentration, effect) after drug administration in a single individual. As depicted in Figure 14.3, the observed outcome may vary in an individual with time. These fluctuations

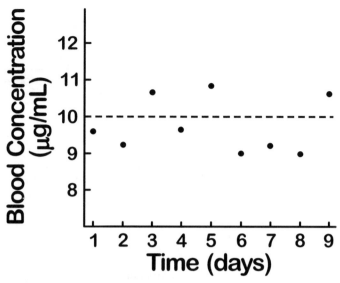

FIGURE 14.3. Drug concentrations collected in an individual at the same time after administration of a nonaccumulating dosage regimen (e.g., samples taken at T_{max} in the regimen from Figure 11.2, see Chapter 11), illustrating how the pharmacokinetic characteristics of a drug may vary within the same individual over time. Transient changes in an individual's physiology or circadian rhythms, or measurement error may be responsible for this component of variability.

could represent steady-state concentrations or measurements of effect after drug administration to a patient. In the effect case, they could be the consequence of intraindividual biochemical changes, such as occurs in the development of tolerance, which affects the pharmacodynamic relationships between drug concentration and effect. They can also result from fluctuations in physiology that affect drug disposition, such as those due to circadian rhythms or induction of metabolism. Finally, measurement errors or temporary changes in the underlying structural pharmacokinetic or pharmacodynamic model also contribute to this random intraindividual variability.

This source of variability is of clinical concern if its magnitude is considerable and it remains unaccounted for in the predictive model. Unknown intraindividual variability would cause an artificial overestimation of the interindividual variability and may lead investigators to erroneously accept as interindividual variability something that is in fact a reflection of methodological shortcomings. Consequently, verifying the stability and reproducibility of the observed response in an individual over time is important in order to place confidence in the estimated interindividual variability. Knowledge of the magnitude of this variability may also be used to set a reasonable threshold on dosage increments in case the observed concentrations indicate the need to increase the dose. For the intraindividual term, another random-effect population parameter is needed; in other words, another variance is needed. This variance combines the random variability afforded by intraindividual changes, as well as measurement error, sampling time recording error, and misspecification of the underlying structural (pharmacokinetic or pharmacodynamic) model fitted to the data.

PHARMACOSTATISTICAL MODELS FOR POPULATION STUDIES

Population methods encompass a series of techniques that allow the study of the pharmacokinetic and/or pharmacodynamic characteristics of a drug in a target population using sparse data obtained from the sampling of only a few plasma concentrations per

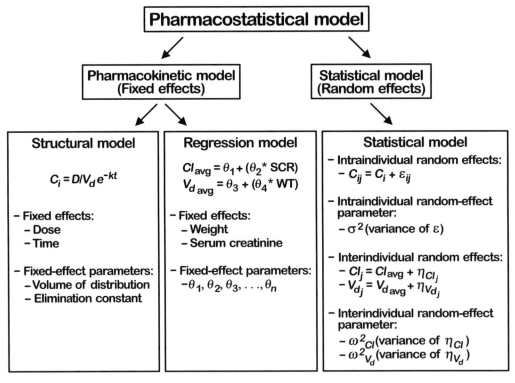

FIGURE 14.4. Pharmacostatistical models can be split into a pharmacokinetic model that accounts for the influence of fixed effects (dose, time, concomitant variables) and a statistical model that accounts for the influence of random effects (interindividual and intraindividual). In the pharmacokinetic model, the fixed-effect parameters (pharmacokinetic parameters and proportionality factors) quantitate the influence of the fixed effects on the model. In the statistical model, the random-effect parameters (variances of the random variables) quantitate the influence of the random effects on the model.

subject, from a large number of subjects. Implementing this methodology allows estimation of average values of pharmacokinetic or pharmacodynamic parameters in a population with determined clinical features. More importantly, information is provided about the interindividual and intraindividual variability of the estimated parameters. Depending on the specific method, the *joint* probability distribution function of the pharmacokinetic or pharmacodynamic parameters and covariates may be estimated. The joint probability distribution reflects the frequency distribution associated with two variables, and consequently provides an indication of the variance of these two variables and their degree of correlation. In the usual clinical setting, there are not enough data points per subject to fully characterize each individual's pharmacokinetic profile. This limitation is overcome by studying a larger number of clinical patients with an average of one to five samples per individual. Given the sampling and design restrictions, population pharmacokinetic methods were conceived to analyze observational rather than experimental data. In order to obtain valid information from this type of data, population methods require an a priori, thorough specification of the pharmacostatistical model (Figure 14.4). This includes specification of the pharmacokinetic or pharmacodynamic model (containing the fixed effects), as well as a complete description of the statistical model (containing the random effects).

The object of study is the entire population; therefore, the outcome of population studies is more representative of the target population than are traditional (STS) studies. One of the most advantageous characteristics of population methods is that they quantify the influence of clinical conditions on the average pharmacokinetic/pharmacodynamic characteristics of the population. Hence, one can explore possible relationships between the therapeutic behavior of drugs and clinical features of patient populations. Another advantage is the explicit estimation of the magnitude of interindividual and intraindividual (residual) variability (parametric methods) or the direct estimation of the joint probability density function of the structural (PKPD) parameters (nonparametric methods). This allows for adequate individual predictions to be made according to their clinical features and an assessment of the degree of uncertainty of those predictions. Furthermore, these estimates can be included as a priori information in Bayesian forecasting techniques to further improve individual predictions (see section on clinical applications).

There are two general types of population pharmacokinetic methods, known as *parametric* and *nonparametric*. A third, intermediate method is the *seminonparametric* approach. In parametric methods, the pharmacokinetic parameters and the error terms are assumed to come from a known probability distribution (normal or log-normal) with unknown parameters (e.g., mean and variance). Parameter estimation is restricted to some structural model. Confidence intervals and standard errors are based on parametric methods. These methods, as implemented by the computer program NONMEM (for nonlinear mixed effects modeling) developed by Beal and Sheiner in 1980 at the University of California, San Francisco, can also handle some multimodal distributions if they are accounted for in the variance model. With seminonparametric methods, the process of parameter estimation is not restricted to a specific structural model, and alternative fitting procedures can be employed. However, estimates of uncertainty about the parameter estimations are confined to parametric procedures. In nonparametric methods, there are no restrictions regarding structural models and distribution of interindividual and intraindividual error terms. The uncertainties about parameter estimates employ nonparametric procedures, such as nonparametric confidence intervals. These methods compute the joint probability density function of the pharmacokinetic parameters, which measures the variance and covariance of two parameters.

Selecting the most appropriate method depends on the original assumptions about the underlying distribution. Parametric methods are usually easier to implement from a modeling standpoint, but they cannot be used to identify evident deviations from normality in the distribution of the pharmacokinetic parameters in the population, such as bimodal or very skewed distributions.

Parametric Methods

Nonlinear Mixed-Effects Modeling.   NONMEM is the most representative parametric procedure, and the first true population pharmacokinetic-pharmacodynamic method to be developed and widely utilized in clinical medicine. The total residual variability is explained in terms of fixed and random effects. A fully specified pharmacostatistical model is fitted to the population data, and estimates of the average population values of pharmacokinetic or pharmacodynamic parameters and their variances as well as the residual variance are obtained. The method of extended least squares (ELS), as applied to a nonlinear mixed-effect statistical model, is used.

This method stems from the ordinary and weighted least squares regression techniques presented in Chapter 13. In ordinary least squares, as applied to a set of individual data, parameter values are estimated that minimize the sum of squared deviations of the observations. The variances of the individual observations are assumed to be equal. If they differ but are known, then weighted least squares techniques can be used. When the differing variances are unknown, the ELS method can be used. This method models the variance as a function of the pharmacokinetic parameters, a vector of independent variables (fixed effects), and some random-effect parameters (interindividual and intraindividual). Although this method has been broadly used, and has the ability to provide adequate estimates of average parameter values and estimates of random variability, it presents some important disadvantages. First, a single set of parameters that may not be appropriate for all the individuals is fit to all of the data. Second, repeated blood drug concentration measures in an individual are treated as independent observations, and in reality they are not since they are statistically nested within an individual.

Figure 14.4 depicts the full pharmacostatistical model divided into pharmacokinetic and statistical components. The pharmacokinetic model (containing the fixed effects) may, in turn, be further subdivided into structural and regression models. The statistical model contains the two types of random effects, namely, interindividual and intraindividual.

Fixed effects are a series of variables and constants (e.g., dose, time, age, weight, serum creatinine) assumed to be measured without error. They are linked by a structural model (e.g., $Cp = [D / Vd] e^{-kt}$) with the dependent variable (plasma concentration) and by a regression model with the pharmacokinetic parameters [e.g., $Cl = f$ (serum creatinine) and $Vd = f$ (weight)]. The fixed effects of the structural model are dose and time. The proportionality constants (fixed-effect parameters) of the structural model are the pharmacokinetic parameters (e.g., Cl, Vd). For example, for the one-compartment open model with intravenous administration, the following expression applies:

$$Cp = (D / Vd) \, e^{-(Cl/Vd)t} \tag{14.1}$$

where Cp is the observation (dependent variable), D is the dose, t is the time at which the observation takes place, and Cl and Vd are, respectively, clearance and volume of distribution. [Note that equation 14.1 is the basic model introduced in equation 7.15 (see Chapter 7), where k_{el} is substituted for Cl / Vd derived by rearranging equation 7.16 to allow these physiologically relevant parameters to be correlated to clinical characteristics, and Cp_0 is expressed in terms of D / Vd.] Cl and Vd quantify the influence of the fixed effects (dose and time) on the dependent variable of the structural model (Cp). As will be seen, many of the basic models presented in earlier chapters may be employed as structural models in population analyses.

If, in turn, the pharmacokinetic parameters can be further explained in terms of patient characteristics (including age, weight, serum creatinine, gender, etc.), then a regression model is specified in which the pharmacokinetic parameters become the dependent variables, the patient characteristics are the fixed effects, and a set of fixed-effect parameters (θ_z) quantify the relationship between patient characteristics and pharmacokinetic parameters. NONMEM computes estimates of the fixed-effect parameters of the regression model. The algebraic form of the equations of the regression model (excluding the random effects) is as follows:

$$Cl_{avg} = \theta_1 + (\theta_2 \times Cov_1) + (\theta_3 \times Cov_2) + \dots \; \dots + (\theta_n \times Cov_{n-1}) \tag{14.2}$$

$$Vd_{avg} = \theta_{n+1} + (\theta_{n+2} \times Cov_n) + (\theta_{n+3} \times Cov_{n+1}) + \dots \; \dots + (\theta_z \times Cov_{z-2}) \tag{14.3}$$

where Cov_z represents the fixed effects (covariates) and θ_z represents the fixed-effect parameters. The intercepts of each regression equation represent the amount of the pharmacokinetic parameter value that is not due to the effect of these concomitant variables (i.e., each covariate value equals zero, for a linear relationship). For example, the term θ_1 in Figure 14.4 represents the population average value of the nonrenal clearance. If no concomitant variable is included in the model for a particular pharmacokinetic parameter, the latter becomes the fixed-effect parameter, not only of the structural but of the regression model as well (i.e., $\theta_1 = Cl_{avg}$).

Random effects are unknown quantities arising from a probability distribution whose shape is assumed in NONMEM to be normal or log-normal. There are two kinds of random effects; namely, interindividual and intraindividual. Interindividual random effects are associated with the pharmacokinetic parameters of the structural model (Cl, Vd) and reflect the between-subject variability in drug disposition. All individuals have a particular value for their pharmacokinetic parameters that will differ from those of the average population by an unknown quantity. This unknown quantity is assumed to arise from a normal or log-normal probability distribution, with a mean of zero and a certain variance w^2 that is estimated by NONMEM. The interindividual random variable is represented in NONMEM by the Greek character eta (η) with a subscript relative to the pharmacokinetic parameter with which it is associated. The relationship between the random variable and the pharmacokinetic parameter is given by the statistical model similar in structure to that presented in Chapter 13, the data analysis chapter (equation 13.1). For example,

$$Cl_j = Cl_{avg} + \eta_{Clj} \tag{14.4}$$

$$Vd_j = Vd_{avg} + \eta_{Vdj} \tag{14.5}$$

where Cl_j and Vd_j represent the clearance and volume of distribution, respectively, in the jth individual, Cl_{avg} and Vd_{avg} are the population averages for clearance and volume of distribution, and η_{Clj} and η_{Vdj} represent the deviations of the individual clearance and volume of distribution, respectively, from their population averages for the jth subject. The error model can be additive (as here) or may adopt other forms (e.g., multiplicative, exponential). Intraindividual random effects represent the residual variability and arise from model misspecification (e.g., fitting a one-compartment model to data that would be better described by a two-compartment model), analytical assay error, sampling time recording error, and time variation in pharmacokinetic parameters within an individual. Formally expressed, the residual variability represents the deviation of the observed concentration from the value that would be expected were the true individual pharmacokinetic parameters known. Algebraically expressed,

$$C_{ij} = C_{ij,true} + \varepsilon_{ij} \tag{14.6}$$

where C_{ij} is the observed concentration in individual j at time i, $C_{ij,true}$ is the true concentration for individual j at time i, and ε is the residual random error or difference between observation and true value for individual j at time i (introduced in Chapter 13). As in the case of the interindividual random effect, the form of this relationship may be other than additive. The random variable ε is assumed to arise from a normal or log-normal probability distribution with mean zero and variance σ^2. NONMEM computes estimates of the variances of the interindividual and intraindividual random effects, namely, w^2_{Cl}, w^2_{Vd}, and σ^2.

Figure 14.5 illustrates the partitioning of the variability that takes place under this mixed-effect modeling strategy. The discrepancy between the observed and predicted outcome (drug concentration in this case) arises from two distinct components. First, the *true residual variability* arises from the difference between the observed (C_{obs}) and the true (C_{true}) blood concentration. The true blood concentration is defined as the concentration that would be expected if the true values of the individual pharmacokinetic parameters were known. The intraindividual variability is a component of the residual variability. Second, the *interindividual variability* arises from the difference between the expected concentrations using the true individual pharmacokinetic parameters (C_{true}) and that

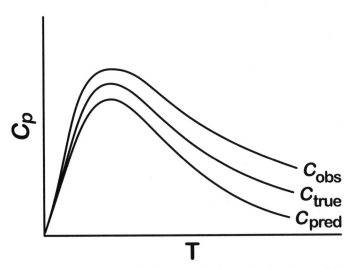

FIGURE 14.5.   Concentration-versus-time profile demonstrating how mixed-effects modeling partitions the *total residual error* ($C_{obs} - C_{pred}$) in terms of *true residual error* ($C_{obs} - C_{true}$), arising from the difference between the observed plasma concentration and the true concentration, and *interindividual error* ($C_{true} - C_{pred}$), arising from the difference between expected concentrations using the true individual pharmacokinetic parameters and those predicted using the values of parameters estimated by the regression model.

expected using the average values of pharmacokinetic parameters estimated by the population model after accounting for the influence of the fixed effects (C_{pred}).

NONMEM uses a variety of algorithms related to nonlinear regression and matrix algebra to obtain estimates of the fixed-effect parameters, the interindividual and intraindividual random-effect parameters (variances), and the standard errors of all these parameter estimates. The covariance and inverse covariance matrices are also computed to show if parameter values are correlated. If the parameters of the model are not independent of each other, the model should be reassessed. The correlation matrix of the parameter estimates is computed as an additional indication of the adequacy of the model, since highly correlated parameter estimates are indicative of model overparameterization. Plots of observations versus predictions, as well as plots depicting the distribution of residuals (or weighted residuals) for different levels of a covariate, are obtained. These kinds of plots can be used to assess the necessity of including a covariate under evaluation in the final regression model.

Figures 14.6 and 14.7 illustrate an example of how to use these scatterplots to develop the regression portion of the population model. Figure 14.6A is the plot of observed versus predicted concentrations for a hypothetical set of data analyzed with NONMEM, which does not account for the influence of concomitant variables (fixed effects). The fit is generally accurate at lower concentrations but inadequate in other regions. Figure 14.6B depicts the plot of residuals versus the covariate body weight (residual plots were introduced in Chapter 13). As we can see, the scatter of the residuals is not homogeneous, and a decreasing pattern is apparent (overprediction in larger individuals). This suggests that weight is related to some structural parameter describing the disposition of the drug in the population and that it should be included in the predictive model.

We explored whether the inclusion of covariates in the regression model would improve the fit. Figure 14.7 represents the model that includes the covariate weight in the predictive model. As one can see in Figure 14.7A, the predictive performance improves dramatically. The residual plot in Figure 14.7B shows homogeneous scattering of the

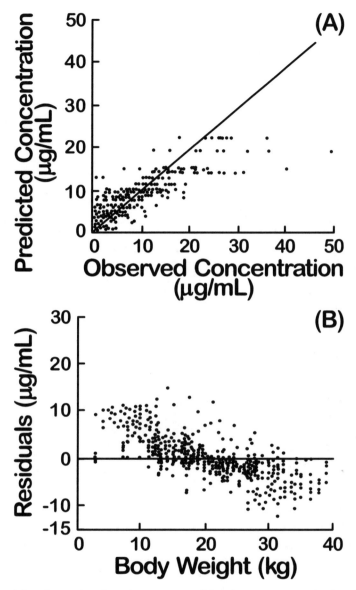

FIGURE 14.6.   Modeling data with NONMEM using a model with no covariates. (A) Plot of observed versus predicted drug blood concentrations after administration of a drug to a hypothetical population. The simplest model is one that does not account for the effect of any pathophysiological covariates. The lack of precision is considerable. (B) Plot of residuals versus the covariate body weight. A plot of the residual (or weighted residual) versus covariates of interest may reveal specific trends that would indicate the necessity to model the effect of such a covariate on the outcome. In this case, there is a pattern of overprediction in large individuals and underprediction in small ones.

residuals as a function of weight, indicating that no further variability in the data seems to be related to weight. The model has been improved.

The model-building procedure (structural and regression model) is conducted in a stepwise fashion. The statistical significance of the reduction in the minimum value of the ELS objective function (MVOF), and the decrease of the interindividual and intraindividual variability when adding a new covariate to the model, are assessed at every step. Each time NONMEM runs a model, it minimizes the value of the ELS objective function. The

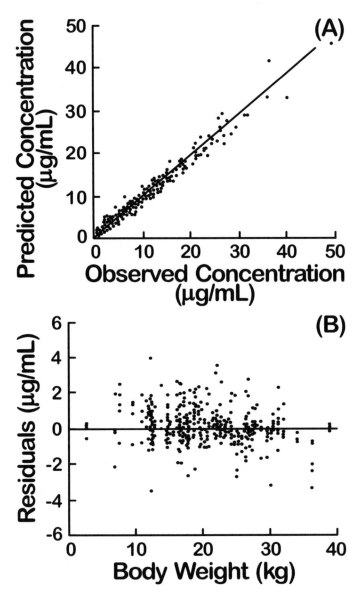

FIGURE 14.7.   Modeling data with NONMEM using a model with body weight as a covariate. (A) Inclusion of the covariate body weight considerably reduces the variability and improves the predictive performance in an observed versus predicted concentration plot compared to the plot in Figure 14.6A. (B) Homogeneous scatter of the residuals in this plot, compared to the plot in Figure 14.6B, indicates that the influence of body weight in the pharmacokinetic profile of this population is adequately modeled.

minimum value of the ELS function is an indicator of the goodness of fit of the model. This value can be used to statistically compare full-reduced regression pairs. The full model is that from which the parameter of the added covariate is estimated. Alternatively, the reduced model is that from which the parameter in question is fixed to the null value. The difference between the MVOF of a full model and a reduced model approximates a chi-square (χ^2) distribution with degrees of freedom equal to the difference in the number of parameters between the full and the reduced model (q). Its statistical significance can be determined by comparing the difference between both MVOF values, with the correspondent value of the χ^2 distribution for q degrees of freedom.

The reader should note the similarity of this modeling strategy to that presented in Chapter 13. Regression plots, supported by statistical tests of fit such as R^2, F test, AIC, and SC are compared against various models (e.g., with one, two, or three compartments) until the proper model is selected. In the case of NONMEN, residual plots and MVOF values are used to arrive at the full model, which is significantly more predictive than the reduced model.

Nonparametric Methods.   Nonparametric methods provide the opportunity for analysis without implicit assumptions as to the population distribution of the random-error terms for interindividual and residual variability. This allows one to visualize the data and determine the best function with which to represent the observed distribution. Due to this feature, nonparametric methods can handle bimodal or multimodal populations, thereby revealing unsuspected clusters of patients (e.g., drug 3 in Figure 14.2), such as those that occur in genetic polymorphisms (e.g., slow and fast acetylators).

These techniques are based on the general method known as *maximum likelihood estimation*. This method, as applied to regression, aims at obtaining parameter values that provide the maximum probability of producing a sample in the neighborhood of the one observed. The maximum likelihood represents a family of statistical procedures used to determine when further iterations are no longer needed to improve the fit between the observed versus the predicted values. Nonparametric methods compute the nonparametric maximum likelihood estimate of the unknown population density function. The differences between the two main types of nonparametric methods reside in the type of algorithm that they utilize. As for the relationships between covariates and structural parameters, nonparametric methods estimate the joint distribution of the parameters (both pharmacokinetic parameters and fixed-effect parameters that describe the relationships between pharmacokinetic parameters and covariates).

Nonparametric Maximum Likelihood (NPML).   This algorithm was first described by Mallet, who showed that the joint probability distribution of parameter values in a population model is discrete as opposed to the continuous nature of a normally distributed parameter. Accordingly, it can be described by some frequency distribution. NPML computes the joint probability density function of the parameter estimates. NPML states the problem of parameter estimation in terms of the probability of obtaining data similar to those actually observed. It relies on the maximum likelihood principle as applied to the estimation of pharmacokinetic parameters. In other words, given a set of unknown terms and a set of data related to the unknowns, the best estimate of the unknowns consists of the values that render the set of data most probable. In the most familiar situation, the unknowns are the pharmacokinetic parameters of an individual and the data set is the individual series of observations. The distribution of the pharmacokinetic parameters in the population can also be unknown, in which case the data are the array of such series of observations within a sample of individuals. In general, nonparametric methods require more mathematical sophistication than the parametric methods, but they allow appropriate parameter estimates to be computed when the distribution of pharmacokinetic parameters in the population departs from normality.

Nonparametric Expectation Maximization (NPEM).   This nonparametric estimator uses an iterative expectation maximization (EM) algorithm with steps utilizing both expectation and maximization. This algorithm as implemented by Schumitzky computes the entire joint probability density function (PDF) of the parameters. During the initial phases of the estimation process, a continuous PDF is calculated. The population fit of the PDF improves with each iteration. With progressive iterations, the spikes of the joint density become narrower. At its limits, discrete distributions are obtained.

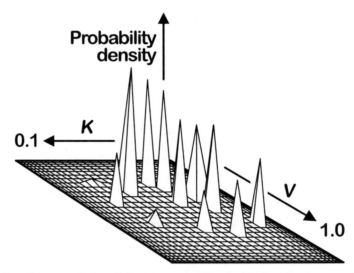

FIGURE 14.8.   Three-dimensional plot of the joint probability density function in a population of patients treated with a drug. K = elimination rate constant (range, 0–0.1 h^{-1}). V = volume of distribution (range, 0–1.0 L/kg). Each spike represents the probability that a subject will have $V = x$ and $K = y$. If all true values for the population were known, this plot would be a scatterplot with a dot per individual (or overlapping dots for individuals with the same values of V and K).

   Figure 14.8 depicts a graphical example of the joint PDF for a patient population. The joint PDF is projected as three-dimensional spikes, the location and height of which represent the estimated values and probabilities of the pharmacokinetic parameters. Together with the joint probability density, it also computes individual density functions for each parameter. This algorithm can operate with a single data point per patient and may be executed on PC-friendly software. It has been integrated as a segment of the USC*PACK software package. As of the writing of this text, this software can handle one-, two- and three-compartment models with repeated oral and intravenous dosing, with a total of seven parameters studied. Different studies have shown similar results when either a nonparametric method or the STS method was used to model blood sample data from populations with normal distribution of the pharmacokinetic parameters. This software also produces estimates of the means, standard deviations, modes, medians, skewness, kurtosis, correlations, and covariances between parameters.

Seminonparametric Methods.   The smooth nonparametric (SNP) maximum likelihood is a seminonparametric method proposed for use in population pharmacokinetic analysis by Davidian and Gallant (1992). This modeling strategy is particularly relevant for population data that can be described with nonlinear mixed-effects model (MEM) strategies. For this type of data, the SNP method simultaneously estimates the fixed effects (by maximum likelihood principles) and the entire random-effects density.

Neural-Net Methods.   Another strategy that has been adopted for many types of modeling problems is the use of neural-nets to define relations between disparate data sets. The input to these programs are dose and any other clinical or patient variable deemed appropriate for predicting concentration and/or effect as outcomes. The data set is divided in half and the neural-net *trained* to predict desired outcome variables from defined input variables. The trained neural-net is then tested on the other half of the input data to see whether the outcome data can be predicted. The process is repeated until convergence occurs. The major criticism of this approach is that the manner in which the neural-net links the input to outcome is not known; however, its use in pharmacokinetics is being explored and no doubt will result in more mechanistically based procedures in the future.

VALIDATION OF THE RESULTS

Many population pharmacokinetic and pharmacodynamic studies are observational rather than experimental. This has led to establishment of appropriate validation methods, to ensure that the parameter estimates obtained can be extrapolated to the general population and results are reasonable and independent of the analyst. Validation procedures are intended to assess how well a population model (obtained from a *study* or an *index* population) describes a set of data (*validation* set) that has not been used to develop the model itself. Whether or not validation of the population study is accomplished depends on the objective of the analysis. When a population model is developed for dosage recommendation, it must be adequately validated. Alternatively, when population models are developed for explaining variability or for providing some descriptive labeling information, validation may not be required.

It is beyond the scope of this review to discuss in detail the different validation methods that have been proposed and the statistics involved in each of them. Selection of the validation method should be justified by the ultimate goal of the population study. The interested reader should refer to the appropriate literature for more comprehensive information on each particular method.

Types of Validation.   The validation of a population model consists of the assessment of its stability and/or predictive performance using a validation data set, different from that used to develop the model. Depending on the availability of validation data, we may distinguish two types of validation, namely, external and internal. In external validation, the validation set consists of an entirely new data set obtained from another study. Alternatively, internal methods use the original data set to derive both the index and validation data sets or use resampling approaches to validate the developed model—much like the scenario described above for training neural-nets. Internal validation techniques include data-splitting and resampling techniques such as cross-validation and bootstrapping.

Data-splitting partitions the available data set into two portions: the index data set (two thirds) and the validation data set (one third). Since the predictive accuracy of the model is dependent on the sample size, it is recommended that after validation of the population model, both sets are pooled together and the final model parameters estimated using this overall data set.

Cross-validation consists of repeated data-splitting. *Bootstrapping* consists of a resampling procedure that allows the evaluation of the stability and performance of a population model by repeatedly fitting the model to the bootstrap samples. The bootstrap samples consist of a large number (e.g., 200) of subsample replicates obtained by resampling the original data with replacement. Subsamples are distributed in a similar manner to that of the original sample and, consequently, the statistical inference of interest can be made as for the original sample. This method is computer-intensive and is an adequate alternative to external validation methods when original sample sizes are too small.

Methods of Validation
Standardized Prediction Errors.   This is one of the first validation methods used in population studies. This method computes the standardized mean prediction error (SMPE) and the variance for each patient. A t-test (actually a z-test) is performed to assess whether the average of $SMPE_j$'s across patients is different from zero; i.e., whether the

prediction is, on the average, biased. Another t-test is conducted to test whether or not the model describes adequately the variability in the validation data set (within and between patients), by comparing the standard deviation of $SMPE_j$ (computed across patients) to 1. The method has received criticism regarding its inadequacy to test the latter hypothesis and the incorrect assumption of lack of error in the estimates of population parameters.

Concentration Prediction Error. This method is based on the prediction error, which is the difference between the predicted and the observed concentrations. This method assesses the predictive performance of a population model by using the mean squared prediction error (MSPE) as an indicator of precision, and the mean prediction error (MPE) as an indicator of bias. This method is inadequate when more than one observation is obtained per subject, because in that case, prediction errors are not independent.

Validation Using Model Parameters. This method accomplishes validation with the parameters of the model, hence avoiding the problems encountered in the previous method. Using the validation set, it assesses both qualitatively and quantitatively the model predictions of individual pharmacokinetic parameters, with or without covariates, and calculates the precision and bias for the predictions.

Graphical Approach. For NONMEM modeling, a graphical approach to the validation of a model may be initiated by plotting the model predicted versus observed concentrations in the validation set. This plot provides one with a visual clue for the degree of agreement between model predictions and validation data. It has been argued that in judging this correlation from a clinical rather than a statistical perspective, the graphical approach may provide as much information, if not more, than that presented by standard statistical comparison approaches. A similar conclusion has been stressed throughout this book concerning the power of data inspection to determine if one's model actually describes the data at hand.

Plots of the residuals (observed minus predicted concentrations) versus some of the covariates provide additional information on the validity of the population predictions. Residuals should be conceptually viewed as the prediction error for every individual in the study. A plot of the residuals versus age may provide an indication of the clinical adequacy of the model for different age groups. Such plots could uncover "age clusters" for which the model fits the validation data with less accuracy and/or precision.

Weighted residuals can be also useful for validation purposes. Weighted residuals are obtained by normalizing the residuals by the standard deviation of the model. Use of weighted residuals is a potential source of bias if inappropriate weighting schemes are used. In computer programs such as NONMEM, the weighted residuals consist of the residuals expressed in population standard deviation units. Consequently, a plot of the weighted residuals versus the individual patient identification number can be useful to assess whether the residuals follow the description established for them under the population model. If the model affords an appropriate description of the validation data, then the weighted residuals should be homogeneously scattered about the zero line on the weighted-residuals axis. Similarly, plots of weighted residuals versus some of the covariates included in the model (e.g., weight, breed, creatinine clearance) may uncover situations in which the influence of the covariate has not been adequately modeled. If a trend or lack of homogeneity is observed in a plot of weighted residuals versus the covariate, instead of a homogeneous scatter, the model is not describing the variability adequately. In this case some changes are necessary regarding the relationship between the covariate and the pharmacokinetic parameter or parameters in the population model.

APPLICATION OF POPULATION PHARMACOKINETICS IN VETERINARY MEDICINE

As presented throughout this text, population pharmacokinetic approaches have been widely applied to problems in human medicine, as indicated in the Selected Readings section of this chapter. However, they have not been widely applied to problems in veterinary medicine.

Clinical Use.   Population pharmacokinetic modeling can be used in the clinical setting in two ways. First, it can be utilized to design initial dosage regimens for new individual patients or patient clusters according to their clinical features. Second, population models can be used as prior information in Bayesian forecasting methods to further improve the accuracy of the predictions in a patient from whom only a few plasma samples can be obtained.

When a drug is used to treat a pathologic condition in a patient (human or animal), the first objective is to optimize the dose for the individual patient. This is the case particularly when the drug has a narrow therapeutic index and/or a large interindividual variability in its disposition or effect. Variability in therapeutic outcome can be partitioned into pharmacokinetic and pharmacodynamic components. Consequently, pharmacokinetic and pharmacodynamic variability in a population will dictate how confidently the clinician will be able to administer an average population dose to an individual subject. The magnitude of this variability and the factors that contribute to it are the critical issues in dealing with dose individualization. When drugs exhibit a large variability in disposition across individuals, poor correlation between plasma concentrations and dose will exist. The consequence of this will depend on the pharmacodynamic characteristics of the drug for both the therapeutic and the toxic effects. By explaining part of this variability in terms of a series of pathophysiological variables (weight, age, renal function, etc.), dosage regimens can be designed that correlate well with serum concentrations for each particular subpopulation since the total residual variability is greatly reduced. If the inclusion of pathophysiological variables in the model reduces the interindividual variability to a relatively small magnitude and the pharmacodynamic variability is not large, one can design an optimum dose for each of these subpopulations derived from their average pharmacokinetic parameter estimated values. This is especially valuable for subpopulations that are more prone to deviate from the general population values (e.g., very young individuals, very old individuals, subjects with impaired renal or hepatic functions).

Bayesian Methods.   The Bayesian approach to the estimation of pharmacokinetic parameters in an individual takes advantage of both the prior information derived from the population as well as the scarce information obtained from the actual patient treated with the drug. First, a population model (accounting for patient clinical conditions) is developed and validated. This model (prior probability) is used to develop an initial dosage regimen. This initial regimen will be based on the average population parameter values of the subpopulation to which the patient belongs (for example, 2-year old beagles with body weight of 13 kg and a serum creatinine level of 1.9). The model (including the estimates of variability) is reassessed (Bayesian feedback) with new data obtained from a few blood samples from the patient. Finally, the probability distribution of the individual parameters is adjusted (posterior probability) in light of the observed patient's plasma concentrations. Iterative fitting procedures continue, selecting those values of individual pharmacokinetic parameters (Bayesian posterior) that minimize the Bayesian objective function:

$$\frac{\Sigma \, (P_{pop} - P_{ind})^2}{\sigma^2 P_{pop}} + \frac{\Sigma \, (C_{obs} - C_{ind})^2}{\sigma^2 C_{obs}} \tag{14.7}$$

where P_{pop} and P_{ind} represent the parameter values of the population pharmacokinetic model and of the patient's individualized model, respectively. C_{obs} and C_{ind} represent the observed plasma drug concentrations and the estimates of those concentrations made with the patient's individualized pharmacokinetic model (for each observation), respectively. $\sigma^2 P_{pop}$ represents the variance for the different population pharmacokinetic parameter values, and $\sigma^2 C_{obs}$ represents the variance of the observed plasma concentrations. Different studies have validated this approach to make individualized pharmacokinetic models of drugs in patients and have shown improvement of the predictive performance (future serum drug concentrations) relative to the traditional methods of linear regression when the number of samples available from each patient was small. As the number of individual samples increases, the Bayesian solution approaches that obtained by the traditional least squares method.

Production Medicine. The use of population pharmacokinetic/pharmacodynamic methods in food animals will most likely improve the conditions of herd drug usage in the near future. The ability of these methods to obtain valuable information from large populations in which each individual is sparsely sampled seems ideal for studying drug therapeutics in food animals. Differences in drug disposition across individuals could be related to disease conditions, nutrition, management practices, lactation status, or breed. This knowledge, together with a better assessment of the sources and magnitude of variance, will allow a more reasonable use of drugs in these animals. Differences in disposition can be related to individual characteristics and to subpopulation characteristics, such as breed of animals or crop groups in fish. Consequently, population pharmacokinetics and pharmacodynamics in production medicine could be applied both to individual and subgroup therapeutics.

Food Animal Residue Avoidance. As pointed out previously, veterinary medicine deals not only with companion species, but also with animal species that will ultimately serve as sources for human food products. In the latter case, the importance of accurately describing the disposition of drugs in animals according to clinical or production variables without designing extensive individual pharmacokinetic studies is clearly evident. This is especially pertinent because of the influence that these variables may bear in the deposition of drug residues in those animals' tissues or food products (milk, eggs).

Although there is great potential for the population approach to address drug tissue disposition and residue avoidance, adequate strategies for its implementation have yet to be explored. One of the obvious limitations of tissue residue studies is the lack of sufficient tissue samples per individual (unless biopsies are performed) to individually characterize tissue-depletion kinetics (only one sample per animal and time point is usually available). To overcome these limitations, population pharmacokinetic studies could be conducted according to a multicompartment experimental protocol. Adequate multicompartmental or hybrid physiological-compartmental models could be analyzed in order to define relationships between plasma and tissue concentrations, taking into account the influence of concomitant pathophysiological or production variables. The outcome would be a model quantifying the relationship between plasma and tissue levels with concomitant variables. Such a model should be able to predict, with a high degree of confidence, tissue concentrations for determined doses and clinical or production conditions. Likewise, withdrawal times (and appropriate confidence intervals) could be determined for specific individuals or subpopulations, depending on the magnitude of their clinical or production parameters.

The ultimate application of this methodology would be the implementation of a Bayesian approach to define therapeutic models useful in the field. Although the initial development of the model would require a relatively large number of animals, these could be the same individuals involved in clinical trials. The strength of the population approach is that data collected from a wide variety of experimental protocols (efficacy, safety, residues) can be pooled into a single model for the drug. The final objective would be to estimate the probability of violative tissue residue levels in a herd undergoing drug therapy by considering the concomitant production variables (e.g., weight, daily gain, disease) and screening a reduced number of animals in the production unit.

The situation for animal food products other than those derived from animal tissues (e.g., milk or eggs) is more straightforward. Serial samples can be obtained from these "compartments," and consequently more accurate pharmacokinetic profiles can be determined for the depletion of drug from these compartments.

Another area worthy of exploration using the population approach is that of allometric interspecies scaling of pharmacokinetic parameters, given that this methodology can be used to directly model large pools of data (often unbalanced) from many individuals. It may not be possible to use population analysis of data from a single species for detecting many covariates that influence the pharmacokinetic-pharmacodynamic profile of a drug or its tissue-depletion characteristics. In contrast, population analysis of data from several species, with body weight and enzymatic composition as covariates, has the potential to unveil allometric relationships that cannot be easily detected by other methods. Studies of this kind would provide veterinarians and comparative pharmacologists with the ability to extrapolate serum and tissue data across species, taking into account the influence of important intraspecies and interspecies clinical factors.

Drug Development. Much can be gained from the application of population pharmacokinetic and pharmacodynamic modeling methods during the process of drug development in veterinary medicine. One of the main goals of drug development is to obtain knowledge about the PKPD characteristics of a drug in populations. First, the dose-blood concentration relationship is defined. Then, the relationship between blood concentration and effect (some clinical output of interest often modeled as an effect compartment) is identified. The resulting PKPD model allows for description of dose-response relationships across a population. This approach can be used to build PKPD models under diverse experimental and nonexperimental conditions, linking them to measurable clinical conditions, which can be a great advantage in the development of veterinary drugs.

In human drug development, strategies involving the population approach have been advocated for assessing pharmacokinetic and pharmacodynamic variability as well as dose-concentration-effect relationships during the drug development process. Combined pharmacokinetic-pharmacodynamic models are used to optimize the completion of phase III studies in humans (clinical trials).

Although the clinical trial phase of the drug development process seems to be best suited to population studies, very valuable information can be derived from the implementation of this approach at earlier stages during drug development. At these early stages, population kinetics can be very useful in targeting the appropriate dose to be used in clinical trials. The interest of the sponsor that develops a drug is to minimize the cost, the time, and the number of experimental subjects and patients that are necessary for completion of these studies; i.e., to minimize the amount of data that has to be obtained to demonstrate safety and efficacy of a drug. Well-defined population PKPD models would help sponsors avoid dose titration studies in which the selected dosages lie on the flat (maximum) portion of the dose-response curve (recall Figure 12.2 in Chapter 12). It would also help the Food and Drug Administration identify situations, based on field trials with diseased animals, in which lower doses may provide comparable efficacy but a reduced potential for toxicity and the occurrence of violative tissue residues.

The main goal of population pharmacokinetics is to identify subpopulations of patients whose responses differ with respect to either location (mean) or variability, and to correlate those differences to some measurable covariate. During field or clinical trials, population pharmacokinetic-pharmacodynamic models would allow identification of subpopulations that may require a different dosage regimen. This would provide a more efficient way to determine dose ranges. Well-defined population PKPD models would be useful to support supplemental applications (e.g., different dosage regimens, alternative indications, new routes of administration). In light of the upcoming implementation of flexible labeling regulations, population PKPD can be a useful tool for sponsors to provide the required information with a minimum expenditure of resources.

Once a drug reaches the market, continued monitoring of the drug and completion of new population studies would provide additional information that, when compiled with previous information in an integrated database system, would help to define even more precisely the pharmacokinetic-pharmacodynamic characteristics of drugs in clinical use. In the case of drugs administered to food animals, this database would provide valuable information on adapting withdrawal times to specific clinical conditions. The extralabel use of drugs in food animals, as implemented by the Animal Medicinal Drug Use Clarification Act (AMDUCA) regulations in 1997, would especially benefit from this approach. Information from different sources on drug pharmacokinetics in edible tissues after different doses and clinical conditions would allow computation of better estimates of preslaughter withdrawal times. Overall, this would improve the safety of animal products destined for human consumption.

SELECTED READINGS

Beal, S.L. 1984. Population pharmacokinetic data and parameter estimation based on their first two statistical moments. *Drug Metabolism Reviews.* 15:173-193.

Beal, S.L., and L.B. Sheiner. 1980. The NONMEM system. *American Statistician.* 34:118-119.

Boeckmann, A.J., L.B. Sheiner, and S.L. Beal. 1994. *NONMEM Users Guide. Part V: Introductory Guide, Technical Report of the Division of Clinical Pharmacology.* San Francisco: University of California.

Chow, H.H., K.M. Tolle, D.J. Roe, V. Elsberry, and H. Chen. 1997. Application of neural networks to population pharmacokinetic data analysis. *Journal of Pharmaceutical Sciences.* 86:840-845.

Davidian, M., and A.R. Gallant 1992. Smooth nonparametric maximum likelihood estimation for population pharmacokinetics, with application to quinidine. *Journal of Pharmacokinetics and Biopharmaceutics.* 20:529-561.

Ette, E.I. 1997. Population model stability and performance. *Journal of Clinical Pharmacology.* 37:486-495.

Ette, E.I., and T.M. Ludden. 1995. Population pharmacokinetic modeling: The importance of informative graphics. *Pharmaceutical Research.* 12:1845-1855.

Frazier, D.L., D.P. Aucoin, and J.E. Riviere. 1988. Gentamicin pharmacokinetics and nephrotoxicity in naturally acquired and experimentally induced disease in dogs. *Journal of the American Veterinary Medical Association.* 192:57-63.

Grasela, T.H., and L.B. Sheiner. 1991. Pharmacostatistical modeling for observational data. *Journal of Pharmacokinetics and Biopharmaceutics.* 19:25S-36S.

Jelliffe, R.W., A. Schumitzky, M. Van Guilder, M. Liu, L. Hu, P. Maire, P. Gomis, X. Barbaut, and B. Tahani. 1993. Individualizing drug dosage regimens: Roles of population pharmacokinetic and dynamic models, Bayesian fitting and adaptive control. *Therapeutic Drug Monitoring.* 15:380-393.

Mallet, A. 1986. A maximum likelihood estimation method for random coefficient regression models. *Biometrika.* 73:645-656.

Martinez, M.N., J.E. Riviere, and G.D. Koritz. 1995. Review of the first interactive workshop on professional flexible labeling. *Journal of the American Veterinary Medical Association.* 207:865-914.

Martín-Jiménez, T., and J.E. Riviere. 1998. Population pharmacokinetics in veterinary medicine: Potential use for therapeutic drug monitoring and prediction of tissue residues. *Journal of Veterinary Pharmacology and Therapeutics.* 21:167-189.

Martín-Jiménez, T., M. Papich, and J.E. Riviere. 1997. Population pharmacokinetics of gentamicin in horses. *Journal of Veterinary Pharmacology and Therapeutics.* 20(Supplement 1):27-28.

Martín-Jiménez, T., M. Papich, and J.E. Riviere. 1998. Population pharmacokinetics of gentamicin in horses. *American Journal of Veterinary Research.* 59: 1589-1598.

Melmon, K.L., H.F. Morrelli, B.F. Hoffman, and D.W. Nierenberg. 1992. *Melmon and Morrelli's Clinical Pharmacology: Basic Principles in Therapeutics,* 3ed. New York: McGraw Hill, Inc.

Riond, J.L., L.P. Dix, and J.E. Riviere. 1986. Influence of thyroid function on the pharmacokinetics of gentamicin in pigs. *American Journal of Veterinary Research.* 47:2141-2146.

Riviere, J.E. 1988. Veterinary clinical pharmacokinetics. Part II: Modeling. *Compendium Continuing Education Practicing Veterinarian.* 10:313-328.

Riviere, J.E., L.P. Dix, M.P. Carver, and D.L. Frazier. 1986. Identification of a subgroup of Sprague-Dawley rats highly sensitive to drug-induced renal toxicity. *Fundamental and Applied Toxicology.* 7:126-131.

Riviere, J.E., T. Martín-Jiménez, S.F. Sundlof, and A.L. Craigmill. 1997. Interspecies allometric analysis of the comparative pharmacokinetics of 44 drugs across veterinary and laboratory animal species. *Journal of Veterinary Pharmacology and Therapeutics.* 20:453-463.

Rosenbaum, A.E., A.A. Carter, and M.N. Dudley. 1995. Population pharmacokinetics: Fundamentals, methods and applications. *Drug Development and Industrial Pharmacy.* 21:1115-1141.

Rowland, M, L.B. Sheiner, and J.L. Steimer. 1985. *Variability in Drug Therapy: Description, Estimation and Control.* New York: Raven Press.

Schumitzky, A. 1991. Nonparametric EM algorithms for estimating prior distributions. *Applied Mathematics and Computation.* 45:141-157.

Sheiner, L.B. 1994. A new approach to the analysis of analgesic drug trials, illustrated with bromfenac data. *Clinical Pharmacology and Therapeutics.* 56:309-322.

Sheiner, L.B., and S.L. Beal. 1980. Evaluation of methods for estimating population pharmacokinetic parameters. I. Michaelis-Menten model; routine clinical pharmacokinetic data. *Journal of Pharmacokinetics and Biopharmaceutics.* 8:553-571.

Sheiner, L.B., and S.L. Beal. 1981. Evaluation of methods for estimating population pharmacokinetic parameters. II. Biexponential model; experimental pharmacokinetic data. *Journal of Pharmacokinetics and Biopharmaceutics.* 9:635-651.

Sheiner, L.B., and S.L. Beal. 1983. Evaluation of methods for estimating population pharmacokinetic parameters. III. Monoexponential model; routine clinical pharmacokinetic data. *Journal of Pharmacokinetics and Biopharmaceutics.* 11:303-319.

Traver, D.S., and J.E. Riviere. 1982. Ampicillin in mares: A comparison of intramuscular sodium ampicillin or sodium ampicillin-ampicillin trihydrate injection. *American Journal of Veterinary Research.* 43:402-404.

Vozeh, S., J.L. Steimer, M. Rowland, P. Morselli, F. Mentré, L.P. Balant, and L. Aarons. 1996. The use of population pharmacokinetics in drug development. *Clinical Pharmacokinetics.* 30:81-93.

15

Dosage Adjustments in Renal Disease

One of the primary and most common factors that affects the disposition of a drug in the body is disease-induced changes in renal function. It is no surprise that renal disease has a profound impact on the disposition of a drug in the clinical setting. Many drugs are excreted primarily in urine as unchanged pharmacologically active drug. Drugs excreted in this manner accumulate in the body during renal insufficiency as a direct result of decreased renal clearance and is the primary manifestation of renal disease, which is compensated for in clinical dosage adjustment regimens. In fact, this approach is implicit to the formulation of many population pharmacokinetic models presented in Chapter 14. Renal disease can also influence drug disposition and effect by additional mechanisms listed in Table 15.1. These effects complicate the establishment of safe and efficacious regimens for drug therapy. As presented in Figure 14.1 (see Chapter 14), a renal disease process not only will affect the mean clearance of the drug but also will often increase the interindividual variability, making treatment of the individual patient a challenge.

PHARMACOLOGIC EFFECTS OF RENAL FAILURE

The degree of protein binding and its alteration by renal disease are important factors in the disposition and activity of a drug during renal insufficiency. The pharmacologic effect of a drug is dependent on the concentration of free drug in plasma. A marked reduction

TABLE 15.1. Possible Effects of Renal Disease on Drug Pharmacokinetics, Pharmacodynamics, and Toxicity

Reduced renal clearance resulting in accumulation of parent drug and/or metabolites
Altered rate of biotransformation
Decreased protein binding
Altered volume of distribution
Altered electrolyte balance
Altered drug disposition and/or activity secondary to acid-base or fluid-balance abnormalities
Reduced activity of urinary tract antimicrobial agents secondary to reduced excretion or dilution in polyuric states
Enhanced drug activity or toxicity secondary to synergy with uremic complications

uremia- accumulation in the blood usu. in severe kidney disease of constituents normally
eliminated in the urine producing a severe toxic condition

284   *Comparative Pharmacokinetics: Principles, Techniques, and Applications*

in protein binding of some drugs can occur in uremia, significantly affecting drug disposition and activity if the fraction of total drug bound is normally greater than 90% and if
the free drug has a relatively small volume of distribution. Examples of drugs that have
decreased binding in human uremics are benzylpenicillin, clofibrate, diazoxide, diazepam, dicloxacillin, fluorescein, pentobarbital, phenobarbital, phenylbutazone, phenytoin, salicylate, sulfonamides, thiopental, thyroxine, triamterene, and warfarin.

The decreased protein binding of drugs in uremia is greater than can be accounted for
by the hypoalbuminemia that may accompany glomerular disease processes. A suspected
mechanism is conformational change in albumin induced by the binding of "uremic toxins," endogenous metabolic by-products that accumulate in the body secondary to reduced renal clearance. These include free fatty acids, amino acids, and unidentified small
dialyzable organic acids. Uremic toxins could also compete with drugs for protein binding sites (recall Figure 4.6 in Chapter 4) as well as alter affinity of the receptor for the
drug secondary to conformational changes. The result of this increased free-drug concentration is an increase in Vd. For any measured concentration of total drug in the blood,
there will be an increased fraction of free drug. Variable effects on the subsequent biotransformation of free drug may also occur. Drugs cleared by glomerular filtration will
show an increased clearance, although subsequent tubular reabsorption may negate this.

The concept of changes in Vd of drugs in renal failure has recently received much attention. In addition to the increased Vd of highly protein-bound drugs in uremia, distributional changes have also been documented for drugs that are not significantly protein
bound. The Vd of digoxin decreases, while that of some aminoglycosides has been shown
to increase. The decreased Vd of digoxin is believed to be, in part, the result of decreased
binding to kidney, liver, and myocardium. As discussed in Chapter 7 (Table 7.2), the decreased excretion of a drug may result in a decreased apparent volume of distribution
(Vd_{area}). This is a result of a mathematical dependence of some estimates of Vd on the
magnitude of k_{el}. Estimates of Vd (i.e., Vd_{ss}) that are independent of k_{el} should be used so
that true volume changes in renal disease states can be detected. The clinical significance
of altered Vd with renal failure is not known, and dosage adjustment regimens generally
do not account for it. True estimates of the magnitude of Vd can be obtained only
through an analysis of drug concentrations in blood.

Changes in the biotransformation of drugs during renal insufficiency and uremia have
been documented. Sharp contrasts among species exist. Glycine conjugation, acetylation,
and hydrolytic reactions are slowed in uremia. Notably, the biotransformation of
cephalothin, cortisol, hydralazine, insulin, isoniazid, procaine, procainamide, salicylate,
succinylcholine, and selected sulfonamides may be decreased in uremia, which could result in a decrease in the nonrenal clearance component of a drug's elimination pattern, a
factor (e.g., decreased k_{nr} from equation 7.24, see Chapter 7) normally assumed to be unchanged in renal insufficiency. The result would be drug accumulation if the overall elimination rate constant, K_{el}, were decreased. Uremia does not appear to alter microsomal
oxidation, reduction, glucuronide synthesis, sulfate conjugation, or methylation pathways. In contrast, some oxidative reactions in human uremics are accelerated. Laboratory animals show markedly different effects of uremia on the disposition of some drugs;
e.g., a study of pentobarbital disposition in nephrectomized dogs did not detect a different drug half-life from that measured in controls. Therefore, species differences are important, necessitating that drug therapy in diseased individuals be evaluated in each case.

An interesting effect of renal insufficiency on drugs eliminated by biotransformation is
the accumulation of active metabolites. Examples of such drugs are allopurinol,
cephalothin, cephapirin, chlorpropamide, clofibrate, digitoxin, doxorubicin, lidocaine,
mephobarbital, primidone, procainamide, and some sulfonamides. Intoxication and enhanced drug activity have been reported to occur by this mechanism.

The uremic patient is in a precarious state of fluid, electrolyte, and acid-base homeostasis. For example, administration of antibiotic drugs containing sodium (ampicillin, 3 mEq/g; carbenicillin, 4.7 mEq/g; cephalothin, 2.5 mEq/g; penicillin G, 1.7 mEq/g); or potassium (penicillin G, 1.7 mEq/g) could result in serious electrolyte overload. Treatment with antacids and laxatives could result in magnesium and aluminum intoxication. Penicillin and carbenicillin, functioning as nonreabsorbable anions in the distal tubules, can cause loss of hydrogen and potassium in the urine. Acidosis of renal insufficiency favors dissociation of salicylate and phenobarbital, thereby increasing drug concentrations in the brain. Acidosis also decreases sensitivity of adrenergic receptors.

Diuretics that produce prolonged polyuric states can decrease antibiotic concentrations in urine to subtherapeutic levels. This dilution effect, coupled with decreased renal clearance of antimicrobial drugs secondary to renal insufficiency, can impair efficacy in treatment of urinary tract infections. Concentrations of antibiotics in renal parenchyma are often lower in severely diseased kidneys than in normal kidneys.

Drug toxicity may be potentiated if the drug's action is synergistic with uremic complications. An example is the administration of anticoagulants, which may induce a bleeding disorder. Untoward gastrointestinal and neurological drug reactions can be more easily elicited when uremia has caused functional changes in these systems. An altered blood-brain barrier in uremia can result in elevated drug concentrations in the cerebrospinal fluid. Sensitivity to opiates, barbiturates, and tranquilizers is increased by this mechanism, and decreased protein binding of these drugs accentuates the effect.

A number of additional complications may also occur with drug therapy in uremics. Erythrocytes collected from human patients who were in renal failure were more sensitive to development of a cephalothin-induced positive Coombs' test than were cells from healthy patients. The antianabolic activity of tetracycline and the catabolic action of corticosteroid hormones may worsen the degree of azotemia. The rate and extent of oral drug absorption can be affected by variation in gastrointestinal motility. Similarly, absorption from alimentary, muscular, and subcutaneous sites may be impaired due to decreased blood perfusion secondary to dehydration.

The prudent course of action in uremic patients is thus to titrate the dose of suspect drugs to the observed response. The clinician must assume normal rates of metabolic clearance in patients until definitive data are available for the specific drug and species being treated. The most obvious approach to accomplish this is to use pharmacokinetic principles to construct modified dosage regimens to compensate for disease-induced alterations in a drug's pharmacokinetic and pharmacodynamic profiles.

DRUG DOSAGE REGIMENS IN RENAL FAILURE

Current guidelines for constructing dosage regimens for renal insufficiency or failure compensate only for decreased renal clearance of the parent drug and are based upon the principles of dosage regimen construction presented in Chapter 11. It is prudent to review these concepts and equations before continuing further with this discussion. There are no published guidelines recommending dosage adjustments to compensate for changes in protein binding, altered drug biotransformation, active metabolite accumulations, or altered Vd. This could only be accomplished using a completely defined pharmacokinetic model for the specific scenario at hand.

The preferred approach would be to construct a population pharmacokinetic model of the drug that directly incorporates parameters of renal dysfunction as concomitant variables in the model (see Chapter 14, equations 14.2 and 14.4). Including appropriate, more complex population models could also directly compensate for changes in Vd or hepatic metabolism.

The best approach to modifying drug therapy is thus to (1) conduct individualized pharmacokinetic studies in patients and monitor progress using therapeutic drug monitoring techniques, (2) utilize Bayesian or population strategies linking dosage regimen construction to observable concomitant physiological variables, or (3) estimate a corrected dose from commonly available renal function tests and then monitor the patient for signs of drug efficacy and toxicity. The latter strategy is the one most often implemented in the clinical setting.

PHARMACOKINETICS IN RENAL IMPAIRMENT

It is appropriate at this point to present an overview of some of the basic pharmacokinetic principles involved in assessing the effects of renal disease on drug disposition. Recall that the total body clearance of a drug can be partitioned into renal and nonrenal parts as previously described. Therefore,

$$Cl_B \text{ (mL / min)} = Cl_r + Cl_{nr} \qquad (15.1)$$

where Cl_r is renal clearance and Cl_{nr} is nonrenal drug clearance. All clearances are normally expressed in terms of body weight or surface area.

The cornerstone of predicting drug disposition during renal failure in a clinical setting is based on the assumption that renal clearance is directly correlated to clinical measures of glomerular filtration rate (GFR) as presented in Chapters 5 and 7 and incorporated as described above in the population pharmacokinetic models of Chapter 14. This assumes that the intact nephron hypothesis holds and that a relative glomerulotubular balance is present. Renal clearance is thus a linear function of GFR, whether the drug is cleared by glomerular or tubular mechanisms.

$$Cl_r \text{ (mL / min)} = M \times GFR \qquad (15.2)$$

where M is a proportionality constant. Substituting in equation 15.1 results in this relation:

$$Cl_B \text{ (mL / min)} = M \times GFR + Cl_{nr} \qquad (15.3)$$

Total body clearance was defined in pharmacokinetic terms throughout Chapters 7 and 8. From this point onward, a one-compartment model will be assumed to simplify discussions. If equation 15.3 is divided by Vd (recall $Cl/Vd = k_{el}$), the generally applicable relationship depicted in equation 15.4 results.

$$k_{el} \text{ (1 / min)} = k_r + k_{nr} = M' \times GFR + k_{nr} \qquad (15.4)$$

This is the equation for a straight line with slope M' and y-axis intercept k_{nr}. Remember that k_{nr} is assumed to be unchanged, as discussed previously. k_{el} represents the fraction of a drug's distribution volume cleared per unit time. Recall that for a one-compartment model, $-k_{el}$ is equivalent to $-k$, the slope of the plasma concentration-time (C-T) profile plotted on semilogarithmic paper (see Chapter 7, Figure 7.4). The relationship defined in equation 15.4 has been shown to hold for most drugs studied when GFR has been estimated by creatinine clearance and actually provides the basis for its use in population pharmacokinetic models.

The relationship in equation 15.4 is graphically depicted on a Cartesian coordinate system in the top of Figure 15.1. Three drugs are shown all having the same k_{nr}. The first is primarily cleared by nonrenal mechanisms ($k_r < k_{nr}$). As creatinine clearance decreases, k_{el}

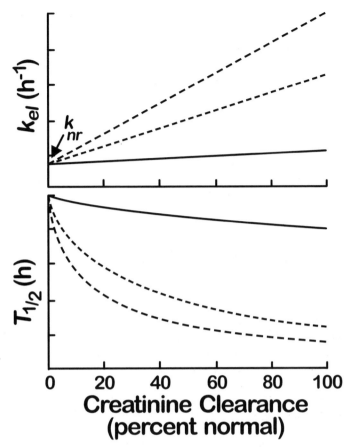

FIGURE 15.1. Relationship between elimination rate constant (k_{el}) or half-life ($T_{1/2}$) and creatinine clearance. The three drugs depicted are dependent on renal elimination (k_r) to varying degrees (— $k_r < k_{nr}$; ---- $k_r > k_{nr}$; --- $k_r >> k_{nr}$).

is seen to remain relatively stable. In the second drug, eliminated from the body by renal and nonrenal mechanisms ($k_r > k_{nr}$), decreases in creatinine clearance result in a steady decline in k_{el}, until $k_{el} = k_{nr}$ at a creatinine clearance of zero (anephric patient). In the third drug, primarily eliminated by renal mechanisms ($k_r >> k_{nr}$), decreases in creatinine clearance result in a great decrease in k_{el}. Note that k_{el} still approaches k_{nr}. If the drug was eliminated solely by renal mechanisms ($k_{nr} = 0$), k_{el} would equal zero in the anephric patient.

A more practical approach to this problem for clinical use is to relate *GFR* to drug elimination half-life ($T_{1/2}$) in a similar fashion. However, this is not a linear relation but rather a hyperbolic function because of the inverse relationships,

$$T_{\frac{1}{2}} \text{ (min)} = \frac{0.693 \, Vd}{Cl_B} = \frac{0.693}{k_{el}} = \frac{0.693}{k_r + k_{nr}} \qquad (15.5)$$

A plot of *GFR* versus $T_{1/2}$ for the same three drugs is depicted in the lower half of Figure 15.1. This plot is clinically applicable because most dosage regimens are expressed in terms of $T_{1/2}$ (Recall equation 11.14 in Chapter 11). If the drug is eliminated primarily by nonrenal mechanisms, $T_{1/2}$ remains relatively constant over varying degrees of renal function. However, if the drug is excreted by renal mechanisms, $T_{1/2}$ is stable until creatinine clearance is 30% to 40% of normal, at which point $T_{1/2}$ drastically increases. This is the basis for the general recommendation that dose adjustment in renal failure is necessary only when more than two thirds of renal function is lost. If a drug is excreted almost entirely by the kidneys, then $T_{1/2}$ approaches infinity as creatinine clearance approaches zero.

An alternative method used to relate $T_{1/2}$ to *GFR* for drugs primarily eliminated by renal mechanisms is through the use of a dose fraction, (K_f), defined as

$$K_f = \frac{\text{Abnormal creatinine clearance}}{\text{Normal creatinine clearance}} = \frac{Cl_B \text{ (abnormal)}}{Cl_B \text{ (normal)}} \tag{15.6}$$

These relationships will now be applied to formulae designed to calculate dosage regimens in animals with renal failure.

CALCULATION OF MODIFIED DOSAGE REGIMENS

The approach in this section will be to modify dosage regimens that are appropriate in normal animals in proportion to decreases in renal function estimated by dose fraction. This method assumes that (1) a standard loading dose is administered; (2) drug absorption, volume of distribution, protein binding, extrarenal elimination, and tissue sensitivity (dose-response relation) are unchanged (major assumptions); (3) creatinine clearance is directly correlated to drug clearance; and (4) renal function is relatively constant over time.

The ultimate aim of dosage adjustment in renal disease is to fulfill the fundamental therapeutic postulate that the C-T profile should be as similar as possible to the normal situation. Recall from Chapter 11 that ε, the ratio $\tau/T_{1/2}$, determines the fluctuation in a multiple dose C-T profile based on its influence on the value of f_{el} from equation 11.5. The dose ratio, D/τ, determines the average steady-state plasma concentration (C_p^{avg}). If τ is not adjusted in the face of an increasing $T_{1/2}$ in a patient with renal failure, C_p^{avg} will dramatically increase, as can be seen from revisiting equation 11.2. This can be compensated for by either reducing D or increasing τ in this equation, which is the basis of the dose modification methods introduced below. However, the fluctuations in these regimens is a function of f_{el}, which in a renal disease patient is dependent upon ε. When constructing dosage regimens for patients with renal disease that have fundamentally altered pharmacokinetic parameters, both D and τ must be modified to achieve C_p^{avg} and f_{el}, which are similar to those parameters in patients with normal renal function.

Dose-Reduction Method.   Let us assume that one has already defined a safe and effective dosage regimen for use in a normal patient. This normal dosage regimen is then adjusted according to the dose fraction by two basic procedures. The first method, termed *constant-interval, dose-reduction (DR)*, reduces the dose (D) by a factor of the dose fraction. Dose interval (τ) is the same as that used in the healthy animal.

$$D_{\text{renal failure}} = D_{\text{normal}} \, K_f$$

$$\tau_{\text{renal failure}} = \tau_{\text{normal}} \tag{15.7}$$

Interval-Extension Method.   The second method, referred to as *constant-dose, interval-extension (IE)*, extends the dosage interval by the inverse of the dose fraction, a value referred to as the *dose-interval multiplier*.

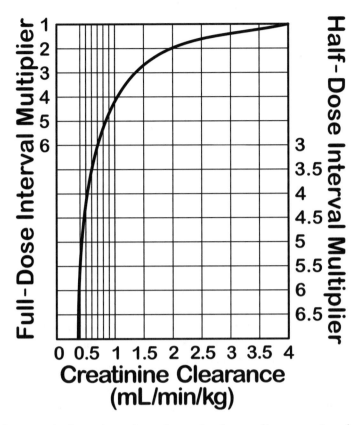

FIGURE 15.2.　Nomogram implementing an interval-extension dosage adjustment regimen based on creatinine clearance in the dog.

$$\tau_{\text{renal failure}} = \tau_{\text{normal}} \, (1 / K_f)$$
$$D_{\text{renal failure}} = D_{\text{normal}}$$

(15.8)

This type of dose adjustment strategy may also be implemented through the use of a nomogram (Figure 15.2), in which the dosage interval multiplier for this *IE* regimen is simply read off a plot of creatinine clearance.

Implementation.　The therapeutic goal is to maintain a constant product of $(T_{1/2} \times D/\tau)$ in healthy animals and those with renal failure. When this product is constant, the average steady-state plasma concentration of drug will remain unchanged. This is the approach followed in the *DR* and *IE* methods. A constant steady-state plasma concentration is achieved by the use of the dose fraction to compensate for decreased $T_{1/2}$ in the following manner:

$$(T_{1/2} \times D / \tau)_{\text{normal}} = K_f \, (T_{1/2} \times D / \tau)_{\text{renal failure}}$$

(15.9)

When repeated doses of a drug are administered, accumulation occurs until steady-state plasma concentrations are achieved. Recall from Chapter 11 that this takes approximately four or five $T_{1/2}$s. *The prolonged $T_{1/2}$ present in patients with renal insufficiency would cause excessive delay in attaining steady-state concentration. Therefore, an appropriate loading dose should always be administered so that a therapeutic concentration of* *the drug is immediately attained.* If the constant-interval method is employed, this can be accomplished by giving the usual dose initially, followed by the calculated reduced dose. If the constant-dose method is used, the initial two doses should be given according to the usual interval.

Equations 15.7 and 15.8 hold for drugs that are excreted solely by the kidney, since the dose fraction adjusts dosages as if K_{nr} equaled zero. For drugs undergoing biotransformation, a measure of the percent nonrenal clearance is necessary. This proportion can be estimated by knowledge of the fraction of the absorbed dose of drug excreted unchanged in the urine (*f*). Recall from Chapter 7 that the ratio $U_\infty / D = k_r / k_{el}$. The constant-interval method then becomes

$$D_{\text{renal failure}} = D_{\text{normal}} \left[(f(K_f - 1)) + 1 \right]$$

$$\tau_{\text{renal failure}} = \tau_{\text{normal}}$$

(15.10)

For the constant-dose, increased-interval method,

$$\tau_{\text{renal failure}} = \tau_{\text{normal}} \div \left[(f(K_f - 1)) + 1 \right]$$

$$D_{\text{renal failure}} = D_{\text{normal}}$$

(15.11)

The fraction excreted unchanged in urine is not currently available for animals for most drugs. Additionally, if it is relatively small, then K_r is less than K_{nr}, and $T_{1/2}$ will remain relatively stable, avoiding the need to adjust dosages.

When creatinine clearance has not been available, the inverse of serum creatinine (mg/dl) has been substituted. Since the relationship between $T_{1/2}$ and serum creatinine is not linear above 4 mg/dl, adjustment formulae may not accurately predict the dose fraction.

Selection of the Appropriate Method of Dosage Adjustment. A great deal of controversy exists over the relative merits of the constant-dose and the constant-interval methods. These two regimens produce different C-T profiles, as is depicted in Figure 15.3. This hypothetical drug, primarily eliminated by renal processes, is dosed every four $T_{1/2}$s. Creatinine clearance is one sixth of normal ($K_f = 1/6$). The constant-dose regimen produces peak and trough concentrations similar to those seen in the healthy patient; however, there are prolonged periods of potentially subtherapeutic serum concentrations. This is preferred for drugs such as aminoglycoside antibiotics, whose toxicity correlates with high trough rather than peak concentrations. If the dose is decreased but the interval held constant, peak concentrations are lower and trough concentrations greater than during the usual regimen. There are no periods of subtherapeutic concentrations. A compromise can be made by multiplying both the dose and the increased interval calculated in equations 15.7 and 15.8 by a constant fraction, a procedure that does not alter the steady-state plasma concentration. An example is the half-dosage *IE* method in the nomogram of Figure 15.2.

The normal drug plasma C-T profile can never be exactly duplicated in a patient with renal failure because the slopes of the elimination curves are not parallel due to different $T_{1/2}$s. *All dosage regimens are only approximations.* This inability to match C-T profiles in normal and diseased animals was the driving force behind using deconvolution techniques to develop the computer controlled infusion profiles depicted in Figure 8.5 (see Chapter 8). This is the only approach that allows one to assess the inherent toxicity of a drug in healthy versus diseased animals independent of accumulation secondary to a prolonged terminal elimination slope.

An advantage of the fixed-dose method is convenience. The recommended dose used in healthy animals is administered less frequently. If drugs available in fixed dosage forms

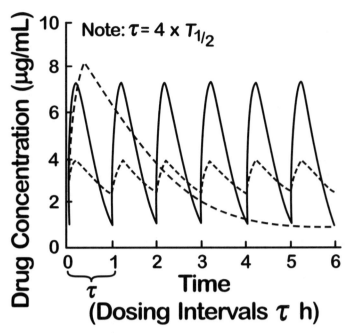

FIGURE 15.3. Comparison of constant-dose (‒‒‒) and constant-interval (‐‐‐‐) regimens in renal failure (Cl_{cr} = one sixth usual) with a normal dosage regimen (—) in a healthy patient. τ is the dosage interval.

are used, the constant-dose method is clearly easier to administer. As discussed in Chapter 11, the clinician should determine if drug efficacy and/or toxicity is correlated to peak, trough, or average plasma concentrations and then select a regimen balancing efficacy against potential toxicity. It should be noted that the most effective means of maintaining a constant plasma concentration of drug is by continuous infusion at a constant rate. Note that in animals with chronic renal failure whose nephrons are undergoing compensatory hypertrophy, the intact nephron hypothesis would predict that each individual surviving nephron would be exposed to a greater tubular load of drug per unit of whole kidney *GFR* than would a nephron in a healthy animal. Therefore, even if a drug dose is appropriately reduced according to decreased *GFR*, the toxic potential of a tubular nephrotoxin could be greater in the renal failure patient.

The most accurate method of adjusting a dosage regimen in renal failure is to calculate a dose, administer it, and monitor the resultant peak and trough serum concentrations by direct assay since interindividual differences in disposition cannot be accounted for using these nonpharmacokinetic approaches. A Bayesian approach can then be used to adjust subsequent drug dosage. The main advantage is that dose can be constantly adjusted so that changes in parameters assumed to be constant in the above formulae will be detected. This procedure, rooted in the principles of therapeutic drug monitoring protocols, is becoming economically feasible, even in veterinary medicine. Chapter 14 should be consulted for details. The methods discussed assume stable renal function. In clinical states in which renal function is constantly changing, drug elimination is also changing, and accurate predictions are difficult.

Rules of Thumb. The following points should serve as guidelines for drug treatment during impaired renal function.

1. Do not use drugs unless definite therapeutic indications are present.

2. If the dosage regimen of a drug in renal failure has been determined via individual clinical pharmacokinetic studies, this should be followed in preference to use of the previously discussed general guidelines.

3. In a situation in which the drug has not been studied but some information on its characteristics are available (e.g., the percentage of its excretion in an unchanged form by the kidney), it is possible by use of the above equations to make an estimate of the proper dose in renal failure.

4. If an assay procedure for the drug is available, the periodic measurement of blood concentrations of the drug is advisable for any schedule.

5. Careful clinical monitoring for toxicity and pharmacologic effect is mandatory in all cases.

6. When ever possible, the clinician should select a drug that is biotransformed by the liver or excreted in the bile rather than eliminated unchanged by the kidneys (e.g., digitoxin rather than digoxin, a fluoroquinolone instead of gentamicin, a barbiturate or inhalant anesthetic in place of ketamine).

Hepatic Disease.   Finally, the same conceptual approach may be used to adjust dosage regimens to compensate for decreased hepatic clearance in the presence of liver disease. In many cases, drug disposition will only be altered with severe liver failure. The easiest rule of thumb is to avoid using any drug cleared by hepatic processes since the complex pharmacokinetics normally associated with such drugs, coupled with the lack of an easily measured clinical indicator of hepatic clearance applicable to all drug types, precludes development of an easy dosage adjustment strategy. Chapter 6 should be consulted to assess how liver disease could impact on hepatobiliary excretion and metabolism before dosage in such patients is attempted.

DRUG CLEARANCE IN DIALYSIS

The importance of considering the effects of dialysis on drug therapy is to determine the dosage required to compensate for increased drug clearance due to peritoneal dialysis and hemodialysis. A simple way to approach this problem is to modify equation 15.1 to include dialyzer clearance (Cl_D), allowing total body clearance to include all clearance mechanisms, both natural and artificial.

$$Cl_B = Cl_r + Cl_{nr} + Cl_D \tag{15.12}$$

The effect of increased elimination during dialysis is depicted in Figure 15.4, in which $T_{1/2}$ during dialysis is a function of the elimination constant and the dialysis rate constant. This approach again assumes unchanged Vd and a one-compartment pharmacokinetic model. If $T_{1/2}$ before and during dialysis is known, the overall elimination constant can be calculated from similar blood C-T plots, and equation 7.16 may be used to calculate total body clearance in dialysis from elimination constant and Vd. This value could then be used to calculate the precise amount of drug removed during dialysis by the following:

$$\text{Drug recovery} = (Cl_B)\,(C_{ss})(\text{dialysis duration}) \tag{15.13}$$

where C_{ss} = steady-state plasma concentration. When this estimate of total body clearance during dialysis is obtained, dose fraction is determined by the following:

$$K_f = \frac{Cl_B}{\text{Normal } Cl_{\text{creatinine}}} \tag{15.14}$$

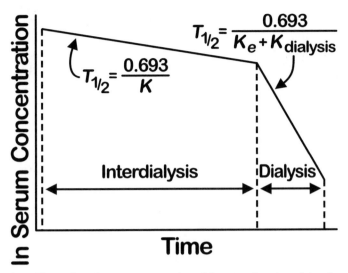

FIGURE 15.4.   Semilogarithmic plot of serum concentration of drug as a function of time in a patient on and off dialysis. K_e is the elimination rate constant and $K_{dialysis}$ is the dialysis rate constant.

If these values are calculated on a daily basis, total body clearance will be the average clearance and will reflect time on and off dialysis. Dose fraction, analogous to dose fraction in renal insufficiency without dialysis, can then be used directly in equations 15.7 and 15.8. Alternatively, the preferred method would be to calculate the amount of drug lost during a dialysis period according to equation 15.13, and then give this dose post-dialysis. The normal dose fraction is then used for interdialysis dosing.

If Vd is not known, but $T_{1/2}$ before and after dialysis is available, the fraction of drug removed during dialysis (F) can be calculated.

$$F' = \frac{T_{1/2}\,(\text{before}) - T_{1/2}\,(\text{dialysis})}{T_{1/2}\,(\text{before})}$$

$$F = F' \times \left[1 - e^{-0.693/T_{1/2\,(\text{dialysis})}\, \times\, \text{duration of dialysis}} \right]$$

(15.15)

Dialyzer clearance can also be calculated solely for the dialysis process independent of body clearance mechanisms. With peritoneal dialysis,

$$Cl_D = \frac{C_D V}{(C_p)\,(\text{dialysis duration})}$$

(15.16)

where C_D is the concentration of drug in the dialysate fluid after exchange, V is the total dialysate drainage volume, and C_p is the plasma concentration of drug at the midpoint of dialysis. Hemodialysis and hemofiltration clearance can be calculated using Fick's law according to the relationship

$$Cl_D = \frac{Q\,(C_{in} \times C_{out})}{C_{in}}$$

(15.17)

where Q is the flow of blood through the dialyzer, C_{in} is the concentration of drug in plasma entering the dialyzer (arterial, inflow), and C_{out} is the concentration of drug in plasma exiting the dialyzer (venous, outflow). Some discrepancies in dialyzer clearance may occur when plasma concentration of drug is not representative of total blood concentration. This results because the concentration of drug is measured for plasma while the flow is measured for blood. Adjustments based on hematocrit can be made, or blood concentrations can be separated into erythrocyte and plasma water concentrations. Equation 15.17 may be written in terms of plasma and blood. The derivation and applications of equations 15.12 through 15.17 are based upon an extension of the basic principles of clearance, volume of distribution, and elimination rate constants developed throughout this text.

CONCLUSION

The application of these principles to specific drugs is discussed in many clinical pharmacology and nephrology texts and should be consulted for the specific data and therapeutic strategies applicable to a drug.

In conclusion, the best approach to adjust dosages in a patient with renal disease is to implement a population pharmacokinetic model that specifically describes drug disposition in terms of clinical parameters that are altered in renal impairment. The proper strategy for dose reduction must still be selected (e.g., *IE* or *DR*) for designing such regimens, taking into account the drug's safety and efficacy administered according to these different approaches. Bayesian approaches can then be used to titrate the drug dosage to the individual patient.

SELECTED READINGS

Anderson, R.J., J.G. Gambertoglio, and R.W. Schrier. 1976. *Clinical Use of Drugs in Renal Failure.* Springfield, IL: Charles C. Thomas, Publisher.

Benet, L.Z. 1976. *Effects of Disease States on Drug Pharmacokinetcs.* Washington, D.C.: Academy of Pharmaceutical Sciences.

Bennett, W.M., G.R. Aronoff, T.A. Golper, G. Morrison, I. Singer, and D.C. Brater. 1987. *Drug Prescribing in Renal Failure. Dosing Guidelines for Adults.* Philadelphia, PA: American College of Physicians.

Bennett, W.M., G.A. Porter, S.P. Bagby, and W.J. McDonald. 1978. *Drugs and Renal Disease.* New York: Churchill Livingstone.

Brater, D.C. 1989. *Pocket Manual of Drug Use in Clinical Medicine,* 4ed. Toronto: B.C. Dekker.

Brater, D.C., S.A. Anderson, and D. Brown-Cartwright. 1986. Response to furosemide in chronic renal insufficiency. Rationale for limited doses. *Clinical Pharmacology and Therapeutics.* 40:134-139.

Bricker, N.S. 1969. On the meaning of the intact nephron hypothesis. *American Journal of Medicine.* 46:1-11.

Frazier, D.L., and J.E. Riviere. 1987. Gentamicin dosing strategies for dogs with subclinical renal dysfunction. *Antimicrobial Agents Chemotherapy.* 31:1929-1934.

Gibson, T.P. Renal disease and drug metabolism: An overview. *American Journal of Kidney Disease.* 8:7-17.

Lee, C.S., T.C. Marbury, and L.Z. Benet. 1980. Clearance calculations in hemodialysis. *Journal of Pharmacokinetics and Biopharmaceutics.* 8:69.

Maher, J.F. 1984. Pharmacokinetics in patients with renal failure. *Clinical Nephrology.* 21:39-46.

Melmon, K.L., H.F. Morrelli, B.F. Hoffman, and D.W. Nierenberg. *Melmon and Morrelli's Clinical Pharmacology: Basic Principles in Therapeutics,* 3ed. New York: McGraw Hill, Inc.

Reidenberg, M.M., and D.E. Drayer. 1984. Alteration of drug protein binding in renal disease. *Clinical Pharmacokinetics.* 9(Supplement 1):18-26.

Riviere, J.E. 1982. A possible mechanism for increased susceptibility to aminoglycoside nephrotoxicity in chronic renal disease. *New England Journal of Medicine.* 307:252-253.

Riviere, J.E. 1984. Calculation of dosage regimens of antimicrobial drugs in animals with renal and hepatic dysfunction. *Journal of the American Veterinary Medical Association.* 185:1094-1097.

Riviere, J.E., and G.L. Coppoc. 1981. Dosage of antimicrobial drugs in patients with renal insufficiency. *Journal of the American Veterinary Medical Association.* 178:70-72.

Riviere, J.E., and L.E. Davis. 1984. Renal handling of drugs in renal failure. In *Canine Nephrology,* ed. K.C. Bovee, 643-685. Media, PA: Harwal Publishers.

Riviere, J.E., and S. Vaden. 1995. Drug therapy during renal disease and renal failure. In *Canine and Feline Nephrology and Urology,* ed. C.A. Osborne and D.R. Finco, 555-572. Baltimore: Williams & Wilkins.

Riviere, J.E., K.F. Bowman, and R.A. Rogers. 1985. Decreased fractional renal excretion of gentamicin in subtotal nephrectomized dogs. *Journal of Pharmacology and Experimental Therapeutics.* 234:90-93.

Riviere, J.E., M.P. Carver, G.L. Coppoc, W.W. Carlton, G.C. Lantz, and J.S. Shy-Modjeska. 1984. Pharmacokinetics and comparative nephrotoxicity of fixed-dose versus fixed-interval reduction of gentamicin dosage in subtotal nephrectomized dogs. *Toxicology and Applied Pharmacology.* 75:496-509.

St. Peter, W.L., K.A. Redic-Kill, and C.E. Halstenson. 1992. Clinical pharmacokinetics of antibiotics in patients with impaired renal function. *Clinical Pharmacokinetics.* 22:169-210.

16
Interspecies Extrapolations

The purpose of this chapter is to address how pharmacokinetic data may be extrapolated across species based on coupling the basic processes of distribution and elimination to physiological factors that vary as a function of body weight. A review of interspecies scaling could easily require multiple books; thus, this chapter will focus on basic principles and techniques that illustrate the strategies employed.

The ultimate aim of any interspecies extrapolation would be to predict drug activity or toxicity in a new species not previously studied. There are two sources of error inherent in such an extrapolation. The first is that a drug's pharmacokinetic profile (especially excretion, metabolism, and distribution) does not extrapolate across species without adjusting for some individual species characteristics. The second, which will always be problematic, is that the pharmacodynamic response of a drug may be very different between species and not at all related to pharmacokinetics. This latter concern may not be important for antimicrobial drugs since the pathogenic organisms being treated should have susceptibilities that are pathogen-dependent and host-independent. However, for drugs that interact with physiological functions that have species-specific receptor types and distributions, an estimate of pharmacokinetic parameters may not be sufficient to predict pharmacodynamic response. Although this issue will be touched upon in this presentation, the emphasis will be on extrapolating pharmacokinetic parameters across species. When such an extrapolation is made, the techniques of pharmacokinetic-pharmacodynamic modeling presented in Chapter 12 could then be applied.

The optimal strategy to make interspecies extrapolations would be to derive a physiologically based pharmacokinetic (PBPK) model for the drug in question, as discussed in Chapter 10. In this case, one models the disposition of a drug in terms of the major anatomical organs responsible for its distribution, metabolism, and excretion from the body. These organs are linked by the rate of blood flow to each organ. As can easily be appreciated, once a PBPK model is obtained for one species, knowledge of the second species' organ weights and blood flows may be input into the process and the disposition of the drug in this species simulated. Likewise, differences in plasma/tissue binding or pathways of biotransformation may be accounted for and input into the model. A PBPK model also lends itself to straightforward pharmacodynamic coupling with *in vitro* data collected in the target species. This approach has not been widely adopted primarily because of the paucity of complete PBPK studies published to date and the overall complexity of conducting such studies at early stages of drug development. Instead, the literature is replete with descriptive compartmental and noncompartmental studies that report on classic pharmacokinetic parameters (Vd, Cl, $T_{1/2}$) collected from individual trials in a species at a specific dose. How can these existing data be used to probe the differences in drug disposition across species?

PHARMACOKINETIC SCALING

There is a wealth of empirical observations that suggest that physiological functions such as O_2 consumption, renal glomerular filtration, and cardiac output, are not linearly correlated to the mass of an individual animal, both within and between species. That is, if one expresses any physiological function on a per kg of body weight basis [e.g., glomerular filtration rate (GFR)/kg], an *isometric* relationship would suggest that the parameter is constant. However, in the case of these physiological functions, such a relationship does not hold since the parameter on a mg/kg basis still is species dependent and not constant. A knowledge of body weight does not allow one to determine the value of the parameter across species with different body weights. However, if these parameters are expressed on a per unit surface area basis, then many parameters, such as GFR, will be equivalent across species. More refined analyses suggest that the optimal scaling factor would be to a species' basal metabolic rate (BMR). Empirical observations suggest that BMR is a function of (body weight in kg) raised to the 0.75 power [$GFR = f\,(BW_{kg})^{0.75}$]; when expressed on body surface area, the exponent is 0.67. An exponent of 0.75 is also theoretically predicted if metabolic functions are based on a model in which substances in the body are transported through space-occupying fractal networks of branching tubes (e.g., the vascular system) that minimize energy dissipation and share the same size at the smallest level of structure (e.g., capillaries). Whatever the mechanism, these approaches are well suited for extrapolating drug disposition across species.

Basis of Allometry.   Equations in which a parameter is related to a mathematical function (in this case a power function) of a metric such as body weight is termed an *allometric* relationship. The extensive literature surrounding the question of how one "collapses" physiological parameters between species has created a field of study called allometry. Since most drug pharmacokinetic parameters are dependent upon some physiological function, they may also be scaled across species using these strategies. The method for doing this is to correlate the parameter of concern (e.g., GFR, Cl_B) with body weight (BW) using the following allometric equation:

$$Y = a\,(BW)^b \tag{16.1}$$

where Y is the parameter of concern, a is the allometric coefficient, and b is the allometric exponent. The data are obtained using simple linear regression on $\log_{10} Y$ versus $\log_{10} BW$ as depicted in Figure 16.1. The slope is the allometric exponent b and the intercept a.

There is uniform agreement that for most physiological processes, the allometric exponent b ranges from 0.67 to 1.0. Note that if the parameter being modeled is an inverse function of a physiological process (e.g., $T_{1/2}$), then the exponent will be $1 - b$ for that process. The coefficient a is actually the value of Y for a 1.0 kg BW animal ($b = 0$).

This is also a good point at which to consider what happens if isometry is assumed. In this case, $b = 1.0$ and the parameter is a function of BW^1, which equals body weight. From this perspective, *if one adjusts dosages across species on the basis of kg of body weight alone, one is implicitly assuming that $b = 1$ for the relationship between parameters,* which we know is not correct from data such as the above.

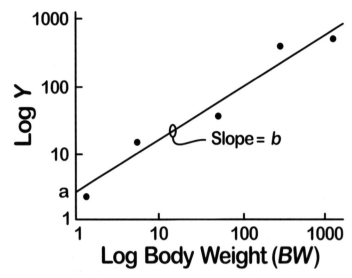

FIGURE 16.1.   Basic log-log allometric plot of a biological parameter (Y) versus body weight (BW) with slope b and intercept a.

Scaling of Half-Life.   An example of an allometric analysis conducted in our laboratory is shown in Figure 16.2, with gentamicin β-elimination phase $T_{1/2}$ data collected after intravenous administration of 10 mg of gentamicin per kg of body weight to animals ranging in size from the mouse to the horse. There is an excellent fit based on analysis of this large data set, with $T_{1/2\beta}(\text{min}) = 42\ BW^{0.249}$. This suggests that knowing the $T_{1/2\beta}$ in any species, the corresponding value of this parameter can be estimated in another. In general, the $T_{1/2}$ will be shorter in small animals with a large BMR and ratio of surface area to body mass than in larger animals, which have a smaller BMR and surface area.

This equation has been extensively applied to numerous sets of pharmacokinetic data. The first was demonstrated by Dedrick and coworkers, who analyzed methotrexate data and achieved results very similar to those of gentamicin, as shown above. This is not surprising, since both compounds are primarily eliminated from the body by renal glomerular filtration, which scales with $b = 0.75$ based on BMR. Thus $T_{1/2}$ scales to 0.25 $(1 - 0.75)$. From the perspective of pharmacokinetics, the important parameters in a pharmacokinetic equation are both the clearance (Cl) and volume of distribution (Vd).

When one scales $T_{1/2}$, one is actually scaling to Vd / Cl in the exponent since $T_{1/2} = 0.693\ Vd / Cl$ (equation 7.20, see Chapter 7). If Vd usually scales with a $b = 1$ and Cl to 0.75, the exponent is now $BW^{1-0.75}$, which equals 0.25. In all of these studies, intravenous dosing must be used since formulation variables and differences in absorption would completely confound the analyses.

Scaling of Volume of Distribution.   The Vd of a drug generally is related to the fraction of body mass occupied by body water (see Chapter 4). If a drug distributes primarily through body water or primarily into one tissue that is a constant fraction of total body water, the allometric exponent is 1.0 since body water is directly proportional to BW. If the drug is limited to extracellular fluid, b becomes 0.67. If one is looking at the volume of distribution at steady-state (Vd_{ss}), which is a function of vascular, extracellular, and total body fluid, b will be between 0.67 and 1.0. If the drug is lipophilic, allometric analysis does not produce consistent predictions. Most workers in this field assume that Vd directly correlates to BW ($b = 1.0$); however, as shown with the macrolide data below, this

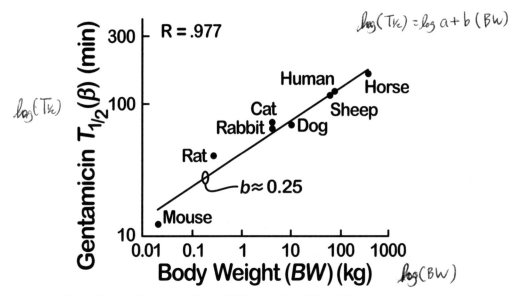

FIGURE 16.2.   Allometric plot of log gentamicin half-life versus log BW in eight species.

may not be accurate. Note that if the species has relatively unique compartments into which drug may distribute and become sequestered or eliminated (e.g., rumen, equine cecum), interspecies extrapolations would fail.

Scaling of Clearance.   For clearances, the situation is more straightforward. Total body clearance (Cl_B) is actually the sum of all clearances $(Cl_B = Cl_{renal} + Cl_{hepatic} + Cl_{other})$ (equation 5.1, see Chapter 5). Most drugs are primarily cleared by either the kidney or the liver. Overall renal and hepatic function are determined by blood flow to these organs, which are dependent upon cardiac output. As mentioned earlier, cardiac output scales to $b \approx 0.75$. Thus, for all drugs cleared by the kidney, renal clearance scales to $b = 0.75$, and thus $T_{1/2}$ should scale to approximately $b = 0.25$. This is even true of drugs excreted by active tubular transport (unless transport is saturated) since renal blood flow governs this function.

For the liver, the hepatic clearance (Cl_h) of a drug has been previously expressed in equation 6.2 (see Chapter 6) as

$$Cl_h = Q_h \, [Cl_{int} / (Q_h + Cl_{int})] \tag{16.2}$$

where Cl_{int} is the intrinsic metabolic clearance of a drug and Q_h the hepatic blood flow, which is a constant fraction of cardiac output. If a drug's Cl_h is "flow limited" when the drug is a "high-extraction drug" $(Cl_{int} >> Q_h)$, its value approaches hepatic blood flow and thus scales with an allometric exponent of $b \approx 0.75$. However, if the drug is "capacity limited" and thus is a "low-extraction drug" $(Cl_{int} << Q_h)$, then clearance is a function of the intrinsic metabolic capability of the individual and species, a value that is very dependent upon isoenzyme expression and other genetic factors. For these drugs, allometric scaling may not be feasible. In fact, these drugs show the greatest interindividual variation in drug disposition.

Relationship Between Parameters.   It is informative to illustrate scaling of all these parameters. An example for a common class of antimicrobials, the macrolides, was reported by Duthu (1985) using data from the mouse, rat, rabbit, dog, and cow. Individual allometric exponents for Vd, Cl, and $T_{1/2}$ were calculated as

	Vd	Cl	$T_{1/2}$
Erythromycin	0.73	0.69	0.14
Oleandomycin	0.64	0.76	0.14
Tylosin	0.75	0.68	0.18

The most robust exponent is $T_{1/2}$, even if Vd and Cl are different (compare erythromycin with oleandomycin). Note for this drug, the b for $Vd \neq 1.0$ (as for gentamicin), and thus the aggregate b was not a simple combination of the allometric exponents for Vd and Cl. By doing studies as above, more confidence can be placed in the allometric extrapolations since data for a specific drug are utilized. Also, allometric techniques are more effective if there is a wide range of BW (e.g., mouse to cow) because of the logarithmic transformation involved. It would not be effective if data were, say, collected in pigs, goats, and sheep.

Protein Binding.   This is a good point at which to consider the extent of protein binding of the drug that was discussed *earlier* in Chapters 4, 6, and 9. The magnitude of protein binding may have a significant effect on drugs cleared by "capacity limited" mechanisms if total protein binding is greater than 85% to 90%. Flow-limited drugs should be insensitive to protein binding, as should capacity-limited drugs with very low protein binding. Secondly, the magnitude of protein binding may also affect the Vd, again with significant levels of protein binding (> 85% to 90%) having the most impact. As will be demonstrated below, allometric scaling should be performed using the free fraction of drug. The major problem with drug protein binding is that there is, at present, no easy way to predict the extent of interspecies binding. As discussed above, many parameters are insensitive to protein binding, and thus allometric relationships are insensitive to changes.

One must also realize that many proteins besides albumin (e.g., α_1-acid glycoproteins, lipoproteins, hormone carrier globulins) may bind to drugs, making interspecies extrapolation problematic in a limited number of cases. For example, our laboratory has studied the disposition of testosterone in pigs as a model for transdermal human drug delivery. Pigs, like rodents and carnivores, are deficient in sex hormone binding globulin compared to humans, primates, rabbits, goats, cows, and sheep. This results in an alteration of the species' ability to metabolize testosterone to dihydrotestosterone and estradiol. This difference in metabolic disposition could not be predicted on the basis of an allometric analysis.

Applications.   There is a great deal of empirical evidence to suggest that the allometric approach of expressing drug dosage scaled to a $(BW)^b$ works. A number of workers allometrically analyzed the maximum tolerated dose (MTD) or LD_{10} of numerous antineoplastic drugs, which relates to the toxic potential of these chemicals across different species. Not surprisingly, b was equal to 0.75. For these compounds, this correlation simply supports the hypothesis that drug action or toxicity is correlated to the area under the curve, as presented throughout this text. This extrapolation holds for most subacute toxicities but does not work for predicting chronic toxicity or carcinogenesis. These effect models are much more complicated and are beyond the scope of the dose extrapolation problem addressed in this chapter (see Chapter 12). Similar types of acute toxicity data have been reanalyzed recently with $b = 0.73$ (95% confidence interval = 0.69 to 0.77).

A similar approach was used by our laboratory to estimate isonephrotoxic doses (i.e., doses that produce the same degree of kidney damage) for gentamicin across species. In this procedure, one essentially calculates a proportion of the dose of drugs in two species based on a ratio of their respective half-lives. In the case of gentamicin, the allometric exponent $b \approx 0.25$ from Figure 16.2 was used in the following equation to estimate species-equivalent doses:

$$D_{Species\ A} = D_{Species\ B}[BW_B / BW_A]^{0.25} \qquad (16.3)$$

where $D_{Species\ B}$ is a dose of known nephrotoxicity in species B. This resulted in the following isonephrotoxic doses (mg/kg–species): 20–rat, 9–dog, 5–human, and 3–horse. These are confirmed by the literature and illustrate why a large species such as the horse would appear more sensitive to a canine dose of 9 mg/kg. Equation 16.3 could be used to extrapolate the dose known to be efficacious in one species and to estimate the therapeutically equivalent dose in another, as suggested for selecting pilot pharmacokinetic trial doses in equation 13.9 (see Chapter 13).

THE CONCEPT OF KALLYNOCHRONS AND SPECIES-INDEPENDENT CONCENTRATION-VERSUS-TIME PROFILES

There is another way to view allometric scaling as simply a method of changing the time coordinates of a serum/blood/plasma concentration-time (C-T) profile from chronological or astronomical time to the more relevant physiological time. Many authors, especially Boxenbaum, strongly argue that physiological processes are linked to an internal biological clock that is a function of *BMR* and body size. This relationship, in turn, is defined by the interaction of the animal with its environment, relative to energy conservation and biomechanical constraints (elasticity), which is related to the surface area of interfacing membranes. Body size can be viewed as a regulating mechanism for a species' internal biological clock. Specifically, each species may have a finite number of heartbeats; thus a mouse, which has a shorter life span (because its *BMR* must be higher due to its small body size), will have a more rapid heart rate when measured in chronological time. Boxenbaum contends that each species also has a finite quantity of "pharmacokinetic stuff" that also is spread over a life span. This is quantitated with a unit of equivalent time across all species equal to the amount of time any species clears the same volume of plasma per unit of *BW*. This is termed a *kallynochron*, which equals

$$\text{Kallynochron} = (\text{time}) / (BW^{1-b}) \qquad (16.4)$$

What this effectively does is scale the time axis of a C-T plot by a measure of physiological time. Thus, if BW scales with $b = 0.75$, then the time axis should be plotted using the above equation. Again, Dedrick and coworkers earlier demonstrated this relationship with methotrexate. Accordingly, this technique is often referred to as a Dedrick plot. However, this assumes that the Y axis (concentration) of a C-T profile also scales "properly"; that is, Vd scales to the same value of b. If this is not true, then the Y axis may also be scaled, and a "complex" Dedrick plot results.

These approaches can best be illustrated using doxycycline pharmacokinetic data generated in our laboratory. In this study, all species were given an intravenous dose of 10 mg/kg. In Figure 16.3, $T_{1/2}$ is plotted against BW using our data and values from the literature. The typical allometric relation is demonstrated. Figure 16.4 is a Dedrick plot of data generated solely from data in our laboratory. In this case, all samples were analyzed by the same high-performance liquid chromatographic assay, which should minimize analytical variation, and parameter estimates obtained by the same pharmacokinetic programs, which should minimize curve-fitting errors. This plot transforms the time axis to

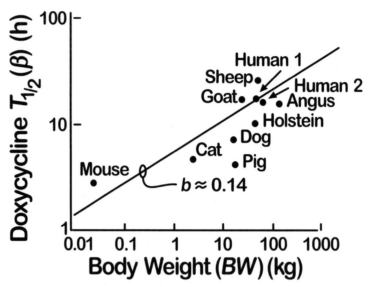

FIGURE 16.3. Allometric plot of log doxycycline half-life versus log BW in nine species.

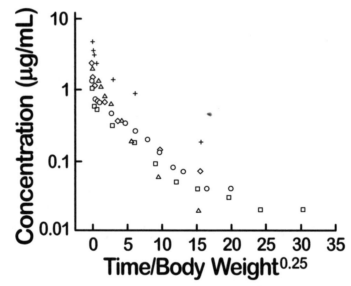

FIGURE 16.4. Dedrick plot of total plasma doxycycline concentrations versus normalized body weight in cats (+), dogs (◊), pigs (△), mature Angus (O), and immature Holstein (□) calves administered a single 10 mg/kg intravenous dose.

kallynochrons and adjusts the plasma concentration (Y axis) to observed concentration divided by dose/kg, thereby normalizing by dose (assumes that b for Vd equals 1.0). Here one can see that the serum concentration-time profile is relatively tight except for the data from cats, which tend to produce higher normalized concentrations than calves, pigs, and dogs. If free doxycycline is plotted (Figure 16.5) from these same five species using ultra-filtered serum to estimate the doxycycline free fraction, a true "species-independent" C-T profile results, which describes the data for all species. The cat is the outlier in the total C-T profile since it uniquely has a very high degree of protein binding ($\cong 98\%$) compared to $\cong 90\%$ for the other species. Thus, the concentration of free drug in the cat is five-fold

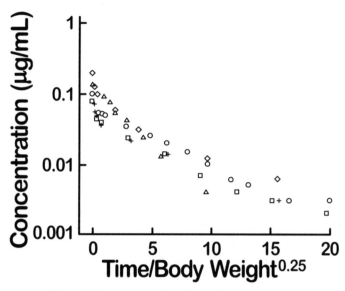

FIGURE 16.5.   Same plot as Figure 16.4 except that free doxycycline concentrations were used, which resulted in better prediction of the cat data. Cats (+), dogs (◊), pigs (Δ), mature Angus (O) and immature Holstein (▢) calves.

higher than other species. The analysis of doxycycline binding to albumin was illustrated in Figures 4.4 and 4.5.

This technique has a tremendous conceptual impact since it clearly indicates that if drug concentrations are expressed in kallynochrons, one C-T profile adequately describes the disposition of drugs across widely disparate species. If one assumes that the action of a drug is correlated to some measure of its C-T profile (e.g., AUC), then if one knows the AUC in one species, one would know it in all species if it was expressed in terms of the more appropriate physiological time. One approach to interspecies scaling is thus to define an effective AUC in species A and calculate a dose per unit BW^b, which could be used for all species. This is another way of generating the isonephrotoxic doses of gentamicin referred to above, for this strategy works if dose is linearly correlated to AUC, an expected finding when the drug has first-order pharmacokinetic properties. Similarly, for the problem of tissue residues presented in Chapter 17, if tissue C-T profiles similarly scale, then withdrawal times for "well-behaved" drugs could be normalized to physiological time and a single parameter used in all species.

EXTRAPOLATION PITFALLS

There are a number of cases, too numerous to outline here, in which interspecies extrapolations would not be expected to work because of complex disposition processes. Our group used the extensive Food Animal Residue Avoidance Databank (FARAD) compilation of 10,300 pharmacokinetic experiments with 419 drugs to assess how well allometry could be used to extrapolate drug disposition for veterinary drugs collected in a database with a wide quality of reported data (Riviere et al, 1997). In this analysis, 44 drugs had sufficient data (intravenous administration, at least four species per drug) to conduct the allometric regression. Three groups of drugs were identified from this meta-analysis.

Eleven drugs (ampicillin, apramycin, carbenicillin, cephapirin, chlortetracycline, diazepam, erythromycin, gentamicin, oxytetracycline, prednisolone, and tetracycline) had statistically significant allometric regressions, with b ranging from 0.1 to 0.415. Significantly, the mean value of the allometric exponent was 0.236 ± 0.09, with 65% of the b's being between 0.19 and 0.32. Thus the rule of thumb quoted above that a *b* for $T_{1/2}$ of 0.25, based on *BMR* scaling factor of 0.75, is a good estimate for most drugs. Plots of these drugs were very similar to the idealization presented in Figure 16.1. These drugs are primarily antibiotics and are eliminated unchanged by the kidney. The only surprise was diazepam since it has a variable degree of protein binding and is cleared by a capacity-limited hepatic metabolic process. Of these well-behaved drugs, the average number of species in the analysis was 6.2 ± 2.2, and the log body weight ratio [log (largest body weight / smallest body weight)] averaged 8. This latter parameter appears to be an excellent metric of how robust the data set is for analysis since a wide spread in log body weights would increase the power of a log-log allometric regression. This analysis suggests that when one has a robust data set covering multiple species of differing masses, and the drug has relatively simple linear pharmacokinetics, allometric scaling is possible even from a multiple-source data set.

Nineteen drugs, although having similarly rich data sets and robust log body-weight ratios, did not have significant allometric regressions. These drugs included many compounds metabolized by capacity-limited hepatic biotransformation. The remainder of the drugs produced equivocal results but were characterized by a smaller species data set. Without further data, it was not possible to determine whether these compounds actually could not be analyzed with allometric principles or if the data set was simply inadequate.

This analysis and those of other workers highlight a number of factors, touched upon in the introduction, which at this point would preclude allometric pharmacokinetic extrapolations.

Biotransformation.   If a drug is eliminated primarily by capacity-limited hepatic biotransformation, total body clearance would be related to $Cl_{intrinsic}$, which is dependent upon the intrinsic ability of that species and individual to metabolize drug. Numerous studies have demonstrated a great deal of heterogeneity in both phase I and phase II drug metabolism reactions. For example, dogs are known to be deficient acetylators, pigs are deficient in sulfation capacity, and cats are deficient in glucuronidation. If a drug is metabolized by one of these phase II pathways, extrapolation might be problematic. However, if the only result is to produce a sulfated rather than an acetylated inactive metabolite, and the C-T profile of the parent drug and active phase I metabolites are not affected, allometry should still work.

Genetic Polymorphism.   The largest and most important species differences relate to genetic differences in cytochrome P_{450} isoenzyme makeup. Although cytochrome content scales to *BW*, species differences in isoenzymes confound one's ability to make predictions. A substantial amount of progress has been made on studying which genes are responsible for controlling P_{450} expression. Chapter 6 should be consulted for specifics. For example, the P_{450} IIIA gene expresses isoenzymes in the rat, dog, and human, which show similar substrate specificity and inhibitor selectivity, with sex differences being expressed only in the rat. If one knew *a priori* that the drug in question was metabolized by an isoenzyme under control of this gene (*N*-demethylation, steroids undergoing 6β hydroxylation), then allometry should work on extrapolating such drugs (flunisolide, cyclosporine, dihydropyridine Ca++ channel blockers). However, the database for which these data are available is sparse at best and, outside of the dog, contains no veterinary species. Secondly, some of these compounds may also be metabolized by isoenzymes controlled by the P_{450} IIC gene which, depending on relative substrate specificities between IIIA and IIC isoenzymes, will produce a different profile of phase I metabolites. The situation becomes very complicated when other genes and non-cytochrome P_{450} enzymes (e.g., flavin monooxygenases) are also considered.

Protein Binding.   As discussed with doxycycline, protein binding is almost impossible to extrapolate across species. Differences in protein binding would be expected to affect *Cl*, *Vd*, and the fraction of a drug dose that can interact with receptors (only free fraction is available). This would be especially evident for orally administered drugs. A similar concern exists with extent of tissue binding.

Saturation.   If the effective dose in any of the species being analyzed produces concentrations that saturate elimination mechanisms, nonlinear pharmacokinetics result, which makes allometry almost impossible. This should not be a problem for most pharmacological doses except where metabolic capacity for a specific pathway is limited (e.g., cats and glucuronidation).

Drug Induces Alterations in Physiology.   Up to this point, we have considered drugs to be pharmacologically inert. If the drug alters physiology (e.g., renal function, hepatic blood flow) in one species and not another, then the allometric relation of physiology to *BW* will be broken and interspecies scaling will not work. In the doxycycline example discussed above, such a situation occurred when single-dose intravenous pharmacokinetic studies were attempted in the horse (note the absence of equine data in these plots). When two horses were injected with this 10-mg/kg dose, they immediately went into cardiac arrest and died, a phenomenon later attributed to the high lipophilicity of the doxycycline, which gave it immediate "access" to cardiac pacemaker cells. This illustrates again that pharmacokinetic data alone are not sufficient to predict pharmacodynamic effect.

Interspecies Differences in Enterohepatic Recirculation.   If a large fraction of a drug is cleared via the bile, and the species differences outlined in Chapter 6 result in changes in the fraction of biliary-excreted drug reabsorbed back into the circulation, pharmacokinetic parameters may not scale well across species. This does not appear to be a major problem since in the FARAD analysis discussed above, many tetracyclines potentially fall into this class, and these drugs were well behaved from the perspective of allometric regression. The same may not hold for drugs cleared primarily by this route.

Renal Tubular Reabsorption Sensitive to Urine pH.   As discussed in Chapter 5, the clearance of some weak acids and bases may be dependent upon distal renal tubular reabsorption, a process that would be sensitive to species differences in urine pH. Carnivores tend to have an acidic urine based on their normal protein-rich diet, while ruminants tend to have an alkaline urine. Depending upon the species included in an allometric analysis and the diets of the animals being studied, one could speculate that weak organic acids with pKa values from 3 to 7 may have a decreased $T_{1/2}$ when urine is alkaline. The opposite would occur with weak bases.

There are probably a number of additional factors that could influence the efficacy of an allometric regression analysis. For example, body weight could be corrected for the volume of the gastrointestinal tract when ruminants and nonruminants are compared since the rumen may represent a substantial fraction of nonavailable body mass into which drug could not distribute.

CONCLUSION

As can be appreciated, scaling pharmacokinetic parameters using allometry is a powerful tool to eliminate the influence of body mass on the value of pharmacokinetic parameters. This technique is applicable to data generated using compartmental and noncompartmental models. One approach that appears useful is to use neural-net techniques, encountered in various sections of this text, to make these extrapolations. However, as presently implemented, the resulting models lack mechanistic foundations and are an example of a purely empirical approach to data analysis.

An optimal approach would be to use PBPK techniques if the relevant experiments could be conducted to generate the necessary input parameters. However, an equally promising approach would be to use population-based models as presented in Chapter 14. If these models are linked to normalized data such as presented in Figure 16.5, the power of this technique could be used to correlate unexplained variance to measurable physiological correlates, such as extent of protein binding, creatinine clearance, markers of hepatic blood flow, and rate of biliary secretion. This approach would also allow interindividual and intraindividual variation to be accounted for and quantitated.

SELECTED READINGS

Boxenbaum, H. 1982. Interspecies scaling, allometry, physiological time, and the ground plan for pharmacokinetics. *Journal of Pharmacokinetics and Biopharmaceutics.* 10: 201-227.

Boxenbaum, H., and C. DiLea. 1995. First-time-in-human dose selection: Allometric thoughts and perspectives. *Journal of Clinical Pharmacology.* 35:957-966.

Boxenbaum, H., and R.W. D'Souza. 1990. Interspecies pharmacokinetic scaling, biological design, and neoteny. *Advances in Drug Research.* 19:139-196.

Brown, S.A., and J.E. Riviere. 1991. Comparative pharmacokinetics of aminoglycoside antibiotics. *Journal of Veterinary Pharmacology and Therapeutics.* 14:1-35.

Calabrese, E.J. 1983. *Principles of Animal Extrapolation.* New York: John Wiley & Sons.

Corvol, P., and C.W. Bardon. Species distribution of testosterone binding globulin. *Biology of Reproduction* 8:277-282.

Davidson, I.W.F., J.C. Parker, and R.P. Beliles. 1986. Biological basis for extrapolation across mammalian species. *Regulatory Pharmacology and Toxicology.* 6:211-237.

Dedrick, R.L., K.B. Bischoff, and D.S. Zaharko. 1970. Interspecies correlation of plasma concentration history of methotrexate (NSC-740). *Cancer Chemotherapy Reports Part 1.* 54:95-101.

Duthu, G.S. 1985. Interspecies correlation of the pharmacokinetics of erythromycin, oleandomycin and tylosin. *Journal of Pharmaceutical Sciences.* 74:943-946.

Hayton, W.L. 1989. Pharmacokinetic parameters for interspecies scaling using allometric principles. *Health Physics.* 57:159-164.

Mordenti, J. 1985. Pharmacokinetic scale-up: Accurate prediction of human pharmacokinetic profiles from animal data. *Journal of Pharmaceutical Sciences.* 74:1097-1099.

Mordenti, J. 1986. Man versus beast. Pharmacokinetic scaling in mammals. *Journal of Pharmaceutical Sciences.* 75:1028-1039.

O'Flaherty, E.J. 1989. Interspecies conversion of kinetically equivalent doses. *Risk Analysis.* 9:587-598.

Reilly, J.J., and P. Workman. 1993. Normalisation of anti-cancer drug dosage using body weight and surface area: Is it worthwhile? *Cancer Chemotherapy Pharmacology.* 32: 411-418.

Riond, J.L., and J.E. Riviere. Allometric analysis of doxycycline pharmacokinetic parameters. *Journal of Veterinary Pharmacology and Therapeutics.* 13:404-407.

Riond, J.L., J.E. Riviere, W.M. Duckett, C.E. Atkins, A.D. Jernigan, Y. Rikihisa, and S.L. Spurlock. 1992. Cardiovascular effects and fatalities associated with intravenous administration of doxycycline to horses and ponies. *Equine Veterinary Journal.* 24:41-45.

Riviere, J.E. 1985. Aminoglycoside-induced toxic nephropathy. In *Handbook of Animal Models for Renal Failure*, ed. S.R. Ash and J.A. Thornhill, 145-182. Boca Raton, FL: CRC Press.

Riviere, J.E., T. Martín-Jiménez, S.F. Sundlof, and A.L. Craigmill. 1987. Interspecies allometric analysis of the comparative pharmacokinetics of 44 drugs across veterinary and laboratory animal species. *Journal of Veterinary Pharmacology and Therapeutics* 20:453-463.

Sawada, Y., M. Hanano, Y. Sugiyama, H. Harashima, and T. Iga. 1984. Prediction of the volumes of distribution of basic drugs in humans based on data from animals. *Journal of Pharmacokinetics and Biopharmaceutics.* 12:587-596.

United States Environmental Protection Agency. 1984. Proposed guidelines for carcinogen risk assessment. *Federal Register.* 49:46294-46301.

Voisin, E.M., M. Ruthsatz, J.M. Collins, and P.C. Hoyle. 1990. Extrapolation of animal toxicity to humans. Interspecies comparisons in drug development. *Regulatory Toxicology and Pharmacology.* 12:107-116.

West, G.B., J.H. Brown, and B.J. Enquist. 1997. A general model for the origin of allometric scaling laws in biology. *Science* 276:122-126.

17

Tissue Residues and Withdrawal Times

The final application of pharmacokinetic principles will be to describe the tissue disposition of drugs after administration to food-producing animals. The concept of a withdrawal time will be developed as essentially an extension of the concept of half-life. This topic is increasing in importance to veterinarians working in food animal medicine and scientists employed in the pharmaceutical and regulatory sectors who are charged with assessing the fate of drugs and chemicals that enter the human food chain via the edible products (meat, milk, eggs) of food-producing animals. As can be appreciated by reexamining Figure 1.3 (see Chapter 1), there is an additional constraint besides efficacy and safety when drugs are used to treat diseases in food-producing animals. When the animal is slaughtered or its edible products collected, there is a legal requirement that drug concentrations not persist at a level greater than those established as safe by the relevant regulatory authority in the country of origin. In the United States, this upper level is termed the *tolerance*, while in many other countries it is referred to as the *maximum residue level* (MRL).

MRLs and tolerances are established by regulatory authorities based on many factors primarily relating to the safety of the animal product to the consumer, the usage pattern of the compound (e.g., pesticide in the field), and analytical methodology. The major determining factor is food safety. However, from the perspective of pharmacokinetics, the method used to arrive at a tolerance or MRL is not important; rather the focus is on the length of time after discontinuation of drug administration or chemical exposure required to allow a tissue to deplete to a concentration below this legal limit. This is the pre-slaughter meat withdrawal time (WDT). If the matrix is milk, then the parameter of interest is the milk discard interval (MDI). Most discussion here will be focused on the WDT as the principles apply equally well to the MDI. Exceptions to this rule will be identified as required.

What is the WDT? As with all pharmacokinetic parameters, the WDT has both kinetic and statistical properties. We will initially focus our discussion on the individual animal and consider the factors that determine the rate of depletion of drug concentrations in specific tissues. The first step is to establish the target concentration in tissue.

ESTABLISHMENT OF A TISSUE TOLERANCE

The tolerance is the target concentration in a residue depletion study. It should be established purely on the basis of safety to the person consuming the tissue and has no pharmacodynamic reality in the animal to which the drug has been administered. Tissue tolerances are normally established in fat, milk, muscle (or sometimes meat by-products), liver, kidney, or skin, or they are combined as edible tissues. The first step in calculating the tolerance is to determine the safe concentration of drug that could be consumed by individuals eating the animal product:

$$\text{Safe concentration} = \frac{(\text{ADI})\,(\text{Body weight})}{\text{Food consumption factor}} \quad\quad (17.1)$$

where ADI is the acceptable daily intake, body weight is the average weight of humans consuming the product (usually assumed to be 60 kg), and the food consumption factor is the amount of edible product estimated to be consumed daily by an individual. The purpose of this equation is to distribute the ADI over different edible tissues on the basis of food consumption patterns.

The food consumption factor is based upon the average individual's daily intake of different types of foods. The Food and Drug Administration (FDA) and other regulatory agencies have tabulated food-specific consumption factors. Examples (kg consumed per day) are 0.3 for muscle, 0.1 for liver, 0.05 for kidney, 0.05 for fat, and 1.5 for milk. The latter is especially high since the total diet for an infant may be entirely milk. An equal amount of the ADI is also assigned independently to milk to protect the infant. Other countries use similar food consumption factors but distribute the ADI based on independent organ consumption data. These factors are then used in equation 17.1 to determine safe concentrations.

The most controversial component of this equation is the establishment of the ADI, which involves a risk assessment extrapolation from laboratory animal toxicology studies. The ADI is the maximum amount of chemical (mg/kg) that may be consumed daily over a lifetime without producing an adverse effect. ADI is estimated as a fraction of the no-observed-adverse-effect-level (NOAEL) determined from standardized long-term laboratory animal toxicological studies conducted in at least two animal species. The NOAEL is then divided by a safety factor ranging from 100 to 1000 depending on the nature of the compound's toxicology or the strength of the data. Part of this factor is to account for the vagaries of interspecies extrapolations (rodent to human) and to be conservative in the face of more acute and serious toxicity (teratogens, hypersensitivity, etc.). The current FDA safety factors are the following:

Type of Toxicology Study	Safety Factor
Chronic	100
90 Day	1000
Reproductive/teratology	100 (only maternal effects)
	1000 (other effects)

As can be appreciated from this tabulation, the safety factor is greater when there is evidence of teratogenic effects or when a more economical subchronic (90-day) study is submitted in place of a more complete chronic study. This latter factor alone could result in a tenfold lower tolerance (and hence longer withdrawal time) being established for a product supported by 90-day studies compared to the identical formulation supported by a chronic study. Thus, a subjective bias is directly built into the analysis that is independent of the actual toxicological properties of the compound. Recently, additional toxicology tests (neurotoxicity, immunotoxicity, hormonal activity, etc.) have also been accepted for assessing potential toxicity (or lack thereof) and are handled similarly to the 90-day data above. Other countries use similar approaches, although the safety factors applied at this stage of the analysis (determination of ADI) generally do not exceed 100.

If the compound is demonstrated to be a carcinogen, a "no-risk" requirement comes into effect. In this case, a risk assessment/extrapolation analysis will be done, using statistical analysis of the laboratory animal tumor data, to derive a concentration of residue (S_0) that *presents no significant risk of cancer*. If there is no information on the compound concerning the mechanism of carcinogenesis, the FDA uses a nonthreshold, linear-at-low dose extrapolation to determine the upper limit of the risk, which is set at 1:1,000,000. An exception to this rule is if the compound is a sex steroid, in which case the agents are assumed not to be genotoxic and at low residue levels do not present a risk for carcinogenesis in the food-consuming public. Other countries adopt different policies for reproductively active compounds.

The final step is to establish the tolerance. The safe concentration is based upon the total concentration of drug (e.g., total residues), which includes the parent drug and any metabolites. Some special regulations apply for covalently bound residues. Depending on the drug, bound residues may be included as either a component of the total or a fraction removed from consideration. A marker residue is now selected that has a defined relationship to the total residues. If the drug is not metabolized, the safe concentration becomes the tolerance. If the drug is metabolized, the tolerance will be a fraction of the safe concentration. Equation 17.1 is then applied for each food source using the organ-specific consumption factors and tolerances established. As discussed below, the tolerance should also not be based on analytical sensitivity, since if the tolerance is below the ability to detect the compound, the resulting withdrawal time will be exceedingly conservative relative to food safety concerns.

The process of establishing MRLs in many other countries is very similar except that, as mentioned earlier, the safe concentration may be partitioned across various organs under the assumption that any one individual could never consume all foods with drug present at the maximum safe concentrations. It must be stressed that tolerances are based on human food safety considerations for the consuming public and not on how long a withdrawal time is required to achieve tolerance. However, in some countries, the concept of good veterinary practices is applied to establish an MRL that may be lower than the ADI safe concentration.

ESTIMATION OF A WITHDRAWAL TIME

The next step is to define the WDT necessary to ensure that the residue being monitored will fall below the established tolerance or MRL. Figure 17.1 illustrates this relationship. Note that if the total residue is the marker residue, then the safe concentration is equal to the tolerance. This process must be repeated with the major organs in which safe concentrations are established, with the final WDT being the longest time at which all tissues will be below the established tolerance. Numerous experimental designs are used to establish the withdrawal time. The FDA presently requires a repeated slaughter experiment in which groups of at least five animals per sex are slaughtered at four time periods in the terminal part of the tissue-depletion curve closest to the established tolerance. A log-linear regression analysis is then performed on the data to determine the withdrawal time such that *the WDT is the upper bound of the 99th percentile of the population established with 95% statistical confidence (α probability of a type I error at 5%)*. As can be appreciated from Figure 17.2, this essentially sets the official withdrawal time such that the 1 in 100 animals with the most persistent residue profile determines the acceptable tolerance.

The many assumptions behind these statistics include a log-linear tissue depletion phase, a log-normal statistical distribution for all residue samples at each time point, homogeneous variance of residues across the various slaughter times, and statistical inde-

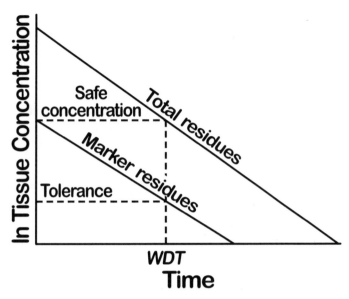

FIGURE 17.1.   Relationship between log-linear tissue depletion of total and marker residues and the established safe concentration and tolerance in that tissue. The withdrawal time (*WDT*) is the time at which total residues are below safe concentrations. This establishes the legal tolerance for monitored marker residue. Note that if the total residue equals the marker residue, the safe concentration becomes the tolerance.

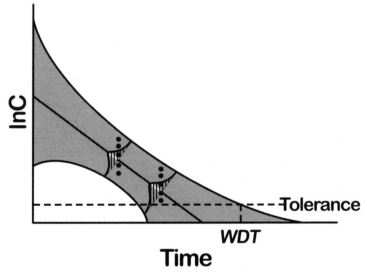

FIGURE 17.2.   Statistical perspective of drug depletion in tissue whereby tolerance is established based on the upper 99% percentile of the distribution centered on the mean tissue depletion profile.

pendence of each residue observation. Many sponsors will increase the number of animals collected at any time point in order to narrow the 99th percentile window, which will result in a shorter WDT.

Based upon the reader's previous exposure to the statistical aspects of drug disposition data presented in Chapters 13 and 14, it is obvious that many of these assumptions may not be valid. The most obvious problem is that a homogenous population of healthy animals is required and, further, that this population is a representative sample of all animals

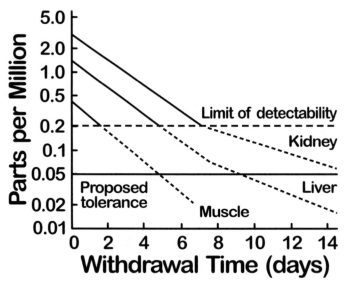

FIGURE 17.3.   Non-parallel tissue depletion profiles and their relationship to the limit of detectability and tolerances. Note that as in this case, if the limit of detectability is greater than the tolerance based on food safety factors, the withdrawal time subsequently established will be conservative.

to which the drug will be administered. As was seen in the discussion of population pharmacokinetic models, most populations of animals are not homogeneous, being composed of various subpopulations based on age, breed, and multiple disease states. Withdrawal studies are done in healthy animals, but drugs are administered to the general population, which would be expected to have a larger variability (recall Chapter 14, Figure 14.1). Log-linear terminal tissue decay is also assumed. Many factors, such as redistribution or enterohepatic recycling, may complicate this decay. Homogenous variance of measured residue concentrations is unlikely since, as analytical sensitivity approaches the tolerance, coefficients of variation are often larger than that seen at more reliably assayed higher concentrations. This scenario was depicted in the bottom panel of Figure 13.3. This is especially troubling when the tolerance is set near the limit of quantitation (LOQ) for the assay being used. Finally, most statistics are based on determining the mean parameter of a distribution, and deviations from normality are minimal due to the operation of the Central Limit Theorem. In contrast, WDTs are estimated based on defining the upper tail of the distribution (1% of the population), which is estimated based on a small number of individuals relative to the population. Unlike the mean, this estimate is sensitive to the nature of the underlying variance model.

Another complicating factor is that the slopes of drug depletion in various tissues are often not parallel, as depicted in Figure 17.3. This is not surprising since most tissues are not in the "central compartment" and thus have a depletion reflecting local distribution processes. This figure also illustrates the dilemma present when the LOQ is greater than tolerance or MRL. Differential rates of tissue decay were discussed in the context of Figure 4.2 (see Chapter 4), which also illustrates the relationship between drug decay in various tissues and the organ-specific tolerances set for each tissue. In this case, using gentamicin, although muscle concentrations fall below tolerance after 72 hours, kidney and liver concentrations never decay in this short time frame due to the extensive tissue binding of aminoglycosides. Thus, WDTs must be set based on the kidney concentrations, which may require up to an 18-month preslaughter WDT. In some countries, an option termed *selective condemnation* has been proposed, whereby the shorter muscle-based WDTs are allowed as long as the liver and kidney are discarded at slaughter.

Some discussion among regulatory authorities outside the United States have focused on non–regression-based determination of WDTs. In these situations, a WDT is established as the slaughter time at which all animals are below tolerance. The actual WDT is being tested, not the slope of the tissue depletion, which is the parameter being modeled with parametric approaches. Other workers have proposed various nonparametric statistics to implement this practice with more statistical confidence. The factors involved in selecting the appropriate approach are actually identical to those used in selecting parametric versus nonparametric methods for population pharmacokinetic studies.

PHARMACOKINETICS APPLIED TO WITHDRAWAL TIMES

Whatever the final method used to establish a WDT in an individual animal, the WDT is closely related to the rate of elimination, and thus the half-life of drug depletion in the specific tissue of interest. *Based on linear pharmacokinetic principles developed in Chapter 7, the problem of estimating a WDT is essentially that of calculating the time for a concentration to decline to a specific target concentration, which in our case is the tolerance.* One can extend the logic presented in equation 11.8 (see Chapter 11), which was used to calculate the length of a dosage interval τ to maintain a concentration-time profile between defined peak (Cp^{max}) and trough (Cp^{min}) concentrations to calculate WDT. In this case, we assume linear first-order decay in the tissue of interest, and we will express the equations in terms of target residue concentrations. Because this relation is central to the concept of *WDT*, we will follow through each step of its derivation. The τ we are thus calculating is the final interval after dosing which is required to achieve a C_t^{min} equal to the established tolerance or MRL. Equation 11.8 may be originally written as

$$\ln \ (Cp^{max} \ / \ Cp^{min}) = (0.693 \ / \ T_{1/2}) \ \tau \tag{17.2}$$

This can be algebraically rearranged to solve for τ as

$$\tau = \ln \ (Cp^{max} \ / \ Cp^{min}) \ / \ (0.693 \ / \ T_{1/2}) \tag{17.3}$$

If we now substitute WDT for τ, C_0 for Cp^{max}, and finally TOL for Cp^{min} (C now represents tissue concentrations), we obtain the relation

$$WDT = \ln \ (C_0 \ / \ TOL) \ / \ (0.693 \ / \ T_{1/2})$$
$$= 1.44 \ \ln \ (C_0 \ / \ TOL) \ T_{1/2} \tag{17.4}$$

Note the similarity to equation 11.9 for dosage interval. Since we know that the slope of the tissue decay, K equals $0.693 \ / \ T_{1/2}$, this equation can be also written as

$$WDT = \ln \ (C_0 \ / \ TOL) \ / \ K \tag{17.5}$$

Therefore, knowing the initial tissue concentration, tissue $T_{1/2}$ or K, and the legal target tolerance, one should be able to calculate the *WDT* for a specific situation. If the disposition of the drug is described by a simple pharmacokinetic model, C_0 can often be estimated from the administered dose using this data. Compilations of plasma and tissue depletion $T_{1/2}$ and C_0 for many common drugs in species of relevance to veterinary medicine have been published in a CRC Handbook Series from data in the Food Animal Residue Avoidance Databank (FARAD).

The problem of using this approach in the field or a regulatory environment is that a priori knowledge of the tissue half-life in a living animal is impossible to determine prior to slaughter. A population estimate (see Chapter 14) of tissue $T_{1/2}$ is required which, according to regulatory philosophy, accurately predicts with statistical confidence of $\alpha <$ 0.05, the $T_{1/2}$ that would be present in the 1% of the target population that has the slowest rate of drug decay in the tolerance-limiting tissue. The reader must realize that the approved *WDT* must account for the *outliers* in the treated animals to ensure that the probability of a violative residue in any animal treated with drug is vanishingly small. One is therefore not interested in the estimate of the *mean* value of $T_{1/2}$ which would be operative in the animal being treated, but rather the upper limit of 99% of the population estimated with a 95% confidence interval of this value. As discussed above, the statistical assumptions used to estimate this limit are prone to error and are heavily dependent upon the yet unknown statistical distributions used to establish the *WDT* in the first place.

GUESSTIMATING WITHDRAWAL INTERVALS AFTER EXTRALABEL USE

The reason that these issues are important relates to the need to have knowledge of the tissue half-life to modify *WDT* in cases in which the drug is used in an extralabel manner. This practice was approved by the FDA under the recently implemented guidelines of the Animal Medicinal Drug Use Clarification Act of 1994 (AMDUCA), which were published in 1997. In this scenario, drugs may be used in an extralabel manner if the veterinarian is able to *establish a substantially extended withdrawal period prior to marketing of milk, meat, eggs, or other edible products supported by appropriate scientific information.* To accomplish this, the veterinarian must have some estimate of the relevant tissue $T_{1/2}$ that governs the *WDT* in the animal being treated and, further, how that $T_{1/2}$ relates to the legal *WDT*.

The most common field scenarios are when the dose is increased in order to improve efficacy and when a disease process is present that prolongs $T_{1/2}$. Figure 17.4 illustrates these relationships assuming that the length of the withdrawal time is directly related to the $T_{1/2}$ according to equation 17.4. If the dose is doubled, C_0 doubles, and the *WDT* should be increased by one $T_{1/2}$. However, if the $T_{1/2}$ doubles due to a systemic disease process, then the *WDT* should also be doubled.

One should immediately realize that the most serious threat to violative residues is when the underlying tissue $T_{1/2}$ changes, since this would most dramatically increase the true *WDT* in that animal. If such a disease process were not present in the animals in which the *WTD* was originally established, then the label-recommended *WDT* may be insufficient to guarantee residues lower than tolerance. In fact, this conclusion is supported by field residue violation data in which a significant number of violative residues are detected either in very young animals, such as veal calves or, alternatively, in culled dairy cows and other emergency slaughtered ruminants that are removed from production because of disease processes. In the immature animal, excretory systems are often not matured, resulting in decreased systemic clearance (Cl_B), and thus a prolonged $T_{1/2}$ (Chapter 7, equation 7.20). As discussed in Chapter 4, volumes of distribution may be greater in very young or diseased individuals, which would likewise prolong $T_{1/2}$. To compound this situation, the culled animals are often treated with drugs to cure their underlying diseases, and thus extralabel drug use would be expected to be greatest in these animals. In the healthy animal not receiving drugs, it is of little surprise that drug residues are not found!

These extrapolations are further complicated when the *WDT* is based on a marker residue and only information about the parent drug's disposition is available. Disease processes that alter the ratio of parent drug to metabolite (in this case the marker residue) may not predict the alteration of withdrawal time necessary to prevent residues. Processes

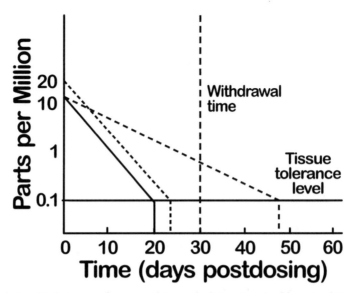

FIGURE 17.4. Relationship between tolerance and tissue depletion. In a healthy animal (—), tissue depletion often occurs at a time point shorter than the withdrawal time established for the 99th percentile of the population. In such an animal, if the dose is doubled, depletion (----) should only require one more half-life and would most likely still be within the established withdrawal time. However, if the half-life is doubled due to disease, depletion (---) would now require double the normal withdrawal time and probably would result in violative residues.

that alter the expression of genes that modulate drug-metabolizing isoenzymes would have similar effects. Problems could exist with changes in protein and/or tissue binding that alter the free fraction of the drug disproportionately to the marker residue.

The only solution to precisely predict these effects is to have a complete pharmacokinetic model defined that adequately predicts tissue concentrations as a function of administered dose. Based on the earlier chapters of this text, physiologically based or population pharmacokinetic models would be optimal due to their sensitivity to physiological and disease factors that might alter disposition. For example, a PBPK model similar to Figure 10.1 (see Chapter 10), incorporating tissue-binding phenomena as depicted in Figure 9.11 (see Chapter 9), would produce data that would be appropriate for estimating when tissue concentrations fall below accepted tolerances. However, these models are generally based on a relatively few individuals, thus making statistical inferences about 1% of the population problematic. In contrast, population pharmacokinetic models can easily integrate the statistical properties of the population and assay methodology; however, they are generally of a simpler inherent structure, which lacks good estimates of plasma to tissue transfer constants. This approach would also allow incorporation of field residue monitoring data to improve the parameterization of the underlying model. Finally, clinical and production variables linked to the proper pharmacokinetic terms could then be used to tailor the withdrawal estimates to individual or herd conditions.

A possible solution is to couple a multicompartment model to either a parametric or nonparametric population approach. One should recall the limitations presented in Chapter 7 and ensure that the model selected actually describes the tissue-concentration profile at the low concentrations relevant for residues (revisit Chapter 7, Table 7.3). The parathion model depicted in Figure 7.24 could serve as the basis for such an approach if specific organs were coupled to compartments. In all probability, the solution will reside in a *hybrid* approach utilizing one of the many pharmacokinetic approaches presented throughout this book. However, this is unlikely to be routinely established as part of the regulatory process since the data requirements would be cost-prohibitive. Bayesian techniques could be adopted that use the pharmacokinetic data as initial estimates in a model to design the regulatory study. The resulting slaughter data would then serve two purposes: (1) to establish the withdrawal time by accepted regulatory standards and (2) to serve as feedback to adjust the parameters of the underlying model. Any additional drug concentrations obtained from field/clinical studies would then further improve the model.

Complexities in tissue depletion profiles such as nonlinearities due to tissue sequestration, extensive tissue binding, or systemic multicompartmental behavior projected on the individual tissue depletion profile thus make the analysis of *WDTs* more complex. However, as discussed in Chapter 8 and illustrated in Figure 8.7, stochastic modeling procedures such as the power function analysis would collapse these more complex kinetics into a scaleable model that would eliminate some of the complexity. The concept of random walk is also mechanistically compatible with tissue residue formation.

If the worker has reliable tissue depletion data available, and has a good estimate of the plasma pharmacokinetic model that would allow estimation of C_0 after any therapeutic dose, equations 17.4 or 17.5 may be directly used to calculate withdrawal time, assuming that the appropriate statistical inferences required by regulatory agencies are taken into consideration.

When an extravascular dose is being administered, an assessment must be made of the rate of absorption and bioavailability to assess whether a *flip-flop* scenario is occurring that would make the absorption $T_{1/2}$ the relevant parameter for use in the above equations. Such adjustments would be expected with extended-release formulations. Similarly, when drug is administered continuously in feed or water, the rate of gastrointestinal input is constant and thus should be modeled by a zero-order rate parameter, much as an intravenous infusion would be handled. However, in this case, the systemic availability would reduce the absorbed dose. Experimental variables that could be shown to alter tissue depletion would provide qualitative feedback to identify scenarios in which withdrawal time may have to be further adjusted.

All of these techniques are more easily applied to milk depletion data because the matrix of food safety concern is easily obtained and directly assayed. This allows the individual animal to be monitored if reliable analytical methodology is available. It allows the veterinarian to estimate a milk withholding interval and test its validity by direct sampling. As of the writing of this text, there are a number of commercially available *screening assays* that are designed to detect milk drug concentrations greater than tolerance levels. These assays, based on enzyme or microbial inhibition strategies, may be applied to the individual animal, dairy, or milk producer cooperative. The problem with these assays, especially those designed to monitor antimicrobial substances, is a lack of specificity for the drugs being monitored and a tendency to produce false-positive readings when correlated back to more specific analytical techniques. False-positives have negative economic implications for the producers and may not be conducive to protecting food safety. Some of these tests are also available to test the urine of treated animals; however, the assumption here is that urine excretion profiles correlate to concentrations of drug in tissues. Without a pharmacokinetic model to quantitate this relationship, extrapolation is difficult.

CONCLUSION

In conclusion, there is nothing unique in the use of pharmacokinetic principles to describe tissue depletion data. The challenge comes in integrating the science with the requirements of regulatory authorities that have preestablished experimental protocols designed to ensure food safety for the consuming public. The design of the experiments discussed above is a result of considerable effort and dialogue among government, industry, and consumer groups. Designs are periodically modified by changing legislative initiatives and public pressure. Although the "governing science" is in the discipline of pharmacokinetics, the experimental procedures practiced are not optimized for defining or solving these models. However, the principles of pharmacokinetics still describe the behavior of drugs in tissues and are fundamentally applicable to interpreting drug-withdrawal information.

SELECTED READINGS

Anonymous. 1994. *General Principles for Evaluating the Safety of Compounds Used in Food-Producing Animals.* Rockville, MD: Center for Veterinary Medicine, Food and Drug Administration.

Bevill, R.F. 1984. Factors influencing the occurrence of drug residues in animal tissues after the use of antimicrobial agents in animal feeds. *Journal of the American Veterinary Medical Association.* 185:1124-1126.

Concordet, D, and P.L. Toutain. 1997. The withdrawal time estimation of veterinary drugs: A non-parametric approach. *Journal of Veterinary Pharmacology and Therapeutics.* 20:374-379.

Concordet, D, and P.L. Toutain. 1997. The withdrawal time estimation of veterinary drugs revisited. *Journal of Veterinary Pharmacology and Therapeutics.* 20:380-386.

Craigmill, A.L., S.F. Sundlof, and J.E. Riviere. 1994. *Handbook of Comparative Pharmacokinetics and Residues of Veterinary Therapeutic Drugs.* Boca Raton, FL: CRC Press.

Fitzpatrick, S.C., S.D. Brynes, and G.B. Guest. 1995. Dietary intake estimates as a means to the harmonization of maximum residue levels for veterinary drugs. *Journal of Veterinary Pharmacology and Therapeutics.* 18:325-327.

Gallo-Torres, H.E. 1990. The rat as a drug residue bioavailability model. *Drug Metabolism Reviews.* 22:707-751.

Lu, A.Y.H., G.T. Miwa, and P.G. Wislocki., 1988. Toxicological significance of covalently bound residues. *Reviews in Biochemical Toxicology.* 9:1-27.

Moats, W.A., and M.B. Medina. 1995. *Veterinary Drug Residues: Food Safety.* Washington, D.C.: American Chemical Society.

Paige, J.C., L. Tollefson, and M. Miller. 1997. Public health impact on drug residues in animal tissues. *Veterinary and Human Toxicology.* 39:162-169.

Rico, A.G. 1986. *Drug Residues in Animals.* New York: Academic Press.

Riviere, J.E. 1991. Pharmacologic principles of residue avoidance for the practitioner. *Journal of the American Veterinary Medical Association.* 198:809-816.

Riviere, J.E., A.L. Craigmill, and S.F. Sundlof. 1991. *Handbook of Comparative Pharmacokinetics and Residues of Veterinary Antimicrobials.* Boca Raton, FL: CRC Press.

Sundlof, S.F. 1989. Drug and chemical residues in livestock. *Veterinary Clinics of North America. Food Animal Practice.* 5:411-447.

Sundlof, S.F. 1994. Human risks associated with drug residues in animal derived food. *Journal of Agrimedicine.* 1:5-22.

Sundlof, S.F., J.E. Riviere, and A.L. Craigmill. 1995. *Handbook of Comparative Veterinary Pharmacokinetics and Residues of Pesticides and Environmental Contaminants.* Boca Raton, FL: CRC Press.

VanDresser, W.R., and J.R. Wilcke. 1989. Drug residues in food animals. *Journal of the American Veterinary Medical Association.* 194:1700-1710.

Weiss, G. The integration of pharmacological and toxicological testing of tissue residues in the evaluation of their human food safety. *Drug Metabolism Reviews.* 22:829-848.

Index

Absorption, 21–45
  bioavailability, 43–45
  curve stripping, 122–23
  gastrointestinal, 21–30
    active transport, 25
    disintegration, 24
    dissolution, 24
    enterohepatic recycling, 25–26
    first-pass metabolism, 27–28
    formulation factors, drug, 29–30
    models, 28–29
    pH effects, 24–25
    regional variations in, 22–24
    species differences in, 26–27
  mean absorption time (MAT), 157
  nonlinear, 180–81
  overview, 11–20
  parameter estimation from urine data, 123–24
  parenteral drug administration, 41–43
  pH partitioning, 15–18
  renal
    active tubular, 67–69
    nonlinearity of, 76–79
    passive tubular, 69–71
  respiratory, 37–41
    aerosols and particulates, 40–41
    structure and function, 37–39
    vapors and gases, 39–40
  topical and percutaneous, 30–37
    body region variations, 36
    metabolism, cutaneous, 36
    models, 37
    modulating factors, 36–37
    pathways, 34–36
    skin structure, 30–31, 33
    species differences in, 36
    stratum corneum barrier, 31–33
  in a two-compartment model, 134–35
  Wagner-Nelson method and, 124–26
Acceptable daily intake, 309
Accumulation, drug. See also Tissue residues
  multiple-dose regimens, 206–7

Acetaminophen and renal metabolism, 71
Acetone, induction by, 93–94
Acids, membrane passage by, 15–17
Active transport, 18
  into bile, 95
  in brain, 51–52
  in renal tubules, 67–69
  in respiratory systems, 41
  in vitro studies of, 28
ADH (antidiuretic hormone), 64
Administration route, 189. See also specific routes
Aerosols and respiratory absorption, 40–41
Age as a variable, 261–62
Ah receptor, 93
Aikake's Information Criterion (AIC), 246–47
Albumin. See also Plasma proteins and drug
        distribution
  drugs binding to, 52, 54–57
  uremia and, 284
Aldosterone, 64
Allometry, 4, 279
  basis of, 297
  scaling, 297–301
Alveoli. See Respiratory system
Aminoglycosides
  nephrotoxicity, 212
  peak concentration and efficacy, 210, 212
  pinocytosis uptake, renal, 70–71
  three-compartment models and, 137
Amount remaining to be excreted (ARE), 118
Amphipathic drugs, bile excretion of, 14, 100
Animal Medicinal Drug Use Clarification Act
        (AMDUCA), 9, 314
Antidiuretic hormone (ADH), 64
Antimicrobials. See also specific drugs
  diuretics and, 285
  efficacy, 210–12
  interspecies extrapolation, 296
  minimum inhibitory concentration, 4, 210–12
Area under the curve (AUC)
  AUMC (moment curve), 150, 152, 155–56
  bioequivalence determination, 157

Area under the curve (AUC) (*continued*)
  defined, 44
  dosage regimens and, 204, 205–6
  integration, 109
  interspecies scaling, 303
  multicompartment models, 139
  nonlinear models and, 177–79
  one-compartment open model, 115–16,
    124–26
  squared curve (AUCC), 160
  testing for nonlinearity, 172
  trapezoidal estimation of, 44–45, 152–56
  two-compartment model, 133
Aspirin
  buffering and absorption, 25
  pH and absorption, 16
ATP-binding cassette proteins, 52
Atropine, biliary excretion of, 100
AUC. *See* Area under the curve (AUC)
Autoradiography, 59

Bacteria. *See* Microbes
Basal metabolic rate (BMR)
  biological clocks, 301
  and pharmacokinetic scaling, 297–98
Bases, membrane passage of, 15–17
Bayesian forecasting, 267, 277–78, 291
Biliary excretion
  mechanism of bile formation, 95–97
  micelle formation, 25
  secretion of bile acids, 97–99
  species differences, 101
  transport pathways, 99–101
Bioavailability, 43–45
  nonlinear models, 178–79
  one-compartment open model, 124–26
  therapeutic equivalence, 212
  Trapezoidal Rule, 152
Bioequivalence determination, 157
Biophase, 215. *See also* Pharmacokinetic–
    pharmacodynamic modeling
Biotransformation. *See* Hepatic biotransformation
Blood-brain barrier
  distribution of drugs, 51
  transport processes, 51–52
Blood flow
  distribution of drugs and, 48–49
  hepatic clearance and, 87, 89
  laser Doppler velocimetry (LDV), 193
Blood urea nitrogen (BUN) as GFR estimate, 75
BMR. *See* Basal metabolic rate (BMR)
Body weight
  scaling and, 297–303
  as a variable, 262
Bootstrapping, 275
Brain
  efflux transport processes, 51–52
  tissue barrier to drug distribution, 51
Bromsulfophthalein (BSP), 100
Bulk-flow, defined, 19

Caco model and gastrointestinal absorption, 28
Calculus, differential, 107–12
Capillary permeability and inflammation, 19
Carbon tetrachloride, renal metabolism of, 71
Carcinogens, 310
Cardiac output, scaling and, 299

Carnivores, urine pH of, 70
Center of gravity of a curve, 160–61
Cephaloridine, active transport in renal tubules, 68
Cerebrospinal fluid and pH partitioning, 17
Chelation
  of tetracycline, 100
  therapy, systemic, 47
Chloroform, renal metabolism of, 71
Ciprofloxacin, biliary excretion of, 100
Circadian rhythms, 182
Cisplatin
  distribution of, 49–51
  plasma protein binding, 52–53
Clearance
  AUC estimation of, 159
  defined, 72
  dialysis and, 292–94
  hepatic, 87–90
    extraction ratios, 104
    hepatic disease and, 292
  interpretation of, 116
  from intravenous infusions, 117
  noncompartmental models and, 159
  nonlinear models, 179
  one-compartment open model, 115–25
  probability distribution, 264
  protein and tissue binding and, 185
  renal, 72–76
    calculation of, 73–76
    definition of, 72, 73
    fractional, 74–76
    one-compartment open model, 117–20
    in renal failure, 286–88
    scaling, 299
  scaling of, 299–300
  two-compartment model, 132–33
Clinical pharmacology, 4
Coefficient of determination (R^2), 242–43
Compartment models, 107–45
  dosage regimen calculations, 209
  multicompartmental, 137–44
    gentamicin example, 138–40
    parathion example, 142–44
  one-compartment open, 114–26
    absorption, 120–26
    intravenous clearance, 117
    parameter interpretation, 116
    renal elimination, 117–20
  two-compartment, 126–37
    absorption, 134–35
    data analysis, 136
    nomenclature, 128–29
    parameter interpretation, 133
    rate equations, 129–31
Compudose®, 43
Concentration-response relationship, 217–33
  C-T profile synchronization, 224–27
  linear models, 218–20
  nonlinear models, 220–23
Concentration-time (C-T) profile. *See* C-T
    (concentration-time) profiles
Conjugation
  of bile acids, 100
  phase II metabolism, 84
CONSAAM software package, 5, 142
Contraceptives, depot preparations of, 43
Covalent binding to tissues, 59

Creatinine clearance, 286–88
    dosage adjustments and, 288–90
    fractional, 75–76
    as GFR estimate, 75–76
Crohn's disease and enteric coated drugs, 24
C-T (concentration-time) profiles
    curve-fitting, 242–45
    dosage adjustment in renal disease and, 288–92
    dosage regimens and, 202–12
    Michaelis-Menten parameter estimation, 173–75
    multicompartment models and, 137–42
    noncompartmental models, 149–63
    NONMEM, 270
    one-compartment open model and, 116–26
    pharmacokinetic-pharmacodynamic modeling,
        223–27
    physiological models, 195
    species-independent, 301–3
    two-compartment models and, 126–36
Curare, biliary excretion of, 100
Curve-fitting, 239–57
    examples, 247–55
    residual plots, 244–46
    rules of thumb, 255–57
    statistical parameters, 246–47
Curve stripping, 8
    absorption and, 123
    two-compartment models, 131
Cytochrome b_5, induction of, 94
Cytochrome P_{450} ($CytP_{450}$), 84–86
    genetic polymorphism, 304
    induction of, 90–93
        Ah receptor-mediated, 93
        mechanisms, 92–93
        by polycyclic aromatic hydrocarbons, 93
    inhibition of, 94–95
Cytotoxicity screens, 4

Data analysis, 239–57
Data-splitting, 275
DDT, plasma protein binding, 56
Dealkylation reactions, 85
Deconvolution analysis, linear system, 161–62
Dedrick plot, 301–2
Dermis, 33. *See also* Skin
Deterministic models, 6
Diabetes and antimicrobial disposition, 263
Dialysis and drug clearance, 292–94
Differential equation and rate determination, 109
Diffusion. *See also* Fick's law of diffusion
    hepatobiliary drug transport and, 99
    passive renal tubular reabsorption, 69
    pH partitioning, 15–18
    physiological model example and, 196–99
    skin, 34
Digoxin, 284
Disintegration, 24, 29–30
Displacement of drugs from plasma proteins, 57–58
Disposition, drug. *See* Distribution, drug
Dissociation constant, acidic, 15–16
Dissolution, 24, 29–30
Distribution, drug, 47–60
    age and, 261
    gender and, 262
    membrane passage, 15–20
    metabolism rate and, 59
    overview, 11–20

physiological determinants, 48–51
plasma protein binding, 52–58
    assessment of, 54–57
    covalent, 53
    displacement, 57–58
    noncovalent, 53–54
    rate in two-compartment model, 127
    steroselective, 58
    storage depots, 47
    tissue barriers to, 51–52
    tissue binding, 58–59
Diuretics, 285
DNA binding screens, 4
Donnan exclusion effect, 19, 66
Dopamine, 102
Dosage regimens, 202–12
    descriptors, 202–4
    efficacy and safety, 209–12
    formulae, 205–9
        accumulation, drug, 206–7
        calculation, 207–8
    population pharmacokinetic modeling, 277
    in renal disease, 283–94, 285–86
    superposition, 204–5
Doxycycline
    binding to albumin, 55–57
    computer curve-fitting examples, 247–55
    species-independent C-T profile, 301–3
Drug development and population pharma-
    cokinetic modeling, 279–80

Effect-compartment. *See* Biophase
Efficacy and dosage regimens, 209–12
Electrical potential, membrane, 19
Electricity and transdermal drug delivery, 37
Electroporation, 37
Empirical models, 6
Endocytosis, 19
Endoplasmic reticulum (ER)
    glucuronyl transferase, 83
    induction and proliferation of, 94
    phase I oxidation enzymes, 83
Enteric coatings, 24
Enterohepatic recycling, 25–26, 100, 139, 305
Enzyme induction and nonlinear models, 181–82
Enzymes. *See* Michaelis-Menten kinetics; *specific
    enzymes*
Epidermis. *See* Skin
Epoxide hydrolase, induction of, 94
Equilibrium dialysis, 54
Esophagus, drug absorption by, 22
Estradiol, depot preparations of, 43
Ethanol
    induction by, 93–94
    zero-order rate clearance, 168–69
Excretion. *See* Biliary excretion; Renal elimination
Exotic/zoo animal medicine and pharmacokinetic
    extrapolation, 4, 9
Expectation maximization algorithm, 273–74
Extended least squares (ELS), 267, 271–72
Extended-release. *See* Dissolution
Extralabel drug use, 9, 280, 314–16
Extrapolations, interspecies, 4–10, 296–306
    kallynochron, 301–3
    physiologically based pharmacokinetic models,
        296–97
    pitfalls, 303–5

Extrapolations, interspecies (*continued*)
  biotransformation, 304
  genetic polymorphism, 304
  protein binding, 305
  saturation, 305
  scaling, 297–301
    applications, 300–301
    clearance, 299–300
    half-life, 298, 300
    protein binding, 300
    volume of distribution, 298–99, 300
  tissue tolerance determinations, 309

Facilitated transport, 18, 67–68
Fanconi syndrome, 70
FDA. *See* Food and Drug Administration (FDA)
Fick's law of diffusion, 15–16
  clearance, 73
  first-order rates, 108
  passive renal tubular reabsorption, 76
  physiological models and, 197
First-order rate elimination, 108, 168–69
  Michaelis-Menten kinetics and, 175–76
First-pass metabolism, 27–28
Flavoproteins, 85–86
Fluid mosaic model, 13–14
Food and Drug Administration (FDA)
  extralabel drug use, 314
  food consumption factors, 309
  toxicology safety factors, 309–10
Food Animal Residue Avoidance Databank
    (FARAD), 303, 313
Fractional clearance, renal, 74–76
F test, 246
Furosemide, renal tubular reabsorption of, 68

Gases and respiratory absorption, 39–40
Gastric emptying time, 26
Gastrointestinal tract
  absorption, 21–30
    disintegration and dissolution, 24
    enterohepatic recycling, 25–26
    first pass metabolism, 27–28
    formulation factors, drug, 29–30
    models, 28–29
    regional variations in, 22–24
    species diversity in, 21–22, 26–27
  transport systems, membrane, 18
Gender as a variable, 262
Genetics
  interspecies scaling and, 304
  as a variable, 262–63
Gentamicin
  deconvolution analysis of nephrotoxicity, 161–62
  multicompartment models and, 138–40
  nonlinear clearance, 182
  power function analysis, 162–63
  scaling, 297–301, 298–99
  two-compartment model and, 132–33
Glomerular filtration. *See also* Renal elimination
  excretion by, 66–67
  rate (GFR)
    estimate of, 74
    half-life, drug elimination, 287–88
Glomerulus, 63–64. *See also* Kidney
Glucuronides, biliary excretion of, 100
Glucuronosyl transferase, induction of, 94

Glucuronyl transferase, 83
Glutathione-S-transferase, induction of, 94
Growth curves, 112
Growth promotants, 43

Half-life ($T_{1/2}$)
  age and, 262
  defined, 112–14
  dependence on distribution and clearance, 116
  dosage regimens and, 202–9
  drug clearance in dialysis, 292–93
  GFR and, 287–88
  interpretation of, 116
  mean residence time compared, 151
  nonlinear models, 176–77
  renal disease and, 289–90
  scaling of, 298, 300
  two-compartment model, 130, 133
  withdrawal times and, 313–16
Henderson-Hasselbalch equation, 16
Hepatic biotransformation, 81–104
  clearance, 87–90
    extraction ratios, 104
    hybrid physiological pharmacokinetic
        models, 88
  induction of metabolism, 90–94
    cytochrome P_{450}, 90–93
    inducers, table of, 91
    mechanisms, 92–93
    non-cytochrome P_{450} enzymes, 94
  inhibition of metabolism, 94–95
  interspecies scaling and, 304
  phase 1 reactions, 82–84
    cytochrome P_{450}, 84–86
    hydrolysis, 83
    oxidation, 83
    pro-drug design and, 102
  phase 2 reactions, 82, 84, 86–87, 102–3
  saturation, 176
  in vitro systems, 83, 101–2
Hepatic clearance, 87–90, 104, 292, 299
Hepatic excretion. *See* Biliary excretion
Herbivores, urine pH of, 70
Hexachlorobutadiene, renal metabolism of, 71
Hill equation, 220–22, 235
Hormones and transport proteins, 52
Horses and gastrointestinal absorption, 26–27
Hybrid physiological pharmacokinetic models, 88
Hydration of skin and drug absorption, 33
Hydrogen binding and plasma proteins, 54
Hydrolysis reactions, 83
Hydrophobic binding and plasma proteins, 54, 56
Hydroxylation reactions, 84–86
Hysteresis, 224–27

Implant-C®, 43
Induction of drug metabolism, 90–94
  $CytP_{450}$, 90–93
  inducers, table of, 91
  mechanisms of, 92–93
  non-$CytP_{450}$ enzymes, 94
Inference space, 6, 7
Inflammation and drug-protein binding, 263
Inhibition of metabolism, 94–95
Integration
  and rate determination, 109–10
  superposition, 161–62

Integument. *See* Skin

Interspecies extrapolations. *See* Extrapolations, interspecies

Interstitial fluid
  microdialysis sampling of, 13
  overview, 13

Interval-extension dosage adjustment regimen, 288–90

Intramuscular (IM) drug administration. *See* Parenteral drug absorption

Intraperitoneal (IP) drug administration, 43

Intravenous (IV) administration
  hysteresis loops, 227
  one-compartment open model and, 117
  two-compartment models and, 128–33

Inulin, fractional clearance of, 75

In vitro diffusion cells, 28

Ionic binding and plasma proteins, 54

Ion pumps, 19

Iontophoresis, 37, 164–65

Ion-trapping, 20
  multicompartment models, 139
  salicylate, 18

Isoproterenol, biliary excretion of, 100

Kallynochron, 301–3

Ketamine, 16

Kidney. *See also* Renal elimination
  aminoglycoside toxicity, 212
  clearance, 72–76, 117–20, 286–88, 299
  disease
    dialysis and drug clearance, 292–94
    dosage adjustments, 288–92
    drug dosage regimens in, 285–86
    guidelines for drug treatment, 291–92
    pharmacokinetics in, 286–88
    pharmacologic effects of, 283–85
  displacement of drugs and toxicity, 57
  drug-tissue binding and withdrawal times, 312
  extraction ratios, drug, 104
  metabolism, drug, 71–72, 284
  physiology, 62–65
  porous endothelium, 19
  structure, 63–64
  transport systems, membrane, 18
  tubular reabsorption, 17–18, 67–71, 76–79, 305

Laboratory animal medicine pharmacokinetic extrapolation, 4, 9

Lactation and drug excretion, 262

Lagrange polynomials, 154

Langmuir equation, 222

Language of pharmacokinetics, 107–12

Laser Doppler velocimetry (LDV), 193

Levodopa, 102

Lidocaine, iontophoretic delivery of, 164–65

Linear pharmacokinetic models and withdrawal times, 313

Lineweaver-Burke equation, 173

Lipids, membrane, 13–14

Liver
  bile formation, 95–97
  bile secretion, 97–101
  biotransformation, 81–104
  clearance, hepatic, 87–90, 104, 292, 299
  drug-tissue binding and withdrawal times, 312

  extraction ratios, drug, 104
  transport systems, membrane, 18

Loading dose
  defined, 202
  half-life of drug and, 208

Loop of Henle, 63–64. *See also* Kidney

Loo-Riegelman method, 134–35

Lung. *See* Respiratory system

Lymph and distribution of compounds, 52

Maintenance dose, defined, 202

Mass action, law of, 55

Mass balance and clearance estimation, 117

Mastitis and pH partitioning, 17

Maximum likelihood estimation, 273

Maximum residue level (MRL), 308, 310. *See also* Tissue residues

Maximum tubular transport, 77

Mean absorption time (MAT), 157

Mean residence time (MRT)
  computer curve-fitting examples, 247–48
  defined, 149–51
  mean absorption time (MAT) compared, 157
  mean transit time (MTT) compared, 157
  topical drug administration and, 164
  variance of residence times (VRT) and, 158

Mean-squared prediction error (MSPE), 276

Mean transit time (MTT), 157

Meat withdrawal time. *See* Withdrawal times, drug

Mechanistic models, 6

Membranes. *See also* Active transport
  as barriers, 13
  compartment definition by, 13
  drug passage across, 15–20
    electrical potential, 19
    endocytosis, 19
    energy and, 19–20
    ion pumps, 19
    pH partitioning, 15–18
    pores, 18–19
    transport systems, 18
  structure, 13–14

Meperidine
  analgesic effect, 222
  PK-PD model, 229–31

Metabolism, drug
  age and, 261–62
  AUC ratio and fraction metabolized, 158
  effects of, 82
  genetic factors, 262–63
  hepatic biotransformation, 81–104
  induction, 90–94
  inhibition, 94–95
  renal, 71–72
  species differences in, 81, 87

Metals
  biliary excretion, 101
  chelation and, 100

MFO (mixed function oxidase) system, 83–86. *See also* Cytochrome P_{450} ($CytP_{450}$)

Micelle formation, 25

Michaelis-Menten kinetics. *See also* Nonlinear models
  Hill equation, 220–21
  parameter estimation from C-T profiles, 173–75
  pharmacokinetic implications of, 175–76

Michaelis-Menten kinetics (*continued*)
  rate laws, overview, 169–75
    Lineweaver-Burke equation, 173
    rate-determining step, 169
    steady-state assumption, 170
    testing for nonlinearity, 172–73
Microbes
  enterohepatic recycling and, 25
  gastrointestinal drug absorption and, 24
  polysaccharide digestion by, 26
  presystemic metabolism, 24
  skin absorption of drugs and, 35–36
Microdialysis probes, 13
Microvilli, renal tubule, 67
Milk and pH partitioning, 17
Milk discard interval (MDI), 308, 316. *See also*
    Withdrawal times, drug
Minimum inhibitory concentration (MIC), 4,
    210–12
Mixed function oxidase (MFO) system, 92
Models, pharmacokinetic. *See also specific models*
  calculus and, 107–12
  compartmental, 107–45
  gastrointestinal absorption, 28–29
  half-life concept, 112–14
  introduction, 5–8
  linear, 218–20
  noncompartmental, 148–65
  nonlinear, 168–87
  pharmacokinetic-pharmacodynamic, 215–37
  physiological, 189–200
  population, 259–80
  structural identifiability, 136
  types, 6
Morphine, 16

NADPH-$CytP_{450}$, 85–86, 94
Na+-K+-ATPase
  bile acid secretion and, 98, 100
  renal tubules, 67–68
Nasal administration, 41
Nephrons, 63–64. *See also* Kidney
Neural-nets, 274–75
Nicotinamide adenine dinucleotide phosphate
    (NADPH)
  NADPH-$CytP_{450}$, 85–96, 94
  phase I oxidation reactions, 84–86
Nitroglycerin, sublingual delivery of, 22–23
Noncompartmental models, 148–65
  center of gravity of a curve, 160–61
  deconvolution analysis, 161–62
  dosage regimen calculations, 209
  power function analysis, 162–64
  statistical moment analysis, 149–60, 164
  usefulness of, 148–49
Nonlinear models, 168–87
  absorption, 180–81
  AUC (area under the curve), 177–79
  bioavailability, 178–79
  clearance, 179, 185
  dosage regimen calculations, 209
  enzyme induction, 181–82
  half-life dynamics, 176–77
  Michaelis-Menten kinetics, 169–75
  NONMEM (Nonlinear Mixed-Effects
    Modeling), 267–73, 276
  protein and tissue binding, 183–87

  renal excretion, 179–80
  volume of distribution, 178–79
NONMEM modeling, 267–73, 276
Nonparametric expectation maximization (NPEM),
    273–74
Nonparametric maximum likelihood (NPML),
    273
Norplant®, 43

Oral cavity drug absorption, 22, 28
Oral drug administration and gastrointestinal
    absorption, 21–30
Ouabain, biliary excretion of, 100–101
Oxidation reactions, 83

Para-amino hippurate, renal clearance of, 77
Paracetamol, 84
Parathion
  AUC determinations of fraction metabolized,
    158
  dermal poisoning, 30
  hepatic clearance, 87
  multi-matrix compartmental analysis, 142–44
  nonlinear absorption, 180
  phase II conjugation, 102–3
  phase I metabolism, 102
  PK-PD model, 235–36
Parenteral drug absorption, 41–43
  depot preparations, 42–43
  injection site physiology, 43
Particulates and respiratory absorption, 40–41
Partition coefficients
  defined, 15
  membrane passage and, 15
  skin penetration and, 32
Penicillin
  biliary excretion of, 100
  dosage regimens and, 212
  pH and absorption, 16
Pentachlorophenol (PCP), 49
Percutaneous absorption, 30–37, 235–36. *See also*
    Skin, absorption
Perfusion. *See* Blood flow
Pesticide. *See specific compounds*
P-glycoproteins, 52, 99
pH
  bile, 95
  drug dissolution and, 24
  gastrointestinal drug absorption and, 24–25
  membrane passage and, 15–18
  renal tubular reabsorption and, 69–70
  skin and hydration, 33
Pharmacodynamics
  defined, 215
  linear models, 218–20
  nonlinear models, 220–23
    Hill equation, 220–23
    sigmoid E_{max}, 221–23
  pharmacokinetic-pharmacodynamic modeling,
    215–37
Pharmacokinetic-pharmacodynamic modeling,
    215–37
  drug disposition modeling strategies, 216–17
  hysteresis, 224–27
  linear pharmacodynamic models, 218–20
  nonlinear pharmacodynamic models, 220–23
  nonparametric approach, 233

parametric approach, 227–33
population based, 217
rate constant determination, 233–35
skin application, 235–36
steps, 236
usefulness of, 224, 236–37
Pharmacokinetics
defined, 3, 6
introduction, 3–10
Phase 1 metabolism
cytochrome P_{450}, 84–86
hydrolysis reactions, 83
overview, 82–84
oxidation reactions, 83
pro-drug design and, 102
Phase 2 metabolism
conjugation reactions, 84, 102–3
overview, 82, 86
parathion and, 102–3
role of, 86
species deficiencies in, 87
Phenobarbitone, inductive effect of, 90, 93
Phenothiazine, 16
Phenylbutazone
pH and absorption, 16
warfarin displacement, 57–58
Phonophoresis, 37
Phospholipids, membrane, 13–14
pH partitioning, 15–18
first-order rates and, 108
tissue barriers to distribution, 51
Physiological models, 189–200
advantages of, 196
analysis, 193–95
application, example, 196–99
construction, 191–93
extralabel drug use and withdrawal estimation, 315
interspecies extrapolations, 296–97
overview, 189–90
Physiology
drug-induced alteration, 305
species differences, 194
Pilot studies, 255–56
Pinocytosis, 19, 70–71
PKAnalyst pharmacokinetic program, 5, 252, 254
Plasma and pH partitioning, 17
Plasma proteins and drug distribution, 52–58
age and, 261
assessing binding, 54–57
covalent binding, 53
displacement, 57–58
ligand-protein interactions, 52–53
noncovalent binding, 53–54
nonlinearity, 183–87
physiological models and, 190
renal disease and, 284
Poisoning, dermal, 30
Polycyclic aromatic hydrocarbons, 93
Population pharmacokinetic models, 4, 259–80
application in veterinary medicine, 277–80
Bayesian methods, 277–78
clinical use, 277
drug development, 279–80
production medicine, 278
residue avoidance, 278–79
drug withdrawal times, 312

extralabel drug use and withdrawal estimation, 315
pharmacostatistical models, 265–75
neural net, 274–75
nonparametric, 273–74
parametric, 267–73
seminonparametric, 274
standard two-stage method, 260–61
validation of results, 275–76
variability, 259–65
biological, 261–63
intraindividual, 264–65
statistical, 263–65
Pores, membrane, 18–19
Power function analysis, 162–64
P-Pharm pharmacokinetic program, 5, 253–54
Pregnancy and drug disposition, 262
Presystemic metabolism, 24, 27
Pro-drug design and phase I metabolism, 102
Production medicine and population pharma-cokinetic modeling, 278
Progesterone depot preparations, 43
Prontosil, 102–3
Protein binding. *See also* Plasma proteins and drug distribution
interspecies extrapolation, 305
scaling, 300
Proteins, membrane, 13–14

Rabbits, gastrointestinal tract of, 21
Ralgro®, 43
Random error, 239–41, 269
Random walk, 162–64, 316
Rates
constant, determination in PK-PD models, 233–35
defined, 108
equation solution, 110–12
first-order, 108
graphic representation of, 109
instantaneous, 109
integration, 109–10
in multicompartment model, 137–42
noncompartmental models and, 149–51, 157, 159–60
in one-compartment open model, 114–26
in two-compartment model, 114–26
zero-order, 108–9
Rats, gastrointestinal tract of, 21
Reabsorption, renal tubular
active, 67–69
interspecies variation, 305
nonlinearity of, 76–79
passive, 69–71
pH and, 17–18
Rectal drug administration, 28
Redistribution
multicompartment models, 139, 141
two-compartment models, 136
Regression analysis, 240–41
allometry, 303–4
maximum likelihood estimation, 273
NONMEM, 268–70
withdrawal time estimation, 310–12
Renal clearance. *See* Clearance, renal
Renal elimination, 62–79
age and, 262

Renal elimination (*continued*)
    anatomy and physiology, kidney, 62–65
    maximum tubular transport, 77
    mechanism of, 65–71
        active tubular secretion and reabsorption, 67–69
        glomerular filtration, 66
        passive tubular reabsorption, 69–71
        pinocytosis, 70–71
    metabolism, drug and, 71–72
    nonlinear, 76–79, 179–80
    one-compartment open model, 117–20
    renal clearance, 72–76, 117–20, 286–88, 299
    species differences, 70
Renal tubular reabsorption. *See* Reabsorption, renal tubular
Residence times
    mean absorption time (MAT), 157
    mean residence time (MRT), 149–51, 164
    mean transit time (MTT), 157, 164–65
    variance of the resident time (VRT), 158
Residual plots, 244–46
    NONMEM, 270–72
    validation and, 276
Residues, tissue. *See* Tissue residues
Respiratory system
    absorption, 37–41
        aerosols and particulates, 40–41
        vapors and gases, 39–40
    as excretory system, 41
    structure and function, 37–39
Risk assessment, 4, 8
Ruminants
    gastrointestinal absorption, 26–27
    pH partitioning, 17
    rumen retention, 27

SAAM-II pharmacokinetic program, 5, 250, 254
Safety and dosage regimens, 209–12
Salicylate
    ion-trapping, 17–18
    uric acid secretion inhibition, 68
    urine pH and excretion of, 70
Saliva as excretion route, 168
Sampling schedule, orthogonal, 255–56
Scaling, interspecies, 296–306
Schwarz's criterion, 246–47
SCIENTIST pharmacokinetic program, 251, 254
Sebum, 31
Secretion. *See also* Renal elimination
    bile, 97–101
    renal tubular, 67–69, 76–79
Serum creatinine (SCR) as GFR estimate, 75–76
Sex-dependent drug disposition, 102
SHAM analysis. *See* Statistical moment analysis
Sheiner model, 227
Sigmoid E_{max}, 221–23
Sinks, 47
Skin
    absorption, 30–37
        body region variation in, 36
        dermis, 33
        dose and, 33
        metabolism, cutaneous, 35
        models, 37
        modulating factors, 36–37
        pathways, 34–36

        physiological model example, 196–99
        species variation, 36
        stratum corneum barrier, 31–33
        transepidermal water loss, 32
    function of, 30
    hydration and drug absorption, 33
    PK-PD model, 235–36
    structure, 30–31, 33
Slow-release. *See* Dissolution
Small intestine
    bile acid reabsorption, 98–99, 100
    drug absorption, 23–24
        active transport, 25
        enterohepatic recycling, 25
        first-pass metabolism, 27
        presystemic metabolism, 24, 27
    first-pass effect, 24, 27
    structure of, 23
Software, 5
    curve-fitting, 241–55
        examples, 247–55
        statistical parameters, 246–47
    dosage regimen calculation, 209, 212
    numerical integration by, 136
    physiological models and, 193
    population pharmacokinetics, 274
Solvents and percutaneous absorption, 36, 235
Species differences. *See also* Extrapolations, interspecies
    biliary excretion, 101
    drug metabolism, 81, 87
    gastrointestinal absorption, 21–22, 26–27
    renal elimination, 70–305
    topical absorption, 36
Spline approximations and moment calculations, 154
Standardized mean prediction error (SMPE), 275–76
Static diffusion cell, 37, 38
Statistical moment analysis
    application example, 164–65
    calculation of moments, 151–56
        end correction, 154
        trapezoidal method, 152–56
    clearance, 159
    mean absorption time (MAT), 157
    mean transit time (MTT), 157
    overview, 149–51
    variance of residence times (VRT), 158
    volume of distribution, 159–60
Statistics, 7–8, 239–57
Stereoselectivity
    distribution, 58
    hepatic drug metabolism, 102
    renal elimination and, 71
Stochastic models, 6
Stomach. *See also* Gastrointestinal tract
    drug absorption, 3, 24–25
    species differences, 26–27
Stratum corneum. *See also* Skin
    barrier, 31–33
    damaging chemicals, 36
    physiological model example and, 197–99
Stripping, curve
    absorption and, 123
    two-compartment models, 131
Strychnine, 16

Study design
 data analysis, 239–55
 guidelines, 255–57
 standard two-stage method, 260–61
Subcutaneous drug administration. *See* Parenteral
  drug absorption
Sublingual drug administration, 22–23
Sulfanilamide, 102–3
Sulfur mustard, 182
Sums of squares (SS), 241–46
Superposition, principle of, 8, 161–62, 205–6
Surfactant and percutaneous absorption, 235
Sustained-release tablets, 26
Sweat as excretion route, 168

Testosterone and protein binding, 300
Tetracyclines
 biliary excretion of, 100
 three-compartment models and, 137
Therapeutic equivalence, 212
Therapeutic window, defined, 210
Thermodynamic activity and membrane passage,
  19–20
Thermoregulation and skin, 30, 33
Tissue binding
 nonlinearity, 183–87
 physiological models and, 190
Tissue residues. *See also* Withdrawal times, drug
 food-producing animals, 47–48
 multicompartment models, 137
 population pharmacokinetic modeling and,
  278–79
 protein and tissue binding, 185
 tolerances, 308–10
Topical administration
 absorption, 30–37, 180
 noncompartmental model and, 164–65
 parathion, 142–44, 180
 physiological models and, 192
Toxicity. *See also* Tissue residues; Withdrawal
  times, drug
 cutaneous metabolism and, 35
 gaseous, 38, 39
 NOAEL (no-observed-adverse-effect-level), 309
 as nonlinear process, 182
 storage depots and, 47
Toxicokinetics, 3–4
Transbuccal drug delivery systems, 23
Transdermal delivery systems, 33, 36
Transport systems, 65, 67–69
Trapping, intracellular, 99
Tubular reabsorption, renal
 active, 67–69
 interspecies variation, 305

 nonlinearity of, 76–79
 passive, 69–71

Ultrafiltration. *See also* Renal elimination
 glomerular filtration as, 66
 ligand-protein interactions, measuring, 54
Ultrasound and transdermal delivery, 37
Urine excretion. *See* Renal elimination
USC*PACK software package, 274

Validation of population studies, 275–76
Van der Waals forces, 54
Vapors and respiratory absorption, 39–40
Variance of residence times (VRTs), 158
Vasodilator and percutaneous absorption, 235
Volume of distribution (*Vd*)
 age and, 261
 body weight and, 262
 defined, 59–60
 dosage regimens and, 202–3, 205–7, 209
 interpretation of, 116
 multicompartment models, 141
 noncompartmental models and, 159–60
 nonlinear models, 178–79
 one-compartment open model, 114–17
  absorption and, 121–22, 125
  intravenous infusion study, 117
 physiological models, 191–92
 pregnancy and, 262
 renal disease and, 284
 scaling of, 298–99, 300
 two-compartment models, 129, 131–35

Wagner-Nelson method, 124–26
Warfarin, 57–58
Weighted sums of squares (WSS), 243–46
Win-Nonlin pharmacokinetic program, 5, 249, 254
Withdrawal times, drug, 9, 11, 308–17
 calculation of, 208
 depot preparations, 42
 estimation of, 310–13
 extralabel use, 314–16
 multicompartment models and, 139
 pharmacokinetics of, 313–14
 tissue tolerance, establishment of, 308–10

Xylazole
 effects, 221
 hysteresis, 226
 PK-PD model, 230, 232

Zeranol, 43
Zero-order rate elimination, 108–9, 168–69